HELICOBACTER PYLORI IN PEPTIC ULCERATION AND GASTRITIS

Supported by an educational grant from
Brocades Pharma BV, Leiderdorp, The Netherlands,
a member of the Yamanouchi Group

Helicobacter pylori in peptic ulceration and gastritis

EDITED BY

BARRY J. MARSHALL MD, MBBS, FRACP, FACG
Assistant Professor of Medicine
Division of Gastroenterology
University of Virginia Health Sciences Center

RICHARD W. McCALLUM MD, FACP, FRACP, FACG
Paul Janssen Professor of Medicine
Chief, Division of Gastroenterology
University of Virginia Health Sciences Center

RICHARD L. GUERRANT MD
Thomas H. Hunter Professor of International Medicine
Head, Division of Geographic Medicine
University of Virginia Health Sciences Center

FOREWORD BY

GERALD L. MANDELL MD
Professor of Internal Medicine
Owen R. Cheatham Professor of the Sciences
Head, Division of Infectious Diseases
University of Virginia Health Sciences Center

BOSTON

BLACKWELL SCIENTIFIC PUBLICATIONS

OXFORD LONDON EDINBURGH

MELBOURNE PARIS BERLIN VIENNA

Editorial offices:
3 Cambridge Center, Cambridge
Massachusetts 02142, USA
Osney Mead, Oxford OX2 0EL, England
25 John Street, London WC1N 2BL
England
23 Ainslie Place, Edinburgh EH3 6AJ
Scotland
54 University Street, Carlton
Victoria 3053, Australia

Other editorial offices:
Arnette SA
2, rue Casimir-Delavigne
75006 Paris
France

Blackwell Wissenschaft
Meinekestrasse 4
D-1000 Berlin 15
Germany

Blackwell MZV
Feldgasse 13
A-1238 Wien
Austria

First published 1991

Set by Excel Typesetters Company, Hong Kong
Printed and bound in Great Britain by
William Clowes Ltd, Beccles, Suffolk

91 92 93 94 5 4 3 2 1

DISTRIBUTORS

USA and Canada
Mosby-Year Book, Inc.
11830 Westline Industrial Drive
St Louis, Missouri 63146
(*Orders*: Tel: 800 633-6699)

Australia
Blackwell Scientific Publications
(Australia) Pty Ltd
54 University Street
Carlton, Victoria 3053
(*Orders*: Tel: 03 347 0300)

Outside North America and Australia
Marston Book Services Ltd
PO Box 87
Oxford OX2 0DT
(*Orders*: Tel: 0865 791155
Fax: 0865 791927
Telex: 837515)

Library of Congress
Cataloging-in-Publication Data

Helicobacter pylori in peptic ulceration and gastritis / edited
by Barry Marshall, Richard W. McCallum,
Richard L. Guerrant.
p. cm. — (Current issues in endocrinology and
metabolism)
Includes bibliographical references and index.
ISBN 0–86542–108–0
1. Peptic ulcer — Pathogenesis. 2. Helicobacter pylori
infections — Pathogenesis. 3. Gastritis — Pathogenesis.
I. Marshall, Barry, 1951– . II. McCallum, Richard W.
III. Guerrant, Richard L. IV. Series.
[DNLM: 1. Gastritis — microbiology. 2. Helicobacter
pylori. 3. Peptic Ulcer — microbiology. WI 310 H475]
RC821.H45 1991
616.3'43 — dc20
DNLM/DLC
for Library of Congress

Contents

List of contributors

MARTIN J. BLASER MD, Director, Division of Infectious Diseases, Department of Medicine, Vanderbilt University School of Medicine, Nashville, TN 37232, USA

SAMY CADRANEL MD, Head, Pediatric Gastroenterology, Queen Fabiola Children's Hospital, Free University of Brussels, 15 rue, JJ Crocq, Brussels 1020, Belgium

STEPHEN H. CALDWELL MD, Division of Gastroenterology, Salem VA Medical Center, Building 4, Room 215 (111G), 1970 Boulevard, Salem, VA 24153, USA

CORNELIUS P. DOOLEY MD, Department of Gastroenterology, 1651 Galisteo St, Suite 12, Sante Fe, NM 87501, USA

LARS N. ENGSTRAND, Department of Clinical Bacteriology, University Hospital, Box 552, S751 85, Uppsala, Sweden

CECILIA M. FENOGLIO-PREISER MD, Chief, Laboratory Services, Veterans Administration Medical Center, Albuquerque, NM, USA, and Professor, Department of Pathology, University of New Mexico School of Medicine, Albuquerque, NM, USA

RICHARD L. GUERRANT MD, Professor and Head, Division of Geographic Medicine, Medicine-Internal Medicine Department, School of Medicine, Box 485, University of Virginia Health Sciences Center, Charlottesville, VA 22908, USA

SVEN GUSTAVSSON, Department of Surgery, University Hospital, Box 552, S751 85, Uppsala, Sweden

STUART L. HAZELL PhD, School of Microbiology and Immunology, University of New South Wales, P.O. Box 1, Kensington, NSW 2033, Australia

MANFRED KIST MD, Institute of medical Microbiology and Hygiene, University of Freiburg, Hermann Herder Str-11, D-7800 Freiburg, Germany

JOHN R. LAMBERT MD, PhD, Department of Medicine and Gastroenterology, Monash University Prince Henry's Hospital, St. Kilda Road, Melbourne 3004, Australia

CLIFF A. LINGWOOD PhD, The Hospital for Sick Children, 555 University Ave, Toronto, Ontario, Canada

RICHARD W. McCALLUM MD, Chief, Division of Gastroenterology, School of Medicine, Box 145, University of Virginia Health Sciences Center, Charlottesville, VA 22908, USA

ALLAN McLEAN MD, PhD, Director, Clinical Pharmacology, Alfred Hospital, Commercial Road, Prahran, Victoria, Australia

BARRY J. MARSHALL MD, Assistant Professor, Division of Gastroenterology, Department of Internal Medicine, Box 145, University of Virginia Health Sciences Center, Charlottesville, VA 22908, USA

WALTER L. PETERSON MD,
Gastroenterology 111B1, VA Medical Center, 4500 S. Lancaster Road, Dallas, TX 75216, USA

ROBERT G. STRICKLAND MD,
Professor and Chairman, Department of Medicine, University of New Mexico, School of Medicine, Albuquerque, NM 87131, USA

NICHOLAS J. TALLEY MBBS, PhD,
Associate Professor of Medicine, Division of Gastroenterology and Internal Medicine, and Department of Health Sciences Research, Mayo Clinic, Rochester, MN 55905, USA

DAVID N. TAYLOR MD,
Department of Bacterial Diseases, Walter Reed Army Institute for Research, Washington, DC 20307, USA

LUCY S. TOMPKINS MD, PhD,
Associate Professor, Department of Medicine, Division of Infectious Diseases, and Department of Microbiology and Immunology, Stanford University Medical Center H1537-J, Stanford, CA 94305, USA

T. ULF WESTBLOM MD, Division of Infectious Diseases, St Louis University School of Medicine, 1402 South Grand Boulevard, St Louis, MO 63104, USA

Foreword

It must be immensely satisfying for those medical scientists involved in the elucidation of the relationship of *Helicobacter pylori* to peptic ulceration and gastritis to see real and tangible benefits to patients in just a few short years. After building a strong basic science base for understanding the pathogenesis of *H. pylori*-induced disease, the expert authors of the chapters in this volume outline approaches to the patient, with practical techniques for diagnosis and therapy.

A few years ago, conventional wisdom (especially in infectious disease and microbiologic circles) held the belief that the stomach was sterile or nearly so. The only known exceptions were patients with enteric fistulas. Any possible relationship of microbes to ulceration or gastritis was not considered, since those conditions were associated with normal or increased levels of gastric acid which is known to kill microbes. In the June 4, 1983 issue of the *Lancet*, there appeared two landmark letters from the Royal Perth Hospital in Perth, Western Australia. Dr JR Warren, a pathologist, reported finding "small curved and S shaped bacilli" in gastric biopsy specimens in association with inflammation (Warren, JR, & Marshall, B. Unidentified curved bacilli on gastric epithelium in active chronic gastritis. *Lancet* 1983; **1**: 1273–5). He stated: "Bacteria in numbers sufficient to see by light microscopy are closely associated with an active form of gastritis, a cause of considerable morbidity (dyspeptic disease). These organisms should be recognized and their significance investigated." This was followed by a letter from Dr Barry Marshall, a young gastroenterologist and colleague of Dr Warren's from the Royal Perth Hospital. Dr Marshall noted that spirochetes had been seen in human stomachs decades previously, but no associa- tion was made with disease and the organisms were never isolated. Marshall was able to grow and characterize the organisms for the first time and these are now known as *Helicobacter pylori*. Marshall stated: "If these bacteria are truly associated with antral gastritis, as described by Warren, they may have a part to play in other poorly-understood gastritis associated diseases (i.e. peptic ulcer and gastric cancer)."

These letters were followed a year later by a more definitive report in the *Lancet* by Marshall & Warren (16 June 1984). An early, burning question was whether the association of organisms with gastritis was causal. Dr Marshall, described in a 1985 paper in the *Medical Journal of Australia* (Marshall, BJ, Armstrong, JA, McGechie, DB, & Glancy RJ. Attempt to fulfill Koch's postulates for pyloric *Campylobacter*. *Med. J. Aust.* 1985; **142**: 436–9), as "a 32-year-old man, a light smoker, and social drinker who had no known gastrointestinal disease or family history of peptic ulceration," underwent endoscopy and gastric biopsy to confirm normal gastric mucosa. About a month later, he "swallowed the growth from a flourishing three day culture of the isolate (10^9 colony-forming units)" and developed symptomatic, biopsy-proven gastritis. From that time on, Marshall was a firm believer, and he and his colleagues and later investigators throughout the world, have attempted to answer the many questions that remain concerning the pathogenesis, diagnosis, and therapy of *H. pylori*-related gastrointestinal disease.

We don't have all of the answers, but we have many of the answers. Fine-tuning of diagnostic techniques and improvements in therapy are goals for the near future. Better understanding of the pathogenesis of the gastric lesion will lead to novel approaches to prevention and treatment of peptic ulceration and gastritis. Questions concerning the role of this microbe in neoplasia would of course alter the approach to patients with asymptomatic infection.

This wonderful medical adventure makes one speculate as to what other poorly-understood diseases of man are caused by microbes. Innovative, adventuresome investigators — you have a challenge.

Gerald L. Mandell MD
Professor of Internal Medicine
Owen R. Cheatham Professor of the Sciences
Head, Division of Infectious Diseases
University of Virginia
Health Sciences Center

Preface

Helicobacter pylori in Peptic Ulceration and Gastritis was conceived by the editors as a book explaining both practical and theoretical aspects of *H. pylori.* My coeditors, Drs Richard McCallum and Richard Guerrant, are authorities in gastroenterology and microbiology, and I thank them for their assistance in the development of the book. We are grateful to the other contributors who are all well known for their original work in *H. pylori*-related fields, and are well able to offer a practical approach to the management of associated gastrointestinal disease. We have included chapters on microbiology, taxonomy, molecular biology, pathogenesis, immunology, and epidemiology as background for the more clinically-oriented sections. Some of the authors have presented previously unpublished data in their chapters and we are especially grateful to them for allowing us to include it here.

For the physician more interested in clinical aspects of *H. pylori,* we have incorporated detailed chapters on peptic ulcer disease and non-ulcer dyspepsia. Authors from both sides of the current controversy have been included, but the reader will easily find practical advice on how to actively manage *H. pylori* patients.

In 1981 Robin Warren brought the new spiral bacterium to my attention, and together we published our first letters in the *Lancet* in June 1983. I thank Robin for his help in those early years, his influence certainly improved the credibility of the initial reports.

H. pylori hit the world stage at the Second International Workshop on *Campylobacter* Infections, in Brussels, during 1983. In my naiveté, I expected *H. pylori* to be immediately accepted as the cause of duodenal ulcer and gastritis, but I did not expect it to be the world's most common bacterial infection. The presence of *H. pylori* in many apparently healthy persons has made its pathogenic role harder to understand, and has delayed wide acceptance of the new bacterium as an important pathogen. For these reasons we may still have a long way to go before eradication of *H. pylori* becomes the "standard of care" in gastroduodenal disease.

This book provides an opportunity to acknowledge several other persons who have facilitated the *H. pylori* story over the past 10 years. Most importantly, my wife Adrienne, who has given me the satisfaction of a wonderful family life while also providing support, encouragement, and protected time for my research. Thanks are due to Drs Robin Warren, Tom Waters, Ian Hislop, and David McGechie who trained me in pathology, gastroenterology, and microbiology between 1981 and 1984, and assisted my early attempts at research when the *H. pylori* story was only an interesting, unfunded hypothesis. I thank Dr Martin Skirrow of Worcester, England, who encouraged the international presentation of *H. pylori,* and promoted its rapid acceptance amongst microbiologists. Our common interest in the antibacterial action of bismuth resulted in the present association with my coeditors, Richard McCallum and Richard Guerrant, who arranged my transfer to the University of Virginia in 1986, and who have since fostered my further studies. I also acknowledge the support of Dr Bruce McCarty, who has been both a good friend and keen advocate for *H. pylori* research in the United States.

I thank Susie Hoffman and Cheryl Boyd for their help with clinical studies at the University of Virginia, and Nancy Noblette who assembled many of the manuscripts. Finally, I commend Victoria Reeders and Mike Snider of Blackwell Scientific Publications Inc for their courtesy, patience, and swift publication of this book.

Barry J. Marshall

1: Gastritis — classification and histology then and now

R.G. STRICKLAND &
C.M. FENOGLIO-PREISER

Introduction

Gastritis "then"

The term "gastritis" has existed in the medical literature for over two centuries. However, until the early part of this century, descriptions of gastritis were all based on post-mortem studies, in which rapid autolysis effectively prevented satisfactory histologic examination of the gastric mucosa. The work of Konjetzny using gastrectomy specimens [1] and of Faber [2] and Magnus [3] using immediate post-mortem preservation of the stomach with formalin, established the basis for an expanded definition and classification of gastritis.

Pioneer studies by Schindler [4] provided early endoscopic–histologic correlations, and the introduction of peroral suction biopsy of the gastric mucosa by Wood *et al.* [5] with its subsequent widespread use in the 1950s and 1960s resulted in a clearer understanding of structural–functional relationships, and recognition of gastritis as a common pathologic change in adult patient populations. Early observations indicating significant associations between chronic gastritis and pernicious anemia, chronic peptic ulcer, and gastric cancer were firmly established during this era. Also, in the 1960s etiologic factors were beginning to be defined, particularly with the discovery of gastric autoimmune phenomena and their association with pernicious anemia and a subpopulation of patients with chronic gastritis [6, 7].

The classification of gastritis "then" was based on gross morphologic features, as observed in surgical or autopsy material and on microscopic examination of peroral mucosal biopsies. The major distinctions were between acute and chronic gastritis, with the chronic form being subclassified into chronic superficial, or chronic atrophic gastritis, or gastric atrophy, on the basis of histologic criteria. Rare miscellaneous forms such as hypertrophic gastritis, and eosinophilic gastritis were also recognized.

Gastritis "now"

Two key advances over the past 20 years have led to increased interest in the field of gastritis. The first was the introduction and widespread use of flexible upper gastrointestinal endoscopy, which has added to the dimension of gross observation of the gastric mucosa and enabled visualization of areas previously hidden from the clinician's view. This procedure also replaced blind peroral suction biopsy, by allowing targeted biopsy sampling of the gastric mucosa. The peroral technique predominantly sampled the corpus mucosa, whereas endoscopic biopsy provides the expanded capability of histologic study of all anatomic regions of the gastric mucosa, enabling evaluation and correlation of histologic features with endoscopic findings.

Endoscopic studies of gastritis have led to a questioning and reappraisal of older classification schemes [8]. It is evident, for instance, that the strict separation of gastritis into acute and chronic forms is frequently not possible, and that acute gastritis may be superimposed on chronic gastritis. Erosive and hemorrhagic mucosal lesions seen grossly are generally thought to represent "acute" disease, even though they may be "chronic" from a temporal view. Moreover, erosive changes may be superimposed on underlying "chronic" histologic gastritis.

Histologic examination of areas of gastritis frequently reveals features of both acute and chronic inflammatory change in individual patients. Additional observations have led to the concept of histologically distinct forms of gastritis, based on the regional distribution of pathologic change in the stomach — so called corpus-predominant (type A), antral-predominant (type B), and pan-gastritis (type AB) patterns of histologic gastritis [9].

The second significant advance in the field of gastritis over the past two decades has been an improved understanding of etiologic factors in these disorders. This area has accelerated particularly since 1983, when Warren & Marshall rediscovered the Gram-negative bacterium, originally termed *Campylobacter pylori* [10], and since reclassified as *Helicobacter pylori* [11]. This organism exclusively colonizes gastric epithelium, is strongly associated with histologic evidence of gastritis, and probably represents a major etiologic factor in gastritis.

Definition, nomenclature, and use

In spite of these significant advances, many gaps remain in our understanding of the biology of gastritis. Accordingly, definitions should continue to be based on descriptive morphology, and to encompass both gross and microscopic observations [12]. Thus, gastritis may be defined as a heterogeneous group of gastric mucosal disorders, characterized by widespread injury at the gross and/or microscopic level, and usually associated with an acute, chronic, or mixed inflammatory response.

Morphologic heterogeneity was recognized in early descriptions of gastritis [1–3], but has become more evident in the endoscopic era. Heterogeneity also extends to functional effects, clinical expression, etiology, and pathogenesis, and probably to natural history and outcome [9].

The nomenclature of gastritis has undergone considerable diversification over the past two decades. Multiple qualifying terms are now used to variously describe general, endoscopic, histologic, and putative etiologic characteristics of these disorders (Table 1.1). In addition, the term gastritis itself continues to be used in a casual fashion by clinicians, radiologists, endoscopists, and even pathologists. Examples of casual use include a tendency of some clinicians to equate all non-ulcer dyspepsia with gastritis, and the use of this term by endoscopists to describe a number of visual mucosal changes (erythema, luster changes, fold changes) that have poorly defined significance as actual indicators of histologic evidence of gastritis, as currently defined. Diverse terminologies and casual use have resulted in significant non-uniformity in the field of gastritis, leading in turn to confusion in interpreting both the published literature, and even clinical communication on a given patient.

Classification and histology, 1990

The ideal classification scheme for gastritis would be one based solely on etiology. However, we do not always know the etiology, or multiple etiologies may affect the gastric histology of a given patient. Thus, despite recent discoveries such as *H. pylori*-associated

Table 1.1 Gastritis — some qualifying terms in current use

General	Morphologic	Clinical–etiologic
Acute	Erosive	Stress
Chronic	Hemorrhagic	Alcoholic
Active	Superficial	NSAID-related
Simple	Atrophic	Reflux (alkaline, bile)
Specific	Gastric atrophy	Autoimmune
Non-specific	Types A, B, AB	Environmental
Primary	Hypertrophic	Hypersecretory
Secondary	Eosinophilic	*H. pylori*-associated
	Granulomatous	

Table 1.2 Gastritis — classification 1990

Category	Diagnostic modality	Etiology
Endoscopic		
	Endoscopy	Alcohol, NSAIDs, stress, chemical agents, physical agents, idiopathic
Histologic		
Specific	Endoscopy, microscopy, special stains	Bacterial, viral, fungal, parasitic, granulomatous, eosinophilic, hypertrophic
Non-specific	Endoscopy, microscopy, special stains, (*H. pylori*), gastric autoantibodies	*H. pylori*, autoimmune, reflux

gastritis, we believe it prudent for the present to retain a classification scheme based on descriptive morphology. The classification should be practical, reproducible, simple, and readily applicable for both clinical and investigative use. The proposed classification of gastritis recognizes that endoscopy with endoscopic biopsy sampling of the mucosa is now the key diagnostic modality (Table 1.2). It combines many of the principles contained in the classification schemes described by Weinstein [12] and Whitehead [13].

The classification scheme uses two separate approaches, one endoscopic and one histologic. The two may not always be concordant in their findings. Histologic evidence of gastritis is a common finding in the general adult population, yet it has not been possible to distinguish between its chance association with grossly visible endoscopic lesions on the one hand, or with clinically significant disease on the other. We view the use of a dual classification scheme as clinically useful, and allowing clearer recording of the gastric findings in an objective and reproducible fashion.

Endoscopic gastritis

Endoscopic gastritis is defined by gross findings of mucosal erosions and focal hemorrhagic lesions. As discussed earlier, other visual mucosal alterations, such as erythema, luster changes, or fold changes, are currently of doubtful significance as true indicators of gastritis [12]. These mucosal alterations should be recorded in a descriptive fashion, but, in the absence of erosive-hemorrhagic lesions, should not be designated as indicative of gastritis. The familiar settings leading to endoscopic gastritis include: alcohol and non-steroidal antiinflammatory drug (NSAID) use, and the stress of serious medical or surgical illness. Less common causes involve injury from chemical (e.g. corrosives, chemotherapeutic drugs), or physical (e.g. irradiation) agents. The major clinical expression of endoscopic gastritis is overt upper gastrointestinal hemorrhage. In addition, there is a group of patients with idiopathic erosive lesions associated with dyspeptic symptoms, usually chronic or recurrent in nature, simulating ulcer disease.

As indicated earlier, histologic gastritis may coexist with grossly visible endoscopic lesions. Until recently, evaluation of microscopic pathology in endoscopic gastritis had been largely confined to patients in whom a specific infectious cause (e.g. viral or fungal), or specific disease process (e.g. Crohn's disease), was suspected. An emerging literature on the association between *H. pylori* colonization and endoscopic gastritis in general may require more routine use of mucosal biopsy in this setting in the future.

Histologic gastritis

The basis for the diagnosis of histologic gastritis is microscopic examination of the gastric mucosa. Histologic gastritis can be separated into specific and non-specific forms.

Specific histologic gastritis

Specific histologic gastritis includes those forms of gastritis with a distinctive morphology, associated with a specific etiologic agent or disease process. Macroscopic mucosal alterations frequently accompany the specific forms of gastritis, but are not themselves diagnostic. Infectious causes of specific histologic gastritis include mucosal invasion by bacteria, viruses, fungi, or parasites. Specific diseases which involve the gastric mucosa and which display characteristic microscopic morphologic features include granulomatous disorders such as Crohn's disease, eosinophilic gastritis, graft-versus-host disease, and hypertrophic gastritis [14]. It should be emphasized that the specific forms of histologic gastritis are uncommon, and that identification is dependent on clinical, microscopic pathologic, and associated observations.

Non-specific histologic gastritis

In contrast to specific histologic gastritis, non-specific histologic gastritis is characterized by variable patterns of microscopic pathology, few of which can be specifically linked to a single etiologic agent or disease process. Identification and full characterization of non-specific histologic gastritis requires multiple stepwise endoscopic biopsies of all anatomic regions of the stomach. Except when endoscopic gastritis coexists, or frank gastric atrophy is present, gross visual mucosal changes are not evident.

Biopsy sampling should include anterior and posterior walls, and both curvatures of the antrum and corpus. Pinch biopsies using standard size biopsy forceps provide adequate samples in approximately 80% of instances [12]. Correct biopsy orientation, and mounting with mucosal surface uppermost on a piece of filter paper or Teflon as is done for small intestinal biopsies, together with diagrammatic

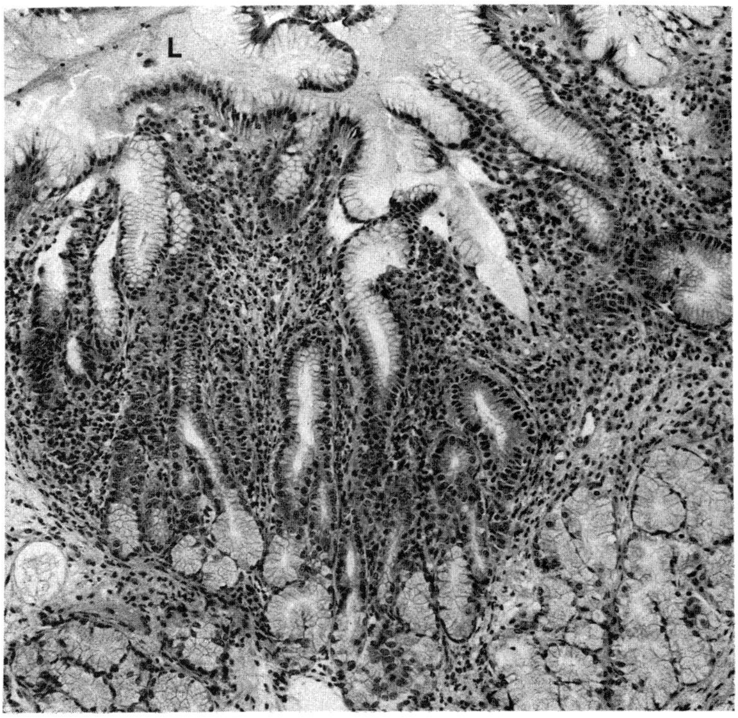

Fig. 1.1 Superficial gastritis. Area of superficial gastritis involving the antrum. The surface foveolar cells lining the luminal surface are intact and not mucin depleted. The inflammation does not extend to involve the antral glands. L, lumen.

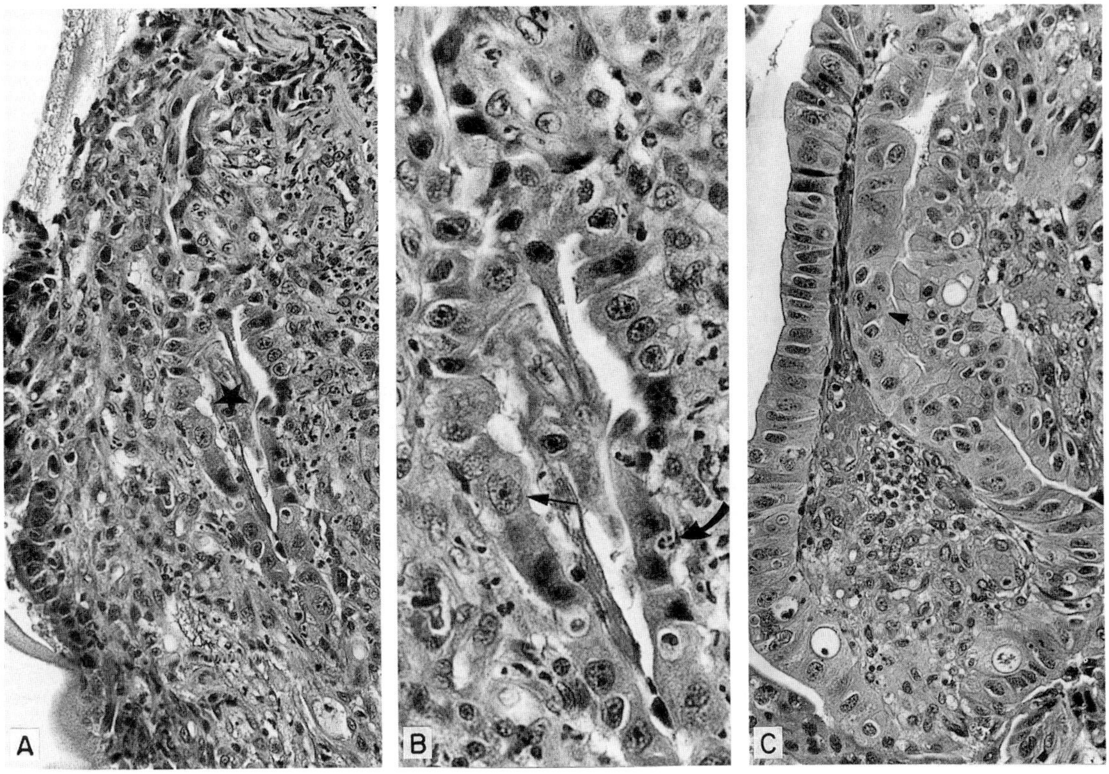

Fig. 1.2 Reactive changes in non-specific gastritis. A, marked reactive epithelial alterations. The lumen is at the left. The lamina propria is infiltrated with polymorphonuclear leukocytes. B, the gland indicated by a star in A is shown at higher magnification. The nuclei are enlarged with a high nuclear : cytoplasmic ratio and prominent nucleoli (←). In addition, the epithelium is infiltrated by polymorphonuclear leukocytes (↷). C, an area of regenerative epithelium which shows prominent nuclei and nucleoli and abundant cytoplasm. In addition, mitoses (◀) are present.

recording of the site of each biopsy, ensure optimal interpretation by the pathologist.

Interpretation of biopsy findings should follow the system developed by Whitehead [13], which includes consideration of the grade of gastritis, the degree of inflammation and its nature (acute, chronic, mixed), and the anatomic distribution of the inflammation.

Grades of non-specific histologic gastritis

The least severe grade is superficial gastritis (Fig. 1.1), in which the inflammation is confined to the gastric pits or foveolar regions. The glandular compartment is unaffected. Reactive changes in the superficial and pit epithelium (mucus depletion, epithelial cell flattening and layering, nuclear hyperchromatism, and increased mitosis) are frequently present (Fig. 1.2). True metaplastic alterations of the epithelium are absent or rare.

In atrophic gastritis, inflammation extends deeper into the mucosa to involve the glandular compartment and variable degrees of glandular atrophy may be present (Fig. 1.3). Mild atrophy refers to focal loss of glands; in severe atrophy diffuse total or subtotal gland loss occurs. Moderate atrophy is intermediate in degree. Atrophic gastritis is usually associated with metaplastic changes in the surface and/or glandular epithelium (Fig. 1.4).

Two primary forms of metaplasia are recognized. Pyloric metaplasia affects only the corpus glands, so that glands normally lined by parietal and chief cells assume the appearance of mucus-secreting antral glands. Intestinal

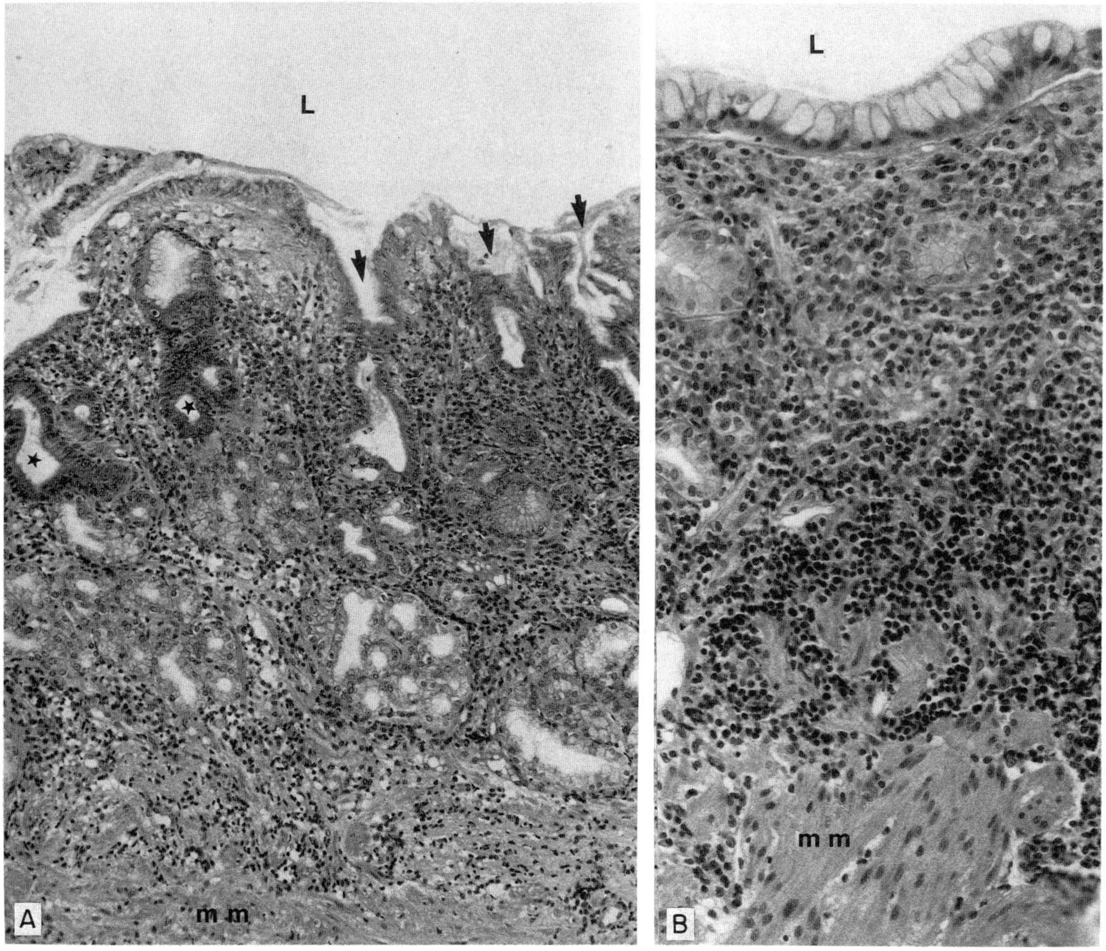

Fig. 1.3 Non-specific gastritis with variable degrees of atrophy. A, antral mucosa with chronic inflammation extending from the lumen (L) to the muscularis mucosa (mm). The height of the mucosa is less than normal and glandular, and foveolar cell loss is noted. In addition, acute changes are superimposed on the chronic ones. The glands indicated by the arrows have acute regenerative changes and are mucin-depleted. The glands indicated by ⋆ are further along in their regenerative pathway and are beginning to reacquire mucin. B, more severe atrophy in which gland loss is severe and foveoli are almost totally absent. The lamina propria contains an infiltrate of mononuclear cells which is most pronounced in the basal portion of the mucosa just overlying the muscularis mucosae (mm). The cells lining the lumen (L) have a normal complement of mucin and represent gastric foveolar cells.

metaplasia (IM) affects the superficial, pit, and glandular epithelium of both corpus and antral mucosa, and can be complete or incomplete (Figs. 1.5, 1.6). Complete IM resembles small or large intestinal mucosa with goblet cells, non-mucus-secreting epithelial cells, and frequently Paneth cells are present (Fig. 1.5); incomplete IM is characterized by the presence of goblet cells admixed with mucus-secreting gastric foveolar cells (Fig. 1.6). Gastric atrophy can be envisaged as the end stage of atrophic gastritis, in which glandular atrophy is diffuse, intestinal metaplasia is widespread, and there is minimal inflammation of the lamina propria.

The differing grades of non-specific histologic gastritis are viewed as a continuum of a single dynamic process. Limited long-term biopsy follow-up studies support this general

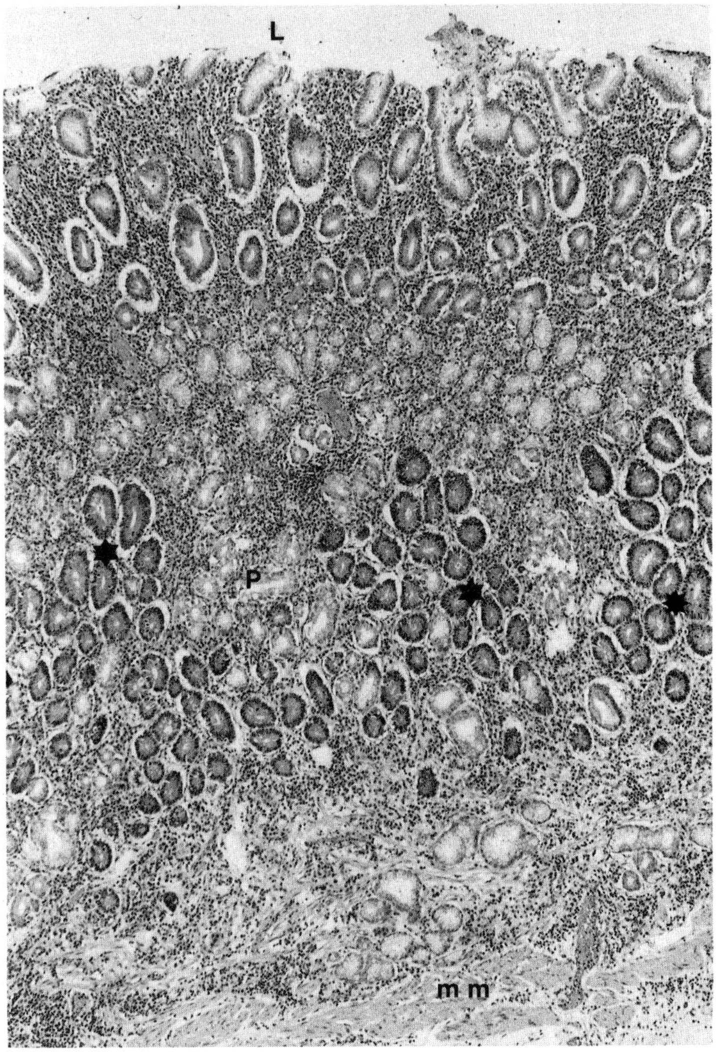

Fig. 1.4 Non-specific gastritis with intestinal metaplasia. Antral gastritis with inflammation extending from the lumen (L) to the muscularis mucosae (mm). Intestinal metaplastic glands (⋆) are interspersed among antral (P) glands. The foveolar epithelium is mucin-depleted and regenerative.

view, and suggest that progression in severity is slow, and measured in decades [15, 16]. However, since histologic gastritis can be patchy, one may see focal areas of all stages in the continuum as it progresses. Studies also, however, indicate that regression may occur, even in advanced grades of atrophic gastritis [16].

Activity of non-specific histologic gastritis

Activity generally refers to the presence of polymorphonuclear leukocytes in the lamina propria, often also seen invading the epithelium and sometimes forming gland abscesses, in a pattern similar to that observed in the colonic mucosa in ulcerative colitis (Fig. 1.7). Such activity may be observed in association with all grades of non-specific histologic gastritis, with the exception of gastric atrophy.

Anatomic distribution of non-specific histologic gastritis

As discussed earlier, the changes of non-specific histologic gastritis, although widespread, may be confined to a particular anatomic region and, rather than being uniformly distributed

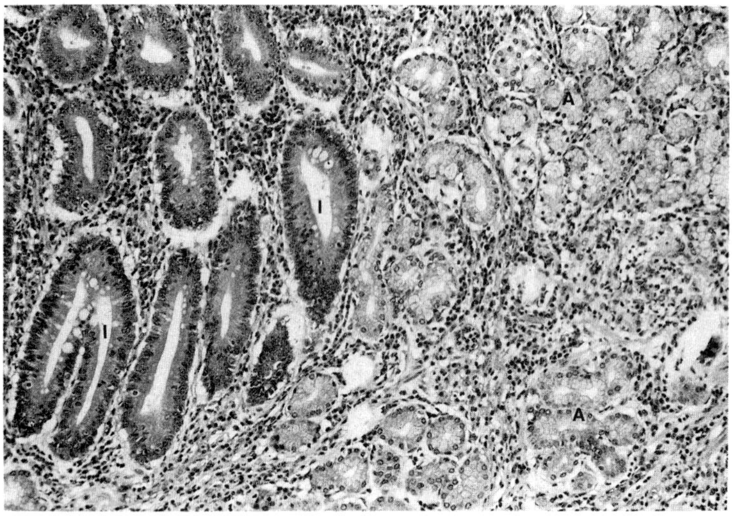

Fig. 1.5 Intestinal metaplasia (complete). Higher magnification of the lesion shown in Fig. 1.4. The intestinalized glands (I) are lined by intestinal epithelium containing Paneth cells and goblet cells. The lamina propria surrounding these contains an increased number of plasma cells relative to the antral mucosa (A) which is also infiltrated, but to a lesser extent.

throughout the stomach, changes may be patchy in severity within an affected area. Population-based studies suggest that the mild grades of non-specific histologic gastritis (superficial, mild atrophic) are often patchy yet involve both antral and corpus mucosa [17]. In contrast, advanced grades of atrophic gastritis appear to segregate into morphologically distinctive anatomic patterns (Fig. 1.8).

These differing patterns of distribution of atrophic gastritis were first identified in the work of Strickland & Mackay [9]. Two distinctive patterns were observed; corpus-predominant (type A) and antral-predominant (type B) forms of atrophic gastritis (Figs 1.9, 1.10). Additional differences were identified [9] including: (1) morphologic (absence of active inflammation in type A, frequent but not universal active inflammation in type B); (2) functional (severe impairment of acid secretion and hypergastrinemia in type A, variable acid secretory impairment and normogastrinemia in type B); (3) immunologic (gastric autoantibodies in type A, no autoantibodies in type B); and (4) differing natural history (type A evolving into Addisonian pernicious anemia,

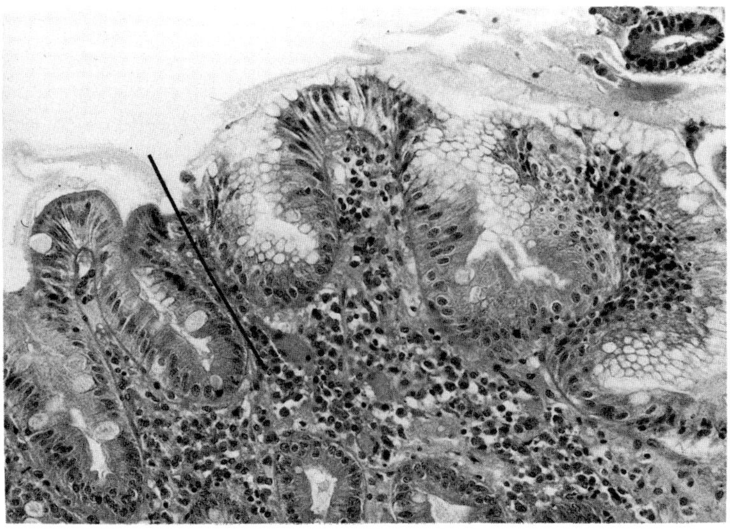

Fig. 1.6 Intestinal metaplasia (incomplete). Non-specific gastritis with intestinal metaplasia involving the surface epithelium. The epithelium to the left of the black line is intestinal in type; to the right there is normal gastric foveolar epithelium. The lamina propria is infiltrated with plasma cells and lymphocytes.

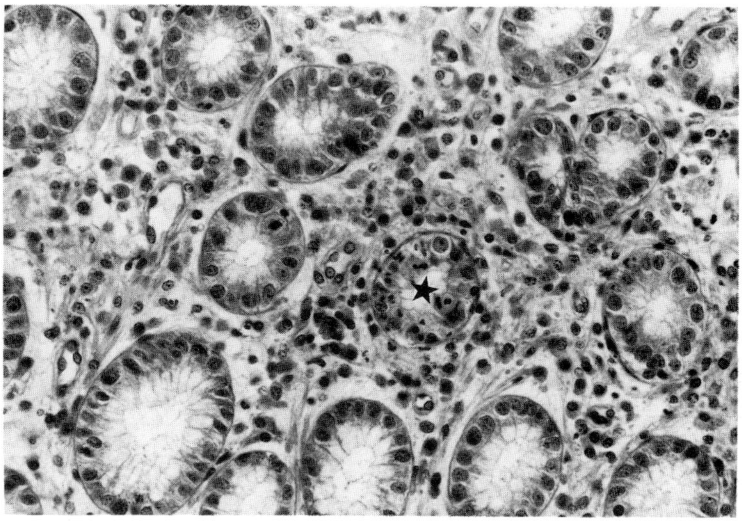

Fig. 1.7 Non-specific gastritis with active inflammation. The lamina propria is infiltrated with numerous plasma cells, as well as lymphocytes. The glandular epithelium is reactive in nature and the gland marked by ★ in the lumen is infiltrated with polymorphonuclear leukocytes. In addition, scattered leukocytes are found in the lamina propria. The patient had *H. pylori* in the lumen.

type B significantly associated with benign peptic ulcer and the development of gastric neoplasia).

It was postulated that these two forms of atrophic gastritis were etiologically distinct; type A gastritis being due to an autoimmune process and type B gastritis caused by luminal environmental injury [9]. Subsequent to this study a third category of atrophic gastritis was proposed — so called type AB or pan-gastritis [18]. Strickland & Mackay [9] had recognized this morphologic pattern in their study, but had suggested that it represented proximal extension of type B gastritis in a majority of instances. As further discussed in the following section it now appears that the major environmental factor causing type B gastritis is *H. pylori*. It is of interest that type AB gastritis is also highly associated with *H. pylori* colonization, thus supporting the original proposal that most pan-atrophic gastritis represents proximal extension of type B gastritis. Further support for the fundamental separation of type A and type B gastritis is that *H. pylori* colonization is not usually identified in type A gastritis.

Prevalence of non-specific histologic gastritis

Non-specific histologic gastritis is exceedingly common in otherwise healthy adults and increases in frequency with advancing age. Its prevalence has been well documented in the adult population in Finland [17]. Whilst equivalent population-based data is lacking in other countries, there is every reason to believe that the general patterns are similar. In the Finnish studies, non-specific histologic gastritis was observed in 68% of a random sample of adults, most of whom were asymptomatic with respect to upper gastrointestinal complaints. The gastritis was mild (superficial and mild atrophic grades) in 80% of the gastritic

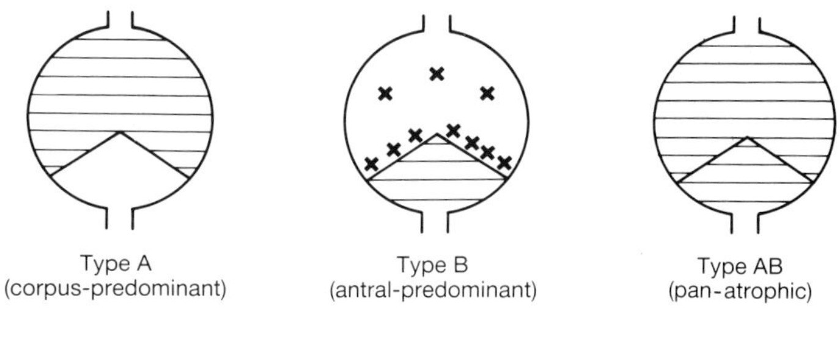

Fig. 1.8 Diagrammatic illustration of patterns of non-specific histologic gastritis in its advanced (atrophic) stage.

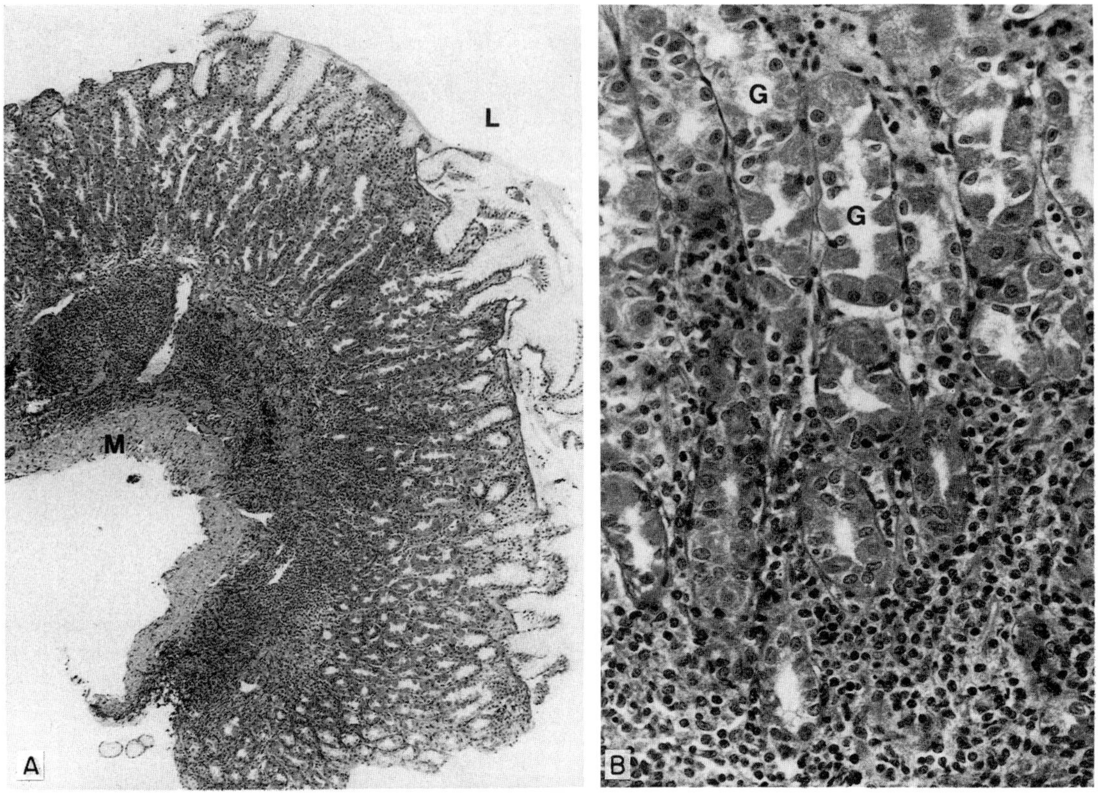

Fig. 1.9 Corpus-predominant (type A) gastritis. A, full-thickness mucosal biopsy demonstrating portion of corpus mucosa. Inflammation is predominantly localized to the area above the muscularis mucosae (M). The corpus glands also show evidence of round cell infiltration around them in the lamina propria. The gastric pits show mild foveolar cell hyperplasia. L, lumen. B, high magnification demonstrating the presence of surviving corpus glands (G) containing chief cells and parietal cells, as well as a mononuclear cell infiltrate containing lymphocytes and plasma cells in the lamina propria surrounding these glands.

population. Advanced atrophic gastritis was observed in 20% of subjects with gastritis, and gastric atrophy was not observed in this population sample. The distribution of morphologic phenotypes in those with advanced atrophic gastritis was: type A, 11%; type B, 51%; and type AB, 38% [17].

These observations, together with limited morphologic follow-up data [15], have led the Finnish workers to hypothesize that non-specific histologic gastritis commences as a generalized process. They proposed that type A gastritis evolves in a susceptible subgroup by healing of antral gastritis and progression of corpus gastritis; determinants of these changes may include genetic predisposition and selective occurrence of gastric autoimmune reactions. Type B atrophic gastritis may similarly evolve from an initial generalized mild gastritis. The determinants of this process or its progression to the AB phenotype are uncertain, but may include persistence of *H. pylori* colonization, variable host–microbial interactions, and perhaps additional cofactors such as alcohol use.

Gastritis and *H. pylori* colonization

The close association between gastric mucosal colonization with *H. pylori* and histologic

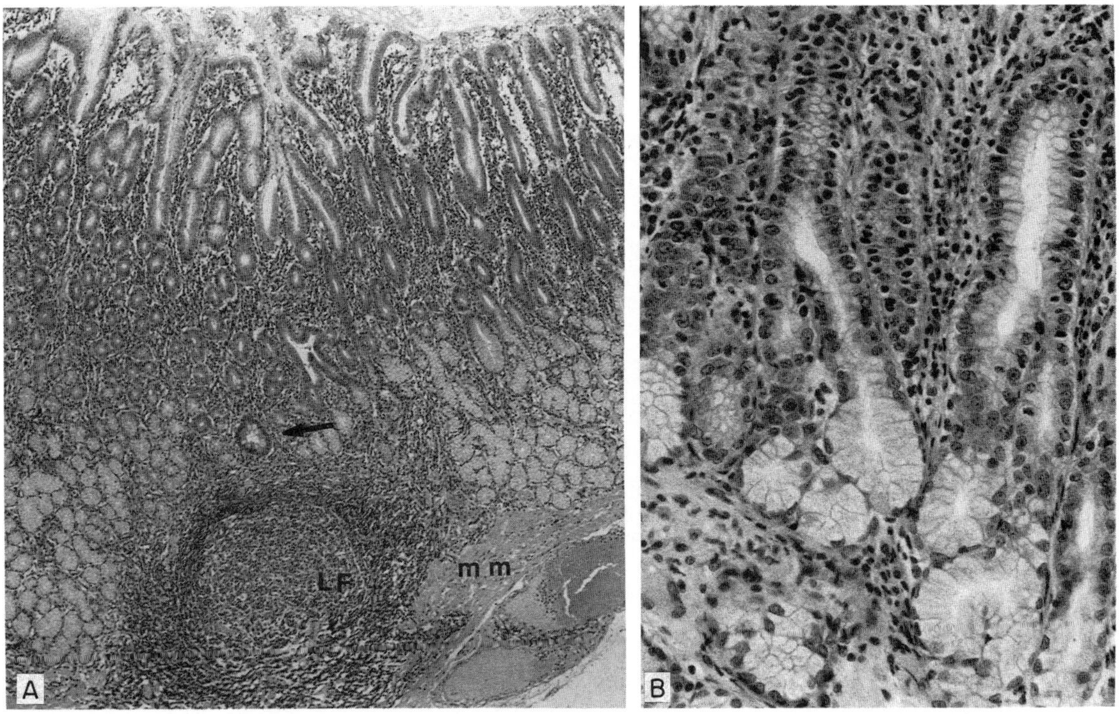

Fig. 1.10 Antral-predominant (type B) gastritis. A, full-thickness biopsy demonstrating the presence of inflammation extending from surface to the muscularis mucosae (mm). In addition to the presence of scattered lymphocytes, numerous lymphoid follicles (LF) are present throughout the mucosa in a pattern also known as follicular gastritis. Early intestinal metaplasia is evident by the presence of single metaplastic gland (←). B, higher magnification demonstrating the atrophic antral glands and the surrounding lamina propria-based mononuclear cell infiltrate.

gastritis was evident in the initial study by Marshall & Warren [19]. Among 100 patients undergoing endoscopy for upper gastrointestinal complaints, 57 showed colonization with *H. pylori*. In this group, 55 (96%) showed histologic gastritis. The prevalence of colonization was higher among patients with active antral gastritis (95%) than in those with quiescent gastritis (62%). Only two of 31 patients with normal antral histology (6%) were colonized with *H. pylori*.

Numerous studies worldwide have amply confirmed these fundamental observations and review of these studies [20, 21] indicates the following characteristics of the gastritis associated with *H. pylori* colonization (Table 1.3). First, the gastritis is largely histologic, although there are isolated case reports of apparent acute *H. pylori* infection that have been associated with impressive gross alterations on upper endoscopic examination [22]. Moreover, preliminary data in patients presenting with endoscopic gastritis, either idiopathic or associated with alcohol use, indicate significant but variable rates of *H. pylori* coloniza-

Table 1.3 Features of *Helicobacter pylori*-associated gastritis

General	Histologic, emerging reports of presence in endoscopic gastritis
Type	Non-specific
Distribution	Pan-gastric, type B, patchy
Grade	Superficial or atrophic
Activity	Active or quiescent, follicular

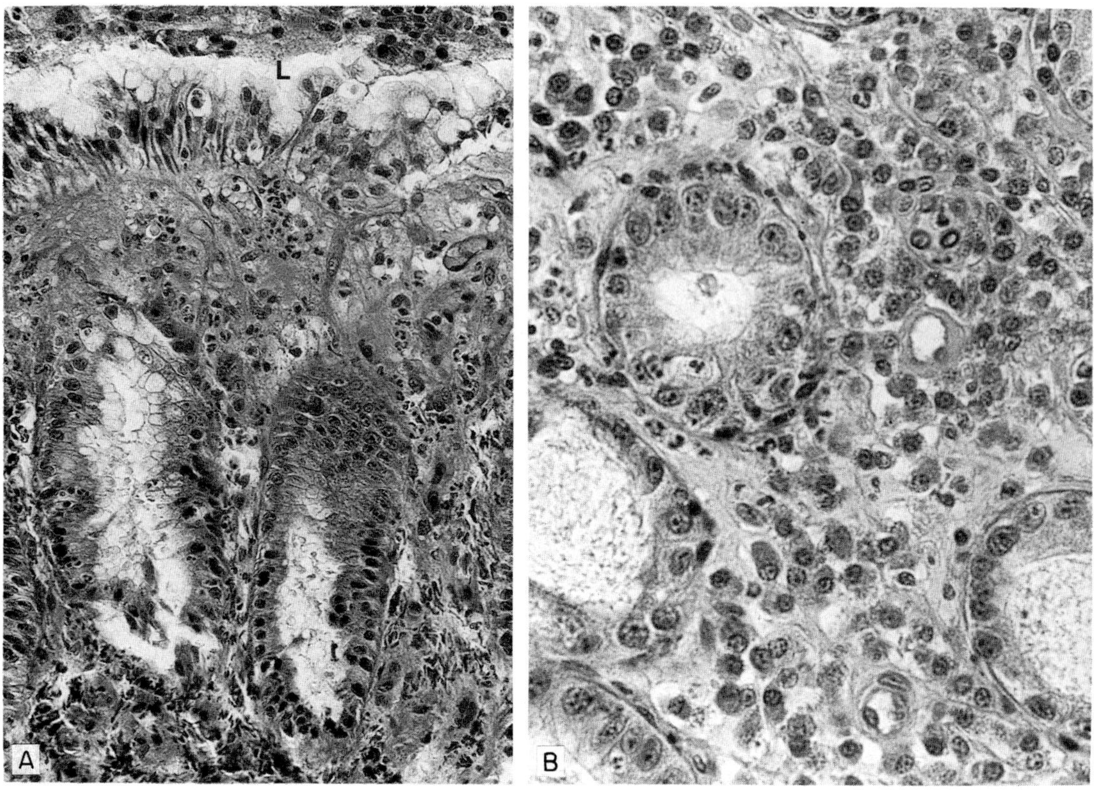

Fig. 1.11 *H. pylori*-associated non-specific gastritis. A, the upper portion of the mucosa in which active inflammation is present. Numerous polymorphonuclear leukocytes are present in the lamina propria underlying the lumen (L). In addition, the gastric pits are infiltrated by the same cell population. B, the glands deeper in the mucosa demonstrate the presence of neutrophilic infiltrates. Within the lumen of the glands numerous microorganisms can be seen. The surrounding lamina propria contains abundant plasma cells and lymphocytes.

tion in these settings [23–25]. It is possible that the observed variation in *H. pylori* colonization relates to variation in the presence of underlying non-specific histologic gastritis.

Second, *H. pylori*-associated gastritis is more frequently superficial than atrophic; the organism does not colonize areas of intestinal metaplasia, but can be present in adjacent non-metaplastic mucosa. Third, while *H. pylori* is seen more frequently in association with active gastritis (Fig. 1.11), it is also observed in quiescent gastritis, and lymphoid follicles may be a prominent finding. Finally, *H. pylori*-associated gastritis may be antral or pan-gastric in distribution, and colonization of normal corpus mucosa has been observed in association with antral gastritis.

These general characteristics have been largely based on observations in selected populations (peptic ulcer, non-ulcer dyspepsia), but in a recent retrospective review of biopsy material, obtained from the random population sample in Finland discussed earlier, the findings are similar [26]. In this study, 60% of the 157 subjects were colonized with *H. pylori*, and a clear correlation existed between colonization and the presence of non-specific histologic gastritis. None of 26 subjects with normal antral and corpus mucosa was colonized. By contrast, *H. pylori* was present in all 30 subjects with pan-superficial gastritis. With regard to advanced atrophic gastritis, the Finnish group found that *H. pylori* was present in 95% of subjects with type B gastritis, 72% of those

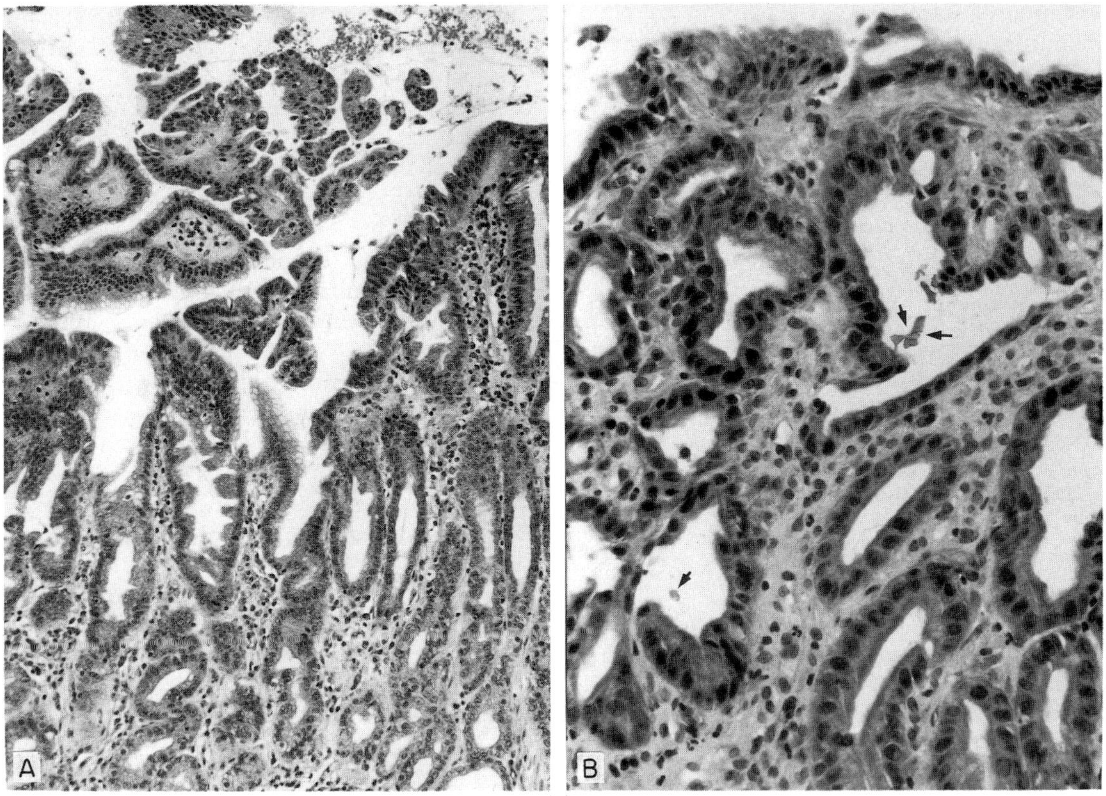

Fig. 1.12 Reflux gastritis in a patient with a Billroth II procedure. A, low magnification showing the presence of atypical gastric glands and prominent syncytial formations in the lumen. The glandular epithelium itself is mucin-depleted. B, higher magnification of the mucin-depleted glands. Within the lumens of several are bile fragments (←). Note the paucity of inflammatory cells within the lamina propria despite the reactive changes in the glandular epithelium.

with gastritis type AB, and 0% of a smaller group with type A gastritis.

It thus appears that a majority of subjects with non-specific histologic gastritis are colonized by *H. pylori*. However, this association is not universal. Patients with pernicious anemia or its antecedent, type A atrophic gastritis, are rarely colonized with this organism [26, 27], and patients with postgastrectomy gastritis believed to be caused by enterogastric reflux also show a lower prevalence of *H. pylori* colonization [28]. It is of interest that reflux gastritis is also characterized by a distinctive morphology [29] — foveolar hyperplasia, lamina propria edema, and capillary dilatation are prominent, whereas inflammation is minimal (Fig. 1.12).

Thus the selective, albeit common, occurrence of *H. pylori* in non-specific histologic gastritis favors an etiologic rather than a secondary role for this organism. More persuasive evidence for this view includes:

1 The occurrence of "epidemics" of *H. pylori*-associated gastritis, apparently related to upper gastrointestinal instrumentation [30–32].

2 Limited human volunteer studies that indicate a cause–effect relationship [33, 34].

3 Studies showing that eradication of *H. pylori* by antimicrobial drug therapy leads to significant healing of histologic gastritis [35, 36].

One unexplained feature of *H. pylori*-associated gastritis is its very wide spectrum of severity and variability in activity. The duration of infection and density of colonization may in part account for this variable morphologic expression but, as discussed in Chapter 12, it may also relate to differing intrinsic properties of *H. pylori* (e.g. toxin production), as well as differences in the local mucosal host response to infection. The possibility of an additive effect of environmental cofactors, such as alcohol, should also be considered.

In general *H. pylori* appears to produce a state of persistent infection. Nevertheless clearance may occur, perhaps in response to antimicrobial therapy given for an unrelated illness, and could account for previous observations of "spontaneous" regression of non-specific histologic gastritis [16].

Summary

In the past two decades, interest in gastritis has greatly accelerated — a direct result of the routine use of endoscopy in the evaluation of upper gastrointestinal symptoms, together with the rediscovery of *Helicobacter pylori*, and the recognition of its probable role as a major etiologic factor in this group of disorders.

Classification of gastritis is currently non-uniform and confused by continued casual application of the term, and by the use of multiple qualifying descriptors in investigative work and in clinical practice. A dual classification into endoscopic and histologic forms of gastritis, with further separation of histologic gastritis into specific and non-specific categories, offers a simple yet practical approach to restoring uniformity to this field.

Non-specific histologic gastritis is the most common pathologic alteration of the gastrointestinal tract. Its high prevalence in otherwise healthy adult populations continues to impede a better understanding of the pathogenic role of non-specific histologic gastritis in benign peptic ulcer, gastric neoplasia, and non-ulcer dyspepsia.

The morphologic expression of non-specific histologic gastritis is quite variable, both in severity and anatomic distribution in the stomach. Less severe grades of gastritis are usually generalized, but frequently are distributed in a patchy fashion. Severe non-specific histologic gastritis segregates into defined anatomic patterns (types A, B, and AB).

Etiologically, most non-specific histologic gastritis appears to be caused by *H. pylori*. This includes the less severe grades (superficial, mild atrophic) and types B and AB atrophic gastritis. Type A atrophic gastritis is a distinctive, though uncommon, form of gastritis due to autoimmune gastric mucosal injury and is the antecedent to Addisonian pernicious anemia.

It is evident from this review that many unresolved questions remain concerning the biology of gastritis. We have proposed a classification scheme of "gastritis now," based on descriptive morphology that can provide a firm basis for application to clinical practice now, and for future clinical and basic studies in this field. Application of these principles is particularly relevant to future studies of *H. pylori*-associated gastritis aimed at gaining a more complete understanding of disease mechanisms caused by this organism.

Appendix: The "Sydney" system, August 1990

At the World Congresses of Gastroenterology held in Sydney, Australia, during August 1990, a working party under the chairmanship of Dr J.J. Misiewicz matured the new thinking on gastritis into a standardized system for classifying, recording, and reporting the changes of gastritis [37]. The stimulus for this exercise was two-fold:

1 The non-uniformity and multiplicity of existing systems of classification.

2 The need to incorporate new information on the role of *Helicobacter pylori* in gastritis.

The new classification was actually an amalgamation of several previous papers, most notably those of Strickland & Mackay [9], who defined types A and B of gastritis; Siurala & Kekki, who described the progression of these changes to atrophic gastritis [17]; Whitehead *et al.* [8], who used precise descriptive terms to convey the histologic appearance; and Warren & Marshall [10, 19], who introduced an ordinal scale for measuring the degree of infiltration

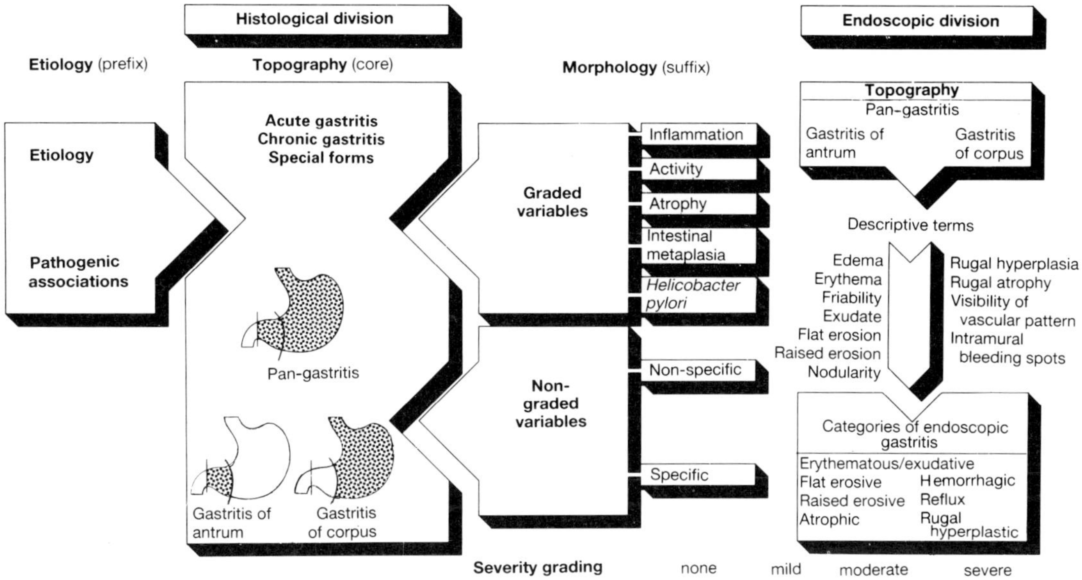

Fig. 1.13 The "Sydney" system of classifying gastritis.

with inflammatory cells, observed the prominent epithelial changes, and recorded the association of these changes with *H. pylori*.

Overview

The new system [38] begins with the premise that endoscopic visualization, together with standardized targeted biopsy of the antral and corpus mucosa, is the only reliable modality to identify and classify gastritis.

There are two major divisions of the classification scheme — endoscopic and histologic. The separate consideration of visual and histopathologic changes is based on the frequent lack of correlation between endoscopic abnormalities and microscopic pathology.

The working party recommends a standardized system (Fig. 1.13), recording in sequence: (1) topography — the core observation; (2) morphology, which provides the suffix for the final report; and (3) etiology or pathogenic association, when known, as a prefix to the final report.

This approach then replaces the multiple and often confusing qualifying terms used in the past to describe various categories of gastritis.

A key element of the new system is the listing of morphologic descriptors, both endoscopic and histologic, and the introduction of a severity grading system (0–3) for certain key changes (Fig. 1.13).

In the histologic division of the new system, only three major categories of gastritis are recognized — acute, chronic, and special forms.

If neutrophils are the dominant inflammatory cell, the gastritis is *acute*. If there is a concomitant or sole increase in chronic inflammatory cells, the gastritis is classified as *chronic*. Special forms of histologic gastritis involve unique pathologic features such as granulomas, eosinophils, or characteristic morphologic patterns such as lymphocytic gastritis or the reactive gastritis of bile reflux. Some examples of application of the "Sydney" system appear in Table 1.4.

Conclusions

The aims of this new system are "to produce a simple, easy to apply, comprehensive and

Table 1.4 The "Sydney" system

		Non-specific histologic gastritis	
	Specific histologic gastritis	Type A	Type B
Topography	Chronic gastritis of antrum	Chronic gastritis of corpus	Chronic gastritis of antrum
Morphology			
Graded variables			
Inflammation	Grade 3	Grade 2	Grade 3
Activity	Grade 2	Grade 0	Grade 2
Atrophy	Grade 0	Grade 3	Grade 0
Metaplasia	Grade 0	Grade 3	Grade 0
H. pylori	Grade 0	Grade 0	Grade 3
Non-graded variables	Non-caseating granulomas	None	Prominent lymphoid follicles Epithelial cell mucus depletion
Etiology/pathogenic association	Crohn's disease with ileocolitis	Pernicious anemia, PcAb+	Recurrent duodenal ulceration
Final report	Crohn's disease-associated granulomatous gastritis of antrum	Autoimmune-associated chronic gastritis of corpus with severe atrophy and metaplasia	*H. pylori*-associated chronic gastritis of antrum with severe inflammation and moderate activity

comprehensible classification which would be flexible and capable of correlation with preexisting ideas" [37].

It remains to be seen whether this new system will be embraced by clinicians, clinical investigators, and histopathologists and whether it will serve to restore order to this advancing field of clinical care and research.

References

1 Konjetzny, GE. Die Entzündung des Magens. In: Henk-Lubarsch (ed), *Handbuch d. Pathol. Anatomie 4, Heft. 2*. Berlin: Springer-Verlag, 1928.

2 Faber, K. *Gastritis and its Consequences*. Oxford: Oxford University Press, 1935.

3 Magnus, HA. Gastritis. In: Jones, FH (ed), *Modern Trends in Gastroenterology*, Ser. 1, pp. 323–5. London: Butterworth, 1952.

4 Schindler, R. *Gastroscopy. The Endoscopic Study of Gastric Pathology*. Chicago: The University of Chicago Press, 1937.

5 Wood, IJ, Doig, RK, Motteram, R, & Hughes, A. Gastric biopsy. Report on fifty-five biopsies using a new flexible gastric biopsy tube. *Lancet* 1949; **i**:18–21.

6 Taylor, KB. Inhibition of intrinsic factor by pernicious anemia sera. *Lancet* 1959;**ii**:106–8.

7 Taylor, KB, Roitt, IM, Doniach, D, Couchman, KG, & Shapland, C. Autoimmune phenomena in pernicious anemia: gastric antibodies. *Br. Med. J.* 1962;**2**:1347–54.

8 Whitehead, R, Truelove, SC, & Gear, MW.

The histological diagnosis of chronic gastritis in fiberoptic gastroscope biopsy specimens. *J. Clin. Pathol.* 1972;**25**:1–11.

9 Strickland, RG, & Mackay, IR. A reappraisal of the nature and significance of chronic atrophic gastritis. *Am. J. Dig. Dis.* 1973;**18**:426–40.

10 Warren, JR, & Marshall, B. Unidentified curved bacilli on gastric epithelium in active chronic gastritis. *Lancet* 1983;**i**:1273–5.

11 Goodwin, CS, & Armstrong, JA. Microbiological aspects of *Helicobacter pylori* (*Campylobacter pylori*). *Eur. J. Clin. Microbiol. Infect. Dis.* 1990; **9**:1–13.

12 Weinstein, WM. The diagnosis and classification of gastritis and duodenitis. *J. Clin. Gastroenterol.* 1981;**3**(suppl 2):7–16.

13 Whitehead R. Gastritis. In: Whitehead, R (ed), *Mucosal Biopsy of the Gastrointestinal Tract*, 3rd edn. Philadelphia: WB Saunders Company, Vol. 3, pp. 41–58, 1985.

14 Fenoglio-Preiser, CM, Lantz, PE, Listrom, MB, Davis, M, & Rilke FO. *Gastrointestinal Pathology. An Atlas and Text.* New York: Raven Press, 1989.

15 Ihamaki, T, Kekki, M, Sipponen, P, & Siurala, M. The sequelae and course of chronic gastritis during a 30–34-year bioptic follow-up study. *Scand. J. Gastroenterol.* 1985;**20**:485–91.

16 Roesch, W, Demling, L, & Elster, K. Is chronic gastritis a reversible process? Follow-up study of gastritis by step-wise biopsy. *Acta Hepat. Gastroenterol.* 1975;**22**:252–5.

17 Kekki, M, Siurala, M, Varis, K, Sipponen, P, Sistonen, P, & Nevanlinna, HR. Classification principles and genetics of chronic gastritis. *Scand. J. Gastroenterol.* 1987;**22**(suppl 141):1–28.

18 Glass, GBJ, & Pitchumoni, CS. Atrophic gastritis. Structural and ultrastructural alterations, exfoliative cytology and enzyme cytochemistry and histochemistry, proliferation kinetics, immunological derangements and other causes, and clinical associations and sequelae. *Hum. Pathol.* 1975;**6**(2):219–50.

19 Marshall, BJ, & Warren JR. Unidentified curved bacilli in the stomach of patients with gastritis and peptic ulceration. *Lancet* 1984;**i**:1311–14.

20 Yardley, JH, & Paul, G. *Campylobacter pylori*: a newly recognized infectious agent in the gastrointestinal tract. *Am. J. Surg. Pathol.* 1988; **12**(suppl 1):89–99.

21 Price, AB. Histological aspects of *Campylobacter pylori* colonization and infection of gastric and duodenal mucosa. *Scand. J. Gastroenterol.* 1988; **23**(suppl 142):21–4.

22 Frommer, DJ, Carrick, J, Lee, A, & Hazell, S. Acute presentation of *Campylobacter pylori* gastritis. *Am. J. Gastroenterol.* 1988;**83**:1168–71.

23 Malfertheiner, P, Stanescu, A, Baczako, K, Bode, G, & Ditschuneit, H. Chronic erosive gastritis — a therapeutic approach with bismuth. *Scand. J. Gastroenterol.* 1988;**23**(suppl 142):87–92.

24 Berstad, A, Alexander, B, Weberg, R, Serck-Hanssen, A, Holland, S, & Hirschowitz, BI. Antacids reduce *Campylobacter pylori* colonization without healing the gastritis in patients with nonulcer dyspepsia and erosive prepyloric changes. *Gastroenterology* 1988;**95**:619–24.

25 Laine, L, Marin-Sorensen, M, & Weinstein, WM. *Campylobacter pylori* in alcoholic hemorrhagic "gastritis." *Dig. Dis. Sci.* 1989;**34**:677–80.

26 Siurala, M, Sipponen, P, & Kekki, M. *Campylobacter pylori* in a sample of Finnish population: relations to morphology and functions of the gastric mucosa. *Gut* 1988;**29**:909–15.

27 Flejou, J-F, Bahame, P, Smith, AC, Stockbrugger, RW, Rode, J, & Price, AB. Pernicious anemia and *Campylobacter*-like organisms; is the gastric antrum resistant to colonization? *Gut* 1989;**30**: 60–64.

28 O'Connor, HJ, Dixon, MF, Wyatt, JI, *et al.* Effect of duodenal ulcer surgery and enterogastric reflux on *Campylobacter pyloridis. Lancet* 1986; **ii**:1178–81.

29 Dixon, MF, O'Connor, HJ, Axon, ATR, King, RFGJ, & Johnston, D. Reflux gastritis — a distinct histopathological entity? *J. Clin. Pathol.* 1986;**39**:524–30.

30 Ramsey, EJ, Carey, KV, Peterson, WL, *et al.* Epidemic gastritis with hypochlorhydria. *Gastroenterology* 1979;**76**:1449–57.

31 Gledhill, H, Leischester, RJ, Lightfoot, N, *et al.* Epidemic hypochlorhydria. *Br. Med. J.* 1985;**290**: 1383–8.

32 Graham, DY, Alpert, LC, Lacey Smith, J, & Yoshimura, HH. Iatrogenic *Campylobacter pylori* infection is a cause of epidemic achlorhydria. *Am. J. Gastroenterol.* 1988;**83**:974–80.

33 Marshall, BJ, Armstrong, JA, McGechie, DB, & Glancy, RJ. Attempt to fulfil Koch's postulates for pyloric *Campylobacter. Med. J. Aust.* 1985; **142**:436–9.

34 Morris, A, & Nicholson, G. Ingestion of *Campylobacter pyloridis* causes gastritis and raised fasting gastric pH. *Am. J. Gastroenterol.* 1987;**82**:192–9.

35 McNulty, CAM, Gearty, J, Crump, B, *et al.* *Campylobacter pyloridis* and associated gastritis: investigator-blind, placebo-controlled trial of bismuth salicylate and erythromycin ethyl succinate. *Br. Med. J.* 1986;**293**:645–9.

36 Rauws, EAJ, Langenberg, W, Houthoff, HJ, Zanen, HC, & Tytgat, GNJ. *Campylobacter pyloridis*-associated chronic active antral gastritis. A prospective study of its prevalence and the effects

of antibacterial and antiulcer treatment. *Gastroenterology* 1988;**94**:33–40.
37 Misiewicz, JJ, Tytgat, GNJ, Goodwin, CS, *et al.* The Sydney system: a new classification of gastritis. *J. Gastro. Hepato.* 1991;**6**:207–52.

2: Microbiology and taxonomy of Helicobacter pylori and related bacteria

S.L. HAZELL

Introduction

In 1982, the spiral bacterium *Borrelea burgdorferi* was identified, thus allowing a major component of the Lyme disease story to be recognized [1, 2]. At about the same time in Australia [3, 4], another spiral bacterium was isolated, the revelation of which has gone on to challenge many of the fundamental doctrines relating to gastroduodenal disease. This bacterium came to be known first as a *Campylobacter*-like organism, then as *Campylobacter pyloridis*, later as *Campylobacter pylori*, and now as *Helicobacter pylori* [5–8].

Whilst *B. burgdorferi* gained acceptance as the etiologic agent of Lyme disease, the road to acceptance of *H. pylori* as an important pathogen has not been easy and in some quarters remains controversial. This may be because *B. burgdorferi* was isolated in circumstances where medical science was looking for a pathogen, whereas *H. pylori* was isolated in circumstances where it was believed no "pathogen" existed.

Whereas other chapters will take up the challenge of addressing the pathogenicity of *H. pylori*, here the focus is the bacterium. There are numerous ways by which this organism can be unveiled; however an understanding of *H. pylori* can readily be achieved by following the path of the microbe as it establishes itself in the gastric environment.

Microbiology

Helicobacter pylori is a spiral-shaped bacterium measuring 2–4 μm × 0.5–1.0 μm, although rod and ox-bow forms are observed *in vitro* [3–5, 9, 10] (Fig. 2.1). The organism grows at 33–40 °C and favors slightly alkaline conditions (pH 6.9–8.0) [11]. Since the first isolation of *H. pylori* there has been only one report of the isolation of the bacterium in humans from sites other than the stomach or immediately associated mucosae. That was from one of 71 human dental plaque specimens [12]. Despite this finding, *H. pylori* does not appear to be associated with periodontal disease [13]. The available evidence points to the human stomach as the normal habitat of this bacterium.

There have been sporadic reports of the isolation of *H. pylori* from non-human primates; however no convincing evidence exists for *H. pylori* infection being a zoonosis [14–19]. A *prima facie* case does exist for person-to-person transmission, possibly by fecal–oral or oral–oral routes, although these assertions require further investigation [20–24]. Thus we shall begin our journey by assuming that the bacterium is ingested, be it by the vehicle of food, water, or another mechanism.

Gastric acidity

The first obstacle faced by *H. pylori* as it enters the gastric lumen is gastric acidity. On first viewing this would appear to represent a significant barrier to the bacterium, as in the two volunteer studies where *H. pylori* cultures were ingested, infection was established only with the aid of acid suppressive therapy [25, 26]. Yet there are reports of apparent transmission of *H. pylori* during the course of gastric analysis in volunteers, the reservoir of microbes presumably being instruments used in these studies

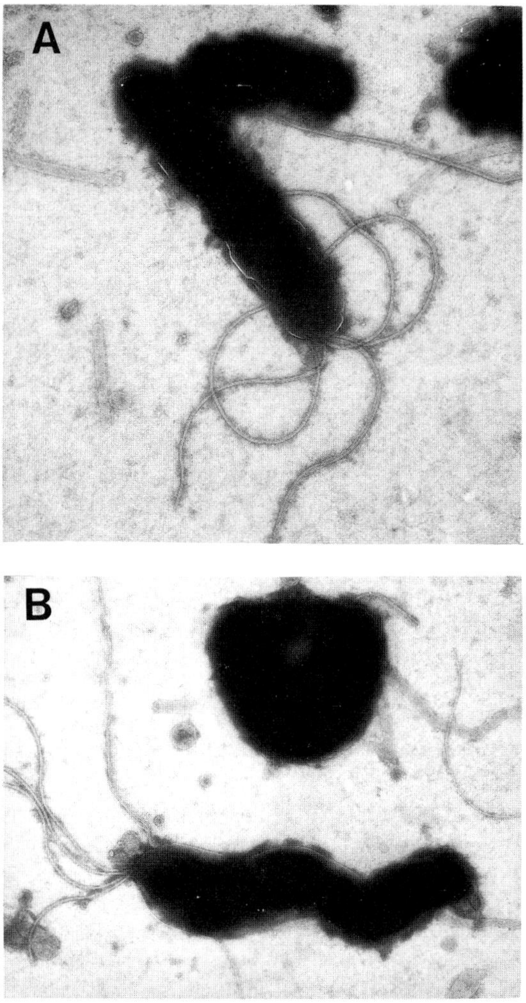

Fig. 2.1 Negative-stained preparations of *Helicobacter pylori* showing variations in morphology. A, rod shaped; B, spiral form and "balled-up" form.

[27–30]. Under such circumstances it remains possible that the bacteria were encapsulated in mucus fragments, and hence could traverse the gastric lumen in relative comfort.

Similarly, bacteria could be carried in food, and hence shielded from the direct effects of gastric acidity [31, 32].

In addition, it has been proposed that the high endogenous urease activity of *H. pylori* could act to protect the bacterium from acid damage, by providing an ammonium buffer between the cell and the environment [33].

Mucus penetration and motility

Between the gastric lumen and the epithelial surface lies the gastric mucus coat. This mucus covering presents an "unstirred" layer of viscoelastic gel that confers some chemical and mechanical protection to the gastric epithelium [34, 35]. The mucus layer also impedes the passage of particulate matter, such as bacterial cells [36], and as such represents a second barrier to the colonization of the mucosa by *H. pylori*.

In vitro studies present data that support the contention that *H. pylori* is adapted to efficient motility in viscous environments by virtue of its spiral morphology [37]. This is in accord with other studies with curved and spiral bacteria derived from gastrointestinal mucus [36, 38, 39]. The ability to transit the mucus efficiently appears a desirable trait, as nearly all other bacteria that colonize the gastric mucosae of man and animals appear spiral [14–17, 40].

An interesting feature of these bacteria is their ability to "track" along mucus strands. This behavior of spiral mucosal colonizers was observed as early as 1896, and has been recorded with *Campylobacter jejuni* and *H. pylori* [37, 38, 41]. A recent study of the mechanisms of pathogenesis in a gnotobiotic piglet model of *H. pylori* infection demonstrated that motility correlated with virulence [42], further evidence that efficient mucus penetration is an important feature in the establishment of *H. pylori* infection.

Flagella

The engines of *H. pylori* motility are the flagella. *H. pylori* has been reported as having up to six flagella [5, 6, 43, 44], although freeze-fracture preparations of the bacterium suggest that the normal configuration is seven [45] (Fig. 2.2). In common with a number of bacteria, e.g. *Vibrio*, *Beneckea*, and *Bdellovibrio* [46], the flagella of *H. pylori* are sheathed.

The function of the flagellar sheath remains to be determined, but may include increasing the effective diameter of each individual flagellum (of little value in the hydrodynamics of motility [47]), protection or epithelial adhesion. That flagella can act as organs of primary

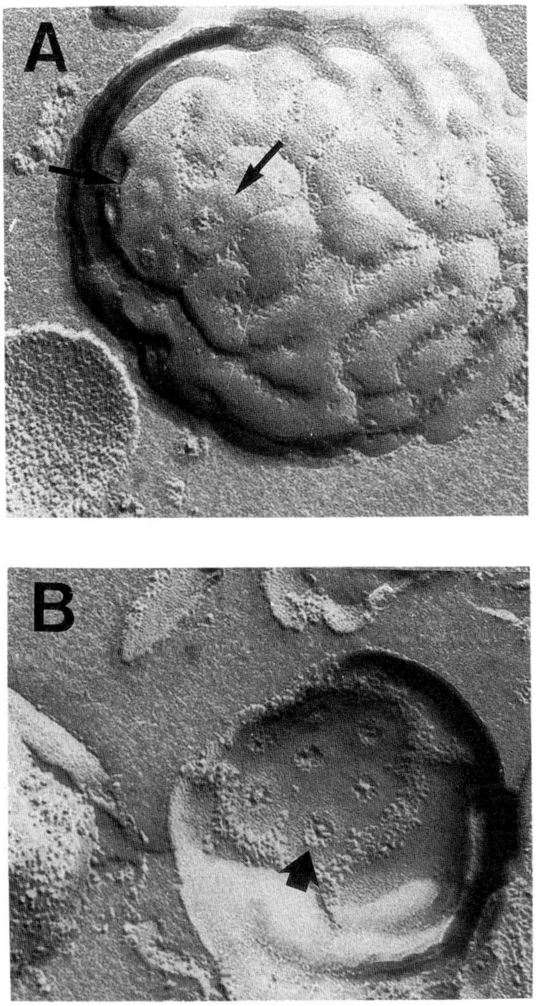

Fig. 2.2 Freeze-fracture preparations of *Helicobacter pylori* showing the flagella insertion sites. A, convex surface; B, the concave surface showing the seven points of attachment of the basal bodies of the flagella, one located centrally and six in a hexagonal array.

attachment has been demonstrated for a range of bacterial species, with the flagella capable of approaching close enough to surfaces for hydrogen or ionic bonds to form [48–50]. However, in the characterization of a putative colonization factor antigen (hemagglutinin) of *H. pylori* it was noted that the flagella were devoid of this antigen [51]. This suggests that the flagellar sheath does not have a colonization-antigen-mediated adhesive function.

Another reported feature of the flagella of *H. pylori* is the presence of a terminal bulb seen on electron microscopy [43, 52]. Such features have been noted in other bacteria with sheathed flagella [46]. As yet no conceivable function has been assigned to these structures. The possibility remains that these "bulbs" are artifacts of processing these bacteria for visualization under the electron microscope.

The flagella of *H. pylori* are constructed of repeating protein units (flagellin) having a molecular weight in the range of 50 000–62 000 [52–54]. Interestingly, the flagella of *H. pylori* are antigenically related to the flagella of *C. jejuni* [54], and also to the flagellar antigens of a diverse range of gastrointestinal spiral bacteria [53]. This suggests either conservation of antigens, or convergent evolution due to some selective advantage in the particular structure of these flagella, possibly related to motility in gastrointestinal mucus.

Mucosal colonization

Having penetrated the mucus, *H. pylori* can be seen to colonize the gastric mucus and to localize at the gastric epithelial intercellular junctions [37, 55, 56]. Although *H. pylori* is not invasive [57], the ability to localize at, and partially penetrate, the intercellular junctions resembles the mechanism of endothelial penetration recently proposed for *Treponema pallidum* [58]. Comparative studies of these bacteria may provide some critical information regarding mechanisms of microbial–tissue relationships.

The localization of *H. pylori* at the mucosal surface presumably proceeds under the influence of some chemotactic factor(s) [37]. Acidic environments can elicit a negative chemotactic response in bacteria [59]. In such a setting, *H. pylori* would be directed away from the gastric lumen to the mucosal surface, where the pH would be nearer to neutral [35]. While little is yet known of the chemotactic factors influencing *H. pylori*, *Campylobacter jejuni* is reported to respond positively to factors contained in mucus [60]. Further research may reveal that elements in gastric mucus may positively affect colonization and even the tissue specificity of *H. pylori*.

Attachment

Once localized at the epithelial surface, primary association leads to specific attachment. Studies aimed at determining the attachment mechanism have drawn investigators to look at the hemagglutination patterns of *H. pylori* strains, using erythrocytes obtained from man and animals [61–63]. These studies have shown some differences in the hemagglutination patterns of *H. pylori*, which may indicate some variation in attachment antigens. It was noted that the hemagglutinin(s) were mannose-resistant and sialic acid-specific [61]. Recently it has been proposed that specific attachment may be mediated by an *N*-acetylneuraminyllactose binding fibrillar antigen [40]. This antigen, a hemagglutinin, appears to be present on the surface of 75% of isolates tested, and so may represent at least one of a potential range of fibrillar antigens that possibly play a role in adhesion of *H. pylori* to the gastric mucosal surface [64]. Whether it is the hemagglutinins or other factors that dictate the observed specificity of *H. pylori* for gastric type epithelia remains to be ascertained.

Table 2.1 Biochemical profile of *Helicobacter pylori* *

Enzyme/activity	Action**
Carbohydrate fermentation	–
Urease	+
Catalase	+
Oxidase	+
Alkaline phosphatase	+
γ-Glutamyl aminopeptidase	+
Leucine aminopeptidase	+
Glutamate dehydrogenase	+
Deoxyribonuclease	+
Protease	+
Esterase	+
Lipase	+
2,3,5-Triphenyltetrazolium reduction	+
H_2S production (lead acetate)	+
H_2S production (triple sugar iron)	–
Nitrate reduction	–
Hippurate test	–
Indole formation	–

* References [5, 67–75].
** Positive result reported for the majority of strains tested. All reports have not agreed upon the biochemical profile of *H. pylori*, and therefore some judgment has been made as to which results may represent the true profile.

Nutritional requirements

Once established on the gastric mucosal surface, it is imperative that the bacterium should grow and propagate. To do this, the bacterium must exploit the available nutrient supply and, where necessary, augment the flux of victuals. *H. pylori* forms a stable population on the mucosal surface that seems not to be influenced by the dietary habits of the host (Professor David Y. Graham, personal communication). Animal studies have demonstrated that where the gastric microbiota (e.g. lactobaccilli and yeasts) is dependent upon the ingesta for nutrition, diet can dramatically alter these populations [65, 66]. The inference here is that *H. pylori* is not dependent upon the lumenal contents for nutrition, but instead derives such from the mucosa. *H. pylori* is non-glycolytic (cannot use sugars as an energy source), but has at its disposal a range of enzymatic mechanisms for obtaining the essentials for growth [5, 67–75] (Table 2.1).

The growing body of information regarding the lipase activity of *H. pylori*, although usually considered from the taxonomic perspective, or as a potential virulence factor [67, 74, 75], points to what may be a primary energy source for the bacterium, i.e. blood-borne or membrane-bound lipids.

Urease

One of the most striking attributes of *H. pylori* is its marked urease activity [37, 71, 76–78]. This high molecular weight (~600 000), apparently surface, enzyme [79], has been proposed as responsible for a number of functions, from aiding survival in acidic environments [33] to augmenting the damaging effects of gastric acidity [80]. The enzyme has two buffer-dependent pH optima (5 and 8), and appears irreversibly inhibited at and below pH 4.5 [81, 82]. This may indicate that protection of the bacterium from gastric acidity may be a secondary function for the urease.

When considering the bacteriologic function of urease, however, it must be remembered that such enzyme activity is shared with some non-gastric *Campylobacter* spp. (e.g. variants of *Campylobacter laridis* and *Campylobacter nitrofigilis*), other spiral bacteria of the bowel, not to mention a diverse range of unrelated bacteria; the urease activity of some of these organisms is as prominent as that of *H. pylori* [76, 78, 83, 84]. Relative to the bacterium, urease may play a vital role in supplying the organism with nitrogen.

It has been proposed that the high endogenous urease activity of *H. pylori* may aid the flux of urea from the blood and across the gastric mucosa to the lumenal side of the gastric mucosa where *H. pylori* is localized [37]. The ammonia liberated by the urease activity of *H. pylori* may be assimilated by glutamate dehydrogenase to form glutamate from α-ketoglutarate for subsequent transamination [71].

Microaerophilicity

A key feature of *H. pylori* is its microaerophilicity [5]. Although recognized, this characteristic of the bacterium has received little attention. It has been proposed that microaerophilicity may be responsible, in part, for the localization of *H. pylori* and *Campylobacter* spp. on the mucosal surface, at the interface between the typically reduced lumenal environment of the gut and the oxygen-enriched blood supply [85].

The reason *H. pylori* and *Campylobacter* species are microaerophiles is not clear. Susceptibility to toxic oxygen metabolites may be part of the story: *C. jejuni* appears to be sensitive to H_2O_2 in the environment, particularly during recovery from freezing or mild heat stress [86]. Recent evidence suggests that *H. pylori* is sensitive to fatty acids or other toxic species *in vitro*, but that in the presence of blood the bacterium may be protected from these toxic effects [87, 88]. This effect can be limited by growing the bacterium on media containing bovine serum albumin and catalase, indicating that an aspect of the toxicity may be mediated by peroxidation of unsaturated fatty acid [88].

The other side of the microaerophilicity story is the presence of CO_2. *H. pylori* will grow in a mixture of air plus 10% CO_2, provided there is a sufficiently humid atmosphere. Heterotrophic bacteria have a requirement for CO_2 in addition to other carbon sources [89, 90]. Some, for example *Neisseria gonorrhoeae*, appear to have a low affinity for CO_2 and so require an increased CO_2 tension or a bicarbonate-rich environment in order to grow [91, 92]. Interestingly, CO_2 is one of the products of urea hydrolysis; in light of this fact, urease activity may be important for providing CO_2 as well as nitrogen to the bacterium *in vivo*. Because of the latter, *H. pylori* may have adapted to a carbon dioxide/bicarbonate-rich environment and so require an increased CO_2 tension for growth *in vitro*.

Host response and *H. pylori*

As discussed in other chapters, *H. pylori* is now established as a major cause of active chronic gastritis. Primary colonization appears to be associated with an acute phase polymorphonuclear cell infiltration which later develops into the more commonly observed active chronic gastritis, wherein mononuclear cells infiltrate the gastric mucosa [26, 93]. As yet, little is known of the mechanism whereby *H. pylori* is able to induce these inflammatory changes, although it appears that activation of complement and endotoxin may play some role [94–97]. In the face of this marked inflammatory response, *H. pylori* not only persists but proliferates. Indeed it has been suggested that the presence of inflammation may actually augment the growth and survival of *H. pylori* by increasing vascular permeability and hence the availability of blood-borne nutrients [37].

Of significance to survival in the presence of an induced inflammatory response is the bacterium's catalase activity. The catalase of *H. pylori* is a tetramer with a subunit molecular weight of 50 000 and has an activity on the order of five times that of *C. jejuni* [98]. This enzyme may function as part of a complex mechanism of bacterial defence against the immune response of the host.

Taxonomy

The naming and classification of a microorganism is of importance to our understanding of the natural history of the species, as well as providing a basis for assessing comparative data from other bacteria. The nomenclature for *H. pylori* was in a state of flux for several years after the initial isolation of the bacterium. For reasons that are outlined below, we can now be confident that the new genus name, *Helicobacter*, will remain.

H. pylori was originally isolated using techniques employed in the isolation of *Campylobacter* spp. [5]. The bacterium's spiral morphology, microaerophilicity, and biochemical profile mean it met most of the criteria of the genus *Campylobacter*. However, *H. pylori* differed from the *Campylobacter* type species, *Campylobacter fetus*, in a number of phenotypic characteristics (e.g. urease activity and multiple sheathed flagella) and so was the subject of continuing taxonomic analysis.

One relatively early study suggested, on the basis of ultrastructural comparisons, that *H. pylori* was more closely related to *Spirillum* (*Aquaspirillum*) spp. than to *Campylobacter* [44].

Taxonomy, DNA and RNA

An important measurement in the classification of bacteria is the determination of mole per cent guanine-plus-cytosine (mol % GC) content of the DNA. This measurement, a guide to the relatedness of bacterial species, has been determined for *H. pylori* and is in the range of 35–38%, which falls into the range of *Campylobacter* species [5, 99]. However, similarities in mol % GC *per se* do not *ipso facto* place a new species of bacteria into a given genus.

Other comparisons placed *H. pylori* on a phylogenetic branch distinct from members of the genus *Campylobacter*. Specifically, comparisons of partial sequences of 16S ribosomal RNA from a range of *Campylobacter* spp. placed *H. pylori* in a taxonomic position closer to, but still distinct from, *Wolinella succinogenes* [100]. This basic finding was confirmed by several groups [101–103], although there was some argument that *H. pylori* should be classified as a *Wolinella* spp. [103]. However, the difference in GC ratio of *Wolinella succinogenes* (42–49 mol % GC) compared to that of *H. pylori* made such a grouping appear unlikely [99, 103].

Quinones

Other indicators of the distinction of *H. pylori* from *Campylobacter* spp. came from biochemical analyses of these bacteria. Analysis of the isoprenoid quinones (electron carriers) of several *Campylobacter* spp. indicated that all such bacteria contain menaquinone-6 and a methyl-substituted menaquinone-6, the latter being considered a useful chemical marker for *Campylobacter* spp. [104]. The absence of thermoplasmaquinones (methyl-substituted menaquinone-6) from *H. pylori* indicated a lack of relatedness between *H. pylori* and species of the genus *Campylobacter* [11].

Cellular fatty acids

Further differences reported for *H. pylori* include a distinct cellular fatty acid profile [44, 105, 106]. The cellular fatty acid composition of bacteria may represent subtle differences in the structure and function of the cell walls of these organisms, and have been recognized as useful taxonomic markers. Study of the cellular fatty acids of *Campylobacter* and related species by gas–liquid chromatography (GLC) has resulted in the tentative arrangement of these bacteria into what are termed GLC groups [105, 106] (Table 2.2).

The results of the GLC analysis, together with DNA–DNA hybridization studies [108, 109] further indicated that *H. pylori* was the member of a group distinct from the *Campylobacter* genus. Thus the transfer of *H. pylori* from the genus *Campylobacter* to a newly created genus was not unexpected [8].

Related bacteria

The isolation of *H. pylori* has reawakened interest in the microbiology of the stomach of animals as well as man. The study of such bacteria has a history reaching back into the 1800s, yet much of this information has lain dormant in forgotten tomes, only to be resurrected in the light of new knowledge.

In 1896 Hugo Salomon was among the

Table 2.2 Classification of *Campylobacter* and *Helicobacter* species by DNA–DNA hybridization[1] and cellular fatty acids (GLC)*

Strain	Group[1]	GLC[2]	GLC[3]
C. jejuni	I	A[a]	
C. jejuni subsp. *doylei*	I		A[b]
C. coli	I	A[c]	
C. laridis	I	B[d]	
"*C. upsaliensis*"	I		
C. fetus subsp. *fetus*	II	C	
C. fetus subsp. *venerealis*	II	C	
C. hyointestinalis	II	B	
C. sputorum subsp. *sputorum*[e]	III	C	H
C. sputorum subsp. *bubulus*[e]	III	C	H
C. fecalis[e]	III	C	
C. concisus	IV		
C. mucosalis	IV		
"*C. fennelliae*"	V	E	E
"*C. cinaedi*"	V	D	D
C. cryaerophila	NR	F	
C. nitrofigilis	NA		
H. pylori	NR	G	
H. mustelae	NA		J
H. pylori ("nemestrina A")	NA		G[f]
H. pylori ("nemestrina B")	NA		K

References: [109][1], [105][2], [106][3]
* Cellular fatty acids determined by gas–liquid chromatography (GLC).
[a] 97% of *C. jejuni* strains tested. [b] Some differences observed between *C. jejuni* and *C. jejuni* subsp. *doylei*. [c] 83% of *C. coli* strains tested.
[d] Contains some *C. jejuni* and *C. coli* strains. [e] Ranked as biotypes of *C. sputorum* [108]. [f] Some differences observed between *H. pylori* and *H. pylori* ("nemestrina A").
NR, considered not related to other *Campylobacter* spp.
NA, not available.

pioneers of gastric microbiology. He reported the presence of "spirochetes" in the gastric mucus of several animal species including cats and dogs [42]. Regaud [110] considered that the organisms of the gastric mucus layer of cats and dogs were morphologically analogous to the syphilis spirochete, and so named them "*Spirochaete regaudi*". Yet Kolmer & Wagner considered that there were three morphologically different spiral bacteria colonizing the gastric mucosa of cats [111].

The studies in animals led others to examine the situation in man, and from the early- to mid-1900s the mucosal microbiota of the human stomach was the subject of sporadic investigation [112–116]. At the end of this period there was neither substantive proof that man was colonized by gastric "spirochetes" nor convincing evidence that gastric "spirochetes" were of any pathogenic significance.

Campylobacter jejuni subsp. *doylei*

History now reveals that what many of these early investigators may have been looking at in man was in fact *H. pylori*. As a result of the interest generated in gastric microbiology, a range of other gastric spiral bacteria has now been isolated or identified from man and animals.

The intense study of the human stomach that followed the isolation of *H. pylori* led almost immediately to the isolation of a second mucosal spiral bacterium, initially termed "the gastric *Campylobacter*-like organism 2" (GCLO2), *H. pylori* being called GCLO1 [117]. The GCLO2 bacterium was later identified as a subspecies of *Campylobacter jejuni* (*C. jejuni* subsp. *doylei*) [118]. This bacterium appears to be a relatively uncommon inhabitant of the human stomach.

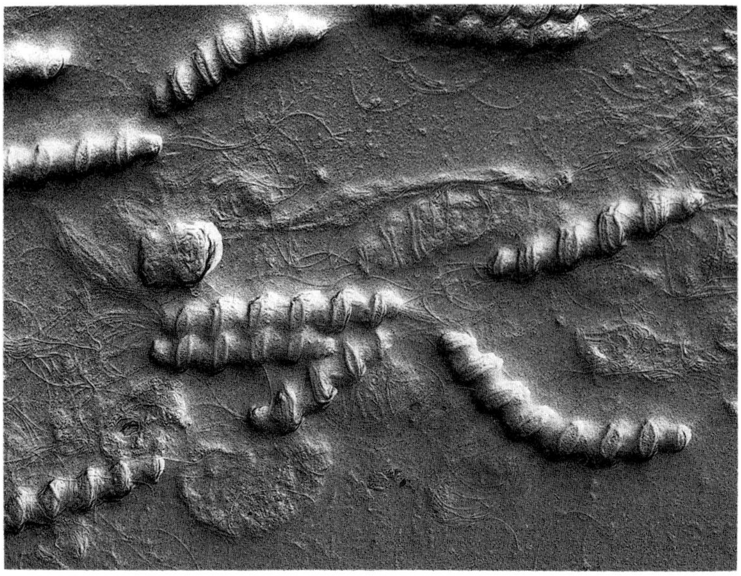

Fig. 2.3 Freeze-dried preparation of the gastric bacterium (*Helicobacter felis*) isolated from the cat showing multiple-sheathed flagella and periplasmic fibrils. (Micrograph courtesy of S. Kouprach.)

Related forms in ferrets

During this period, the focus of numerous investigators turned to the gastric microbiota of animals in the quest for a model of the human condition. Among the first bacteria isolated from animals was a bacterium found in ferrets, now designated *Helicobacter pylori* subsp. *mustelae* [119, 120]. This bacterium shares many phenotypic characteristics with *H. pylori*, has a GC content of 38 mol %, but differs from the latter in that it has lateral as well as polar flagella, grows at 42 °C, is deficient in leucine arylamidase, and reduces nitrates [119, 120].

Recent analysis of the cellular fatty acids of *H. pylori* subsp. *mustelae* have led to the suggestion that although the ferret organism is related to *H. pylori*, it is in fact a species distinct from *H. pylori* [106] (see Table 2.2). *H. pylori* subsp. *mustelae* has been isolated from ferrets in different parts of the world, although not all animals appear colonized, and there remains some debate as to the significance of these bacteria relative to disease in ferrets [119, 121, 122].

Related forms in the cat

Others have isolated from the gastric mucosa of the cat a bacterium that is morphologically distinct from *H. pylori*, yet shares a number of biochemical properties with the latter (urease, γ-glutamyl transpeptidase, leucine amino-peptidase, and alkaline phosphatase, as well as being non-glycolytic) [40]. The cat isolate, designated CS1, was spiral in shape with an average length of 5 μm and width of 0.4 μm (Fig. 2.3). Typically there were five helical turns per cell, with two periplasmic fibrils usually visible on the cell surface. The cells regularly had 10–17 terminal sheathed flagella. The cat isolate resembles in some respects a spiral bacterium isolated from the bowel of rodents by the same group [123] (Fig. 2.4).

This bacterium, designated ST1, is also microaerophilic and urease positive, and exists in a similar niche (i.e. on the mucosal surface and beneath the mucus of the bowel). The final classification of CS1 is pending; however, the name *Helicobacter felis* has provisionally been assigned to the bacterium.

Humans and non-*H. pylori* gastric spiral bacteria

The cat gastric bacterium resembles organisms seen in biopsies from three of 1300 patients involved in a prospective study of *H. pylori* infection in England [124].

Serologic examination of these patients,

using *H. felis* or *H. pylori* as antigen, demonstrated that most of these unusual "human" spiral forms were more closely related to the cat isolate than to *H. pylori* [125]. The presence of these unusual spiral bacteria in the human stomach has been demonstrated by several other groups [40, 126–129]. In one of these, the non-*H. pylori* spiral bacterium was detected in two of 600 patients, confirming a low incidence of colonization with this bacterium [128]. Some of these bacteria appear different to *Helicobacter felis* and the name *"Gastrospirillum hominis"* has been proposed [130], although the latter has not been isolated. Ultrastructurally, these organisms have multiple spirals, smooth cell walls, and numerous sheathed flagella (more than *H. pylori*) (Fig. 2.5).

As pathologists become more aware of these bacteria, and when some are eventually isolated, then the true rate of colonization with such microbes and their significance will be determined.

Related forms in primates

The search for a suitable animal model of *H. pylori* infection in man has also resulted in a reexamination of non-human primates. In the "pre-*H. pylori*" days, as early as 1919 and as late as 1982, there were observations of "spirochetes" and "spirilla" in the stomachs of these animals [114, 131, 132]. Retrospective examination of the data presented in these reports, and new reports on animals such as the baboon [133], indicate that the bacteria these investigators were seeing were morphologically similar to the bacterium recently isolated from the cat (*H. felis*) rather than *H. pylori*. However, there have been reports of the isolation of *H. pylori* from rhesus monkeys maintained in near natural environments or in animal research facilities [14–16]. The gastric microbiota in these situations has usually been mixed, with the "cat like" bacterium also being present.

Other monkeys, such as pigtailed macaques

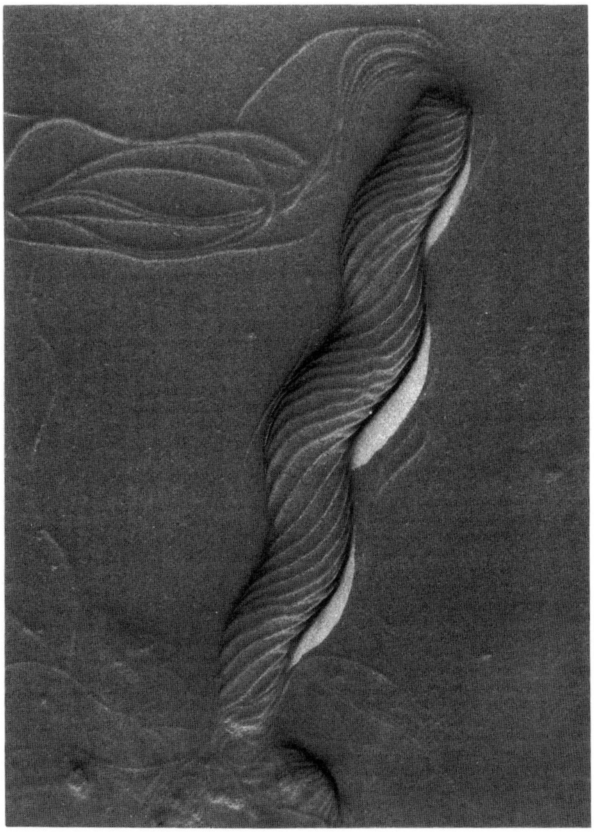

Fig. 2.4 Freeze-dried preparation of a urease-positive spiral-shaped bacterium isolated from the rat gastrointestinal tract (ST1). (Micrograph courtesy of Dr M. Phillips & S. Kouprach.)

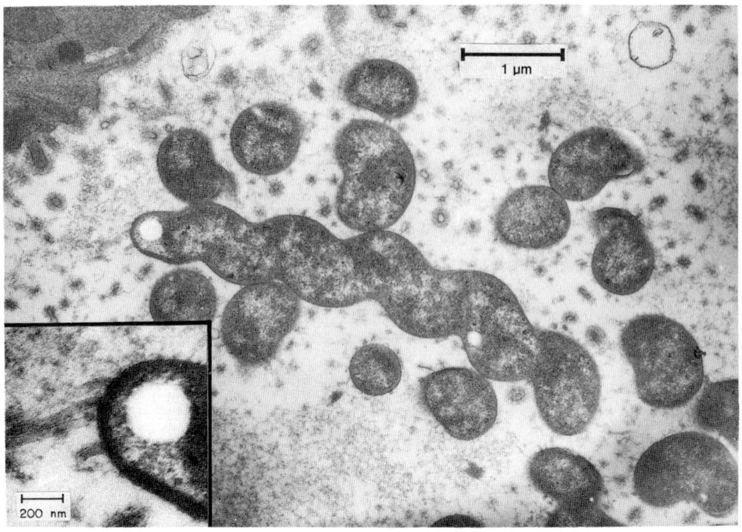

Fig. 2.5 Electron micrograph showing a spirillum cut in longitudinal section with adjacent transverse cuts of other spirilla. Note the smooth cell wall. Inset shows several sheathed flagella emerging from the end of the organism. The patient was a 77-year-old white male with long-standing dyspeptic symptoms. He kept two Irish setters as house pets.

(*Macaca nemestrina*), have been reported as being colonized by *H. pylori* [17]. Cellular fatty acid analysis of some of the strains of *H. pylori* isolated from the pigtailed macaques reveals that there are at least two types [106]. One, designated "nemestrina type A," has a fatty acid profile similar to human isolates of *H. pylori*. The second type, designated "nemestrina type B," has a distinct fatty acid profile and may in the future form the nucleus of a new species (Table 2.2).

Conclusions

Much basic microbiological research remains to be done on *H. pylori*. We know for instance that some strains of this bacterium contain plasmids [134, 135]; what is their function? Further, only basic studies have been conducted into the typing of these bacteria [135–137]. This area may hold the key to why some people develop ulcer disease in the presence of *H. pylori* and others do not. Although there has been progress since 1982, we need to know more of how this bacterium functions.

The intense interest in the non-*H. pylori* gastric bacteria should provide a wealth of comparative information that will aid our understanding of the mechanisms of pathogenicity of *H. pylori*, as well as providing basic information on the adaptation of bacteria to the environment of gastric mucosae.

Acknowledgment

The author would like to acknowledge the help of Ms Jani O'Rourke in the preparation of the photographs for this chapter.

References

1 Anderson, LF, Magnarelli, LA, Burgdorfer, W, & Barbour AG. Spirochetes in *Ixodes dammini* and mammals from Connecticut. *Am. J. Trop. Med. Hyg.* 1983;**32**:818–24.
2 Steere, AC, Grodzicki, RL, Kornblatt, AN, *et al.* The spirochetal etiology of Lyme disease. *N. Engl. J. Med.* 1983; **308**:733–40.
3 Warren, JR. Unidentified curved bacilli on gastric epithelium in active chronic gastritis (letter). *Lancet* 1983;**ii**:1273.
4 Marshall, BJ. Unidentified curved bacilli on gastric epithelium in active chronic gastritis (letter). *Lancet* 1983;**ii**:1273–5.
5 Marshall, BJ, Royce, H, Annear, DI, *et al.* Original isolation of *Campylobacter pyloridis* from human gastric mucosa. *Microbios Lett.* 1984;**25**:83–8.
6 Validation of the publication of new names and new combinations previously effectively published outside IJSB. *Int. J. Syst. Bacteriol.* 1985;**35**:223–5.
7 Marshall, BJ, & Goodwin, CS. Revised nomenclature of *Campylobacter pyloridis*. *Int. J. Syst. Bacteriol.* 1987;**37**:68.
8 Goodwin, CS, Armstrong, JA, Chilvers, T, *et al.* Transfer of *Campylobacter pylori* and *Campylobacter mustelae* to *Helicobacter* gen. nov. as

Helicobacter pylori comb. nov. and *Helicobacter mustelae* comb. nov., respectively. *Int. J. Syst. Bacteriol.* 1989;**39**:397–405.
9 Buck, GE, Gourley, WK, Lee, WK, Subramanyam, K, Latimer, JM, & DiNuzzo, AR. Relation of *Campylobacter pyloridis* to gastritis and peptic ulcer. *J. Infect. Dis.* 1986;**153**:664–9.
10 Jones, DM, Lessells, AM, & Eldridge, J. *Campylobacter*-like organisms on the gastric mucosa: culture, histological, and serological studies. *J. Clin. Pathol.* 1984;**37**:1002–6.
11 Goodwin, CS, Collins, MD, & Blincow, E. The absence of thermoplasmaquinones in *Campylobacter pyloridis*, and its temperature and pH growth range. *Microbios Lett.* 1986; **32**:137–40.
12 Krajden, S, Fuksa, M, Anderson, J, *et al.* Examination of human stomach biopsies, saliva, and dental plaque for *Campylobacter pylori*. *J. Clin. Microbiol.* 1989; **27**:1397–8.
13 Rosenthal, LE, Smoot, D, Mobley, HL, & Guisbert, W. *Campylobacter pylori* gastritis not related to periodontal disease (letter). *Am. J. Gastroenterol.* 1988;**83**:202.
14 Baskerville, A, & Newell, DG. Naturally occurring chronic gastritis and *C. pylori* infection in the rhesus monkey: a potential model for gastritis in man. *Gut* 1988;**29**:465–72.
15 Reed, KD, & Berridge, BR. *Campylobacter*-like organisms in the gastric mucosa of rhesus monkeys. *Lab. Animal Sci.* 1988;**38**:329–31.
16 Newell, DG, Hudson, MJ, & Baskerville, A. Naturally occurring gastritis associated with *Campylobacter pylori* infection in the rhesus monkey (letter). *Lancet* 1987;**ii**:1338.
17 Bronsdon, MA, & Schoenknecht, FD. *Campylobacter pylori* isolated from the stomach of the monkey, *Macaca nemestrina*. *J. Clin. Microbiol.* 1988;**26**:1725–8.
18 Vaira, D, D'Anastasio, C, Holton, J, *et al.* *Campylobacter pylori* and abattoir workers: is it a zoonosis? *Lancet* 1988;**ii**:725–6.
19 Goodwin, S, Armstrong, J, Bronsdon, M, & Sly, L. Is *Campylobacter pylori* a zoonosis? (letter). *Lancet* 1988;**ii**:968.
20 Berkowicz, J, & Lee, A. Person-to-person transmission of *Campylobacter pylori* (letter). *Lancet* 1987;**ii**:680–81.
21 Mitchell, HM, Bohane, TD, Berkowicz, J, Hazell, SL, & Lee, A. Antibody to *Campylobacter pylori* in families of index children with gastrointestinal illness due to *C. pylori*. *Lancet* 1987;**ii**:681–2.
22 Jones, DM, Eldridge, J, & Whorwell, PJ. Antibodies to *Campylobacter pyloridis* in household contacts of infected patients (letter). *Br. Med. J.* 1987;**294**:615.
23 Mitchell, HM, Lee, A, Berkowicz, J, & Borody, T. The use of serology to diagnose active *Campylobacter pylori* infection. *Med. J. Aust.* 1988;**149**:604–9.
24 Graham, DG, Adam, E, Klein, PD, *et al.* Epidemiology of *Campylobacter pylori* infection. *Gastroenterol. Clin. Biol.* 1989;**13**:84B–89B.
25 Marshall, BJ, Armstrong, JA, McGechie, DB, & Glancy, RJ. Attempt to fulfil Koch's postulates for pyloric *Campylobacter*. *Med. J. Aust.* 1985; **142**:436–9.
26 Morris, A, & Nicholson, G. Ingestion of *Campylobacter pyloridis* causes gastritis and raises fasting gastric pH. *Am. J. Gastroenterol.* 1987;**82**:192–9.
27 Gledhill, H, Leischester, RJ, Lightfoot, N, Barnard, J, Viney, N, Darkin, D, & Hunt, RH. Epidemic hypochlorhydria. *Br. Med. J.* 1985; **290**:1383–8.
28 Hunt, RH, & Darkin, D. Epidemic hypochlorhydria (letter). *Br. Med. J.* 1985;**291**:53.
29 Ramsey, EJ, Carey, KV, Peterson, WL, *et al.* Epidemic gastritis with hypochlorhydria. *Gastroenterology* 1979; **76**:1449–57.
30 Graham, DY, Alpert, LC, Smith, JL, & Yoshimura, HH. Iatrogenic *Campylobacter pylori* infection is a cause of epidemic achlorhydria. *Am. J. Gastroenterol.* 1988; **83**:974–80.
31 Park, CE, Stankiewicz, ZE, & Lior, E. Survival of *Campylobacter pylori* (*pyloridis*) in foods and water. *Abstracts of the Annual Meeting of the American Society for Microbiology, Washington, D.C., 1987*, p. 275.
32 Giannella, RA, Broitman, SA, & Zamcheck, N. Gastric acid barrier to ingested microorganisms in man: studies *in vivo* and *in vitro*. *Gut* 1972; **13**:251–6.
33 Goodwin, CS, Armstrong, JA, & Marshall, BJ. *Campylobacter pyloridis*, gastritis, and peptic ulceration. *J. Clin. Pathol.* 1986;**39**:353–65.
34 Williams, SE, & Turnberg, LA. Retardation of acid diffusion by pig gastric mucus: a potential role in mucosal protection. *Gastroenterology* 1980;**79**:299–304.
35 Williams, SE, & Turnberg, LA. Demonstration of a pH gradient across mucus-adherent rabbit gastric mucosa: evidence of a mucus–bicarbonate barrier. *Gut* 1981;**22**:94–6.
36 Greenberg, EP, & Canale–Parola, E. Relationship between cell coiling and motility of spirochetes in viscous environments. *J. Bacteriol.* 1977; **131**:960–69.
37 Hazell, SL, Lee, A, Brady, L, & Hennessy, W. *Campylobacter pyloridis* and gastritis: association with intercellular spaces and adaption to an environment of mucus as important factors in colonization of the gastric epithelium. *J. Infect. Dis.* 1986;**153**:658–63.

38 Lee, A, O'Rourke, JL, Barrington, PJ, & Trust, TJ. Mucus colonization as a determinant of pathogenicity in intestinal infection by *Campylobacter jejuni*: a mouse cecal model. *Infect. Immun.* 1986;**51**:536–46.
39 Ferrero, RL, & Lee, A. Motility of *Campylobacter jejuni* in a viscous environment: comparison to conventional rod-shaped bacteria. *J. Gen. Microbiol.* 1988;**134**:53–9.
40 Lee, A, Hazell, SL, O'Rourke, J, & Kouprach, S. Isolation of a spiral-shaped bacterium from the cat stomach. *Infect. Immun.* 1988;**56**:2843–50.
41 Salomon, H. Über das Spirillum des Säugetiermagens und sein Verhalten zu den Belegzellen. *Centralbl. Bakt. Parasit. Infekt.* 1896;**19**:433–41.
42 Eaton, KE, Morgan, DR, & Krakowka, S. *Campylobacter pylori* virulence factors in gnotobiotic piglets. *Infect. Immun.* 1989; **57**:1119–25.
43 Goodwin, CS, McCulloch, RK, Armstrong, JA, & Wee, SH. Unusual cellular fatty acids and distinctive ultrastructure in a new spiral bacterium (*Campylobacter pyloridis*) from the human gastric mucosa. *J. Med. Microbiol.* 1985; **19**:257–67.
44 Jones, DM, Curry, A, & Fox, AJ. An ultrastructural study of the gastric campylobacter-like organism *"Campylobacter pyloridis"*. *J. Gen. Microbiol.* 1985;**131**:2335–41.
45 Hazell, SL. Factors influencing the colonization of the gastric mucosa by *Campylobacter pyloridis* and the influence of the bacterium on gastric pathology. PhD Thesis, University of New South Wales, Australia, 1987.
46 Allen, RD, & Baumann, P. Structure and arrangement of flagella in species of the genus *Beneckea* and *Photobacterium fisheri*. *J. Bacteriol.* 1971; **107**:295–302.
47 Holwill, MEJ, & Burge, RE. A hydrodynamic study of the motility of flagellated bacteria. *Arch. Biochem. Biophys.* 1963;**101**:249–60.
48 Meadows, PS. The attachment of bacteria to solid surfaces. *Arch. Mikrobiol.* 1971;**75**:374–81.
49 Rogers, HJ. Adhesion of microorganisms to surfaces: some general considerations of the role of the envelope. In: Ellwood, DC, Melling, J, & Rutter, P (eds), *Adhesion of Microorganisms to Surfaces*. London: Academic Press, 1979, pp. 28–55.
50 Belas, MR, & Colwell, RR. Adsorptive kinetics of laterally and polarly flagellated vibrio. *J. Bacteriol.* 1982;**151**:1568–80.
51 Evans, DG, Evans, DJ Jr, Moulds, JJ, & Graham, DY. *N*-Acetylneuraminyllactose-binding fibrillar hemagglutinin of *Campylobacter pylori*: a putative colonization factor antigen. *Infect. Immun.* 1988;**56**:2896–906.
52 Geis, G, Leying, H, Suerbaum, S, Mai, U, & Opferkuch, W. Ultrastructure and chemical analysis of *Campylobacter pylori* flagella. *J. Clin. Microbiol.* 1989;**27**:436–41.
53 Lee, A, Logan, SM, & Trust, TJ. Demonstration of a flagellar antigen shared by a diverse group of spiral-shaped bacteria that colonize intestinal mucus. *Infect. Immun.* 1987;**55**:828–31.
54 Newell, DG. Identification of the outer membrane proteins of *Campylobacter pyloridis* and antigenic cross-reactivity between *C. pyloridis* and *C. jejuni*. *J. Gen. Microbiol.* 1987;**133**: 163–70.
55 Steer, HW. Surface morphology of the gastroduodenal mucosa in duodenal ulceration. *Gut* 1984;**25**:1203–10.
56 Chen, XG, Correa, P, Offerhaus, *et al.* Ultrastructure of the gastric mucosa harboring *Campylobacter*-like organisms. *Am. J. Clin. Pathol.* 1986;**86**:575–82.
57 Katchaki, JN, Bronkhorst, FB, & van Berge Henegouwen, GP. Lack of invasiveness of *Campylobacter pylori* (letter). *Eur. J. Clin. Microbiol. Infect. Dis.* 1987;**6**:500.
58 Thomas, DD, Navab, M, Haake, DA, Fogelman, AM, Miller, JN, & Lovett, MA. *Treponema pallidum* invades intercellular junctions of endothelial cell monolayers. *Proc. Natl. Acad. Sci. USA* 1988;**85**:3608–12.
59 Doetsch, RN, & Seymour, WFK. Negative chemotaxis in bacteria. *Life Sci.* 1970; **9**:1029–37.
60 Hugdahl, MB, Beery, JT, & Doyle, MP. Chemotactic behavior of *Campylobacter jejuni*. *Infect. Immun.* 1988;**56**:1560–66.
61 Emody, L, Carlsson, A, Ljungh, A, & Wadstrom, T. Mannose-resistant haemagglutination by *Campylobacter pylori*. *Scand. J. Infect. Dis.* 1988;**20**:353–4.
62 Huang, J, Smyth, CJ, Kennedy, NP, Arbuthnott, JP, & Napoleon Keeling, PW. Haemagglutinating activity of *Campylobacter pylori*. *FEMS Microbiol. Lett.* 1988;**56**:109–12.
63 Nakazawa, T, Ishibashi, M, Konishi, H, Takemoto, T, Shigeeda, M, & Kochiyama, T. Haemagglutination activity of *Campylobacter pylori*. *Infect. Immun.* 1989;**57**:989–91.
64 Evans, DJ Jr, Evans, DG, Smith, KE, & Graham, DY. Serum antibody responses to the *N*-acetylneuraminyllactose-binding hemagglutinin of *Campylobacter pylori*. *Infect. Immun.* 1989; **57**:644–7.
65 Decuypere, J, & van der Heyde, H. Study of the gastro-intestinal microflora of suckling piglets and early weaner piglets reared using different feeding systems. *Zbl. Bakt. Hyg.*, I Abt., Orig. A, 1972;**221**:492–510.
66 Tannock, GW, & Savage, DC. Influences of

dietary and environmental stress on microbial populations in the murine gastrointestinal tract. *Infect. Immun.* 1974;**9**:591–8.
67 Megraud, F, Bonnet, F, Garnier, M, & Lamouliatte, H. Characterization of "*Campylobacter pyloridis*" by culture, enzymatic profile, and protein content. *J. Clin. Microbiol.* 1985;**22**:1007–10.
68 McNulty, CAM, & Dent, JC. Rapid identification of *Campylobacter pylori* (*C. pyloridis*) by preformed enzymes. *J. Clin Microbiol.* 1987; **25**:1683–6.
69 Swiatlo, AL, Attar, B, Levendoglu, H, Go, B, & Kocka, FE. Identification of *Campylobacter pylori* by using the RapID NH system. *J. Clin. Microbiol.* 1989;**27**:341–2.
70 Taylor, DE, Hargreaves, JA, Ng, L-K, Sherbaniuk, RW, & Jewell, LD. Isolation and characterization of *Campylobacter pyloridis* from gastric biopsies. *Am. J. Clin. Pathol.* 1987;**87**:49–54.
71 Ferrero, RL, Hazell, SL, & Lee, A. The urease enzymes of *Campylobacter pylori* and a related bacterium. *J. Med. Microbiol.* 1988;**27**:33–40.
72 Slomiany, BL, Bilski, J, Sarosiek, J, *et al. Campylobacter pyloridis* degrades mucin and undermines gastric mucosal integrity. *Biochem. Biophys. Res. Comm.* 1987;**144**:307–14.
73 Queiroz, MM, Mendes, EN, & Rocha, GA. Indicator medium for isolation of *Campylobacter pylori. J. Clin. Microbiol.* 1987;**25**:2378–9.
74 Slomiany, BL, Okazaki, K, Zalesna, G, & Slomiany, A. Effect of colloidal bismuth subcitrate (CBS) on the protease and lipase activities of *Campylobacter pylori* towards gastric mucus (abstract). *Gastroenterology* 1989;**96**:A478.
75 Raedsch, R, Stiehl, A, Pohl, S, & Plachky, J. Quantification of phospholipase A2-activity of *Campylobacter pylori* (abstract). *Gastroenterology* 1989;**96**:A404.
76 Langenberg, ML, Tytgat, GN, Schipper, MEI, Rietra, PJGM, & Zanen, HC. *Campylobacter*-like organisms in the stomach of patients and healthy individuals (letter). *Lancet* 1984;**i**:1348.
77 Owen, RJ, Martin, SR, & Borman, P. Rapid urea hydrolysis by gastric *Campylobacters* (letter). *Lancet* 1985;**i**:111.
78 Mobley, HLT, Cortesia, MJ, Rosenthal, LE, & Jones, BD. Characterization of urease from *Campylobacter pylori. J. Clin. Microbiol.* 1988; **26**:831–6.
79 Evans, DJ Jr, Evans, DG, Graham, DY, & Klein, PD. A sensitive and specific serologic test for detection of *Campylobacter pylori* infection. *Gastroenterology* 1989;**96**:1004–8.
80 Hazell, SL, & Lee, A. *Campylobacter pyloridis*, urease, hydrogen ion back diffusion, and gastric ulcers. *Lancet* 1986;**ii**:15–7.
81 Taylor, M, & Karim, QN. Urease activity of *Campylobacter pylori* (letter). *J. Clin. Pathol.* 1988;**41**:112.
82 Taylor, MB, Goodwin, CS, & Karim, QN. Two urease activities with different pH optima in *Campylobacter pylori* and similar organisms. *FEMS Microbiol. Lett.* 1988;**55**:259–62.
83 Megraud, F, Chevrier, D, Desplaces, N, Sedallian, A, & Guesdon, JL. Urease-positive thermophilic campylobacter (*Campylobacter laridis* variant) isolated from an appendix and from human feces. *J. Clin. Microbiol.* 1988;**26**:1050–1.
84 McLung, CR, Patriquin, DG, & Davis, RE. *Campylobacter nitrofigilis* sp. nov., a nitrogen-fixing bacterium associated with roots of *Spartina alterniflora* Loisel. *Int. J. Syst. Bacteriol.* 1983; **33**:605–12.
85 Lee, A, & Hazell, SL. *Campylobacter pylori* in health and disease: an ecological perspective. *Microbiol. Ecol. Health Dis.* 1988;**1**:1–16.
86 Humphrey, TJ. Peroxide sensitivity and catalase activity in *Campylobacter jejuni* after injury and during recovery. *J. Appl. Bacteriol.* 1988; **64**:337–43.
87 Buck, GE, & Smith, JS. Medium supplementation for growth of *C. pylori. J. Clin. Microbiol.* 1987; **25**:597–9.
88 Hazell, SL, Markesich, DC, Evans, DJ Jr, Evans, DG, & Graham, DY. Influence of media supplements on growth and survival of *Campylobacter pylori. Eur. J. Clin. Microbiol. Infect. Dis.* 1989; **8**:597–602.
89 Dangley, S, & Hinshelwood, CN. Quantitative dependence of growth rate of Bact. *Lactis aeroogenes* on the carbon dioxide content of the gas atmosphere. *J. Chem. Soc.* 1938;**1938**: 1936–42.
90 Wood, HG, & Werkman, CH. The relationship of bacterial utilization of carbon dioxide to succinic acid formation. *Biochem. J.* 1940;**34**: 129–38.
91 Jones, RT, & Talley, RS. Effects of CO_2 and bicarbonate on the growth of *Neisseria gonorrhoeae. J. Clin. Microbiol.* 1977;**5**:427–32.
92 Potter, LD, Lewis, JS, Wentworth, BB, & Larsen, EH. Ammonium bicarbonate as a replacement for carbon dioxide in transgrow bottles for primary isolation of *Neisseria gonorrhoeae. J. Clin. Microbiol.* 1983;**18**:1258–9.
93 Frommer, DJ, Carrick, J, Lee, A, & Hazell, SL. Acute presentation of *Campylobacter pylori* gastritis. *Am. J. Gastroenterol.* 1988;**83**: 1168–71.
94 Hazell, SL, & Lee, A. *Campylobacter pyloridis*, urease, and gastric ulcers (letter). *Lancet* 1986; **ii**:626.
95 Pruul, H, Lee, PC, Goodwin, CS, & McDonald, PJ. Interaction of *Campylobacter pyloridis* with human immune defence mechanisms. *J. Med.*

Microbiol. 1987;**23**:233–8.
96 Das, SS, Karim, QN, & Easmon, CS. Opsonophagocytosis of *Campylobacter pylori*. *J. Med. Microbiol.* 1988;**27**:125–30.
97 Fumarola, D, & Miragliotta, G. Possible pathogenic mechanisms of *Campylobacter pylori* (letter). *Eur. J. Clin. Microbiol. Infect. Dis.* 1988; **7**:579–80.
98 Hazell, SL, Evans, DJ Jr, Evans, DG, & Graham, DG. *Helicobacter pylori* catalase *J. Gen. Microbiol.* (submitted).
99 Beji, A, Megraud, F, Vincent, P, Gavini, F, Izard, D, & Leclerc, H. GC content of DNA of *Campylobacter pylori* and other species belonging to the genus *Campylobacter*. *Ann. Inst. Pasteur/Microbiol.* 1988;**139**:527–34.
100 Romaniuk, PJ, Zoltowska, B, Trust, TJ, *et al.* *Campylobacter pylori*, the spiral bacterium associated with human gastritis, is not a true *Campylobacter* sp. *J. Bacteriol.*1987;**169**: 2137–41.
101 Lau, PP, De Brunner-Vossbrinck, B, Dunn, B, *et al.* Phylogenic diversity and position of the genus *Campylobacter*. *Syst. Appl. Microbiol.* 1987;**9**: 231–38.
102 Paster, BJ, & Dewhirst, FE. Phylogeny of *Campylobacter, Wolinella, Bacteroides gracilis*, and *Bacteroides ureolyticus* by 16S ribosomal ribonucleic acid sequencing. *Int. J. Syst. Bact.* 1988;**38**:56–62.
103 Thompson, LM III, Smibert, RM, Johnson, JL, & Krieg, NR. Phylogenic study of the genus *Campylobacter*. *Int. J. Syst. Bact.* 1988;**38**: 109–200.
104 Moss, CW, Kai, A, Lambert, MA, & Patton, C. Isoprenoid quinone content and cellular fatty acid composition of *Campylobacter* species. *J. Clin. Microbiol.* 1984;**19**:772–6.
105 Lambert, MA, Patton, CM, Barrett, TJ, & Moss, CW. Differentiation of *Campylobacter* and *Campylobacter*-like organisms by cellular fatty acid composition. *J. Clin. Microbiol.* 1987;**25**: 706–13.
106 Goodwin, CS, McConnell, W, McCulloch, *et al.* Cellular fatty acid composition of *Campylobacter pylori* from primates and ferrets compared with those of other campylobacters. *J. Clin. Microbiol.* 1989;**27**:938–43.
107 Roop, RM II, Smibert, RM, Johnson, JL, & Krieg, NR. DNA homology studies of the catalase-negative campylobacter and *"Campylobacter fecalis,"* an amended description of *Campylobacter sputorum*, and proposal of the neotype strain of *Campylobacter sputorum*. *Can. J. Microbiol.* 1985;**31**:823–31.
108 von Wulffen, HV. Low degree of relatedness between *Campylobacter pyloridis* and enteropathogenic *Campylobacter* species as revealed by DNA–DNA blot hybridization and immunoblot studies. *FEMS Microbiol. Lett.* 1987;**42**:129–33.
109 Chevrier, D, Larzul, D, Megraud, F, & Guesdon, J–L. Identification and classification of *Campylobacter* strains by using nonradioactive DNA probes. *J. Clin. Microbiol.* 1989;**27**: 321–6.
110 Regaud, cited by Kolmer & Wagner [112].
111 Kolmer, W, & Wagner, RJ. Über eine in Magenfundus des Hundes vorkommende saprophytische Spirochate. *Centralbl. Bakt. Parasit. Infekt.* 1916;**78**:383–4.
112 Krientz, W. Über das Auftreten von Spirochaeten verschiedener Form im Mageninhalt bei Carcinoma Ventriculi. *Deutsche Med. Wchnschr.* 1906;**32**:872.
113 Luger, A, & Neuberger, H. Über Spirochaetenbefunde im Magensaft und deren diagnostische Bedeutung für das Carcinoma Ventriculi. *Zeit. Klin. Med.* 1921;**92**:54.
114 Doenges, JL. Spirochetes in gastric glands of Macacus rhesus and humans without definite history of related disease. *Proc. Soc. Exp. Biol. Med.* 1938;**38**:536–8.
115 Freedberg, AS, & Barron, LE. The presence of spirochetes in human gastric mucosa. *Am. J. Dig. Dis.* 1940;**7**:443–5.
116 Palmer, ED. Investigation of the gastric mucosa spirochetes of the human. *Gastroenterology* 1954;**27**:218–20.
117 Kasper, G, & Dickgiesser, N. Isolation from gastric epithelium of *Campylobacter*-like bacteria that are distinct from *Campylobacter pyloridis* (letter). *Lancet* 1985;**i**:111–2.
118 Steele, TW, & Owen, RJ. *Campylobacter jejuni* subsp. *doylei* subsp. nov., a subspecies of nitrate-negative campylobacters isolated from human clinical specimens. *Int. J. Syst. Bacteriol.* 1988; **38**:316–8.
119 Fox, JG, Cabot, EB, Taylor, NS, & Laraway, R. Gastric colonization by *Campylobacter pylori* subsp. *mustelae* in ferrets. *Infect. Immun.* 1988; **56**:2994–6.
120 Fox, JG, Taylor, NS, Edmonds, P, & Brenner, DJ. *Campylobacter pylori* subsp. *mustelae* subsp. nov., isolated from the gastric mucosa of ferrets (*Mustela putorius furo*), and an amended description of *Campylobacter pylori*. *Int. J. Syst. Bacteriol.* 1988;**38**:367–70.
121 Tompkins, DS, Wyatt, JI, Rathbone, BJ, & West, AP. The characterization and pathological significance of gastric *Campylobacter*-like organisms in the ferret: a model for chronic gastritis? *Epidemiol. Infect.* 1988;**101**:269–78.
122 Tasman-Jones, C. Failure to detect gastric *Campylobacter*-like organisms in a group of ferrets in New Zealand (letter). *N. Z. Med. J.*

1988;**101**:275.

123 Phillips, MW, Lee, A, & Leach, WD. The mucosa-associated microflora of the rat intestine: a study of normal distribution and magnesium sulphate induced diarrhoea. *Aust. J. Exp. Biol. Med.* 1978;**56**:649–62.

124 Dent, JC, McNulty, CAM, Uff, JC, Wilkinson, SP, & Gear, MWL. Spiral organisms in the gastric antrum (letter). *Lancet* 1987;**ii**:96.

125 Lee, A, Dent, J, Hazell, S, & McNulty, C. Origin of spiral organisms in human gastric antrum (letter). *Lancet* 1988;**i**:300–1.

126 Morris, A, Ali, MR, Thompson, L, & Vanderwee, M. Tightly spiral shaped bacteria in gastric antrum: are they urease positive? *J. Clin. Pathol.* 1989;**42**:216.

127 Lee, A, Dick, E, Eckstein, RP, Kellow, JE, & Fevre, DI. Non-*Campylobacter pylori* spiral organisms in the gastric antrum. *Aust. N. Z. J. Med.* 1989;**19**:156–8.

128 Dye, KR, Marshall, BJ, Frierson, HF Jr, Guerrant, RL, & McCallum, RW. Ultrastructure of another spiral organism associated with human gastritis. *Dig. Dis. Sci.* 1989;**34**:1787–91.

129 Fischer, R, Samisch, W, & Schwenke, E. "*Gastrospirillum hominis*": another four cases (letter). *Lancet* 1990;**ii**:335–59.

130 McNulty, CAM, Dent, JC, Curry, A, *et al.* New spiral bacterium in the gastric mucosa. *J. Clin. Pathol.* 1989;**42**:585–91.

131 Kasai, K, & Kobayashi, R. The stomach spirochete occurring in mammals. *J. Parasitol.* 1919;**6**:1–10.

132 Sato, T, & Takeuchi, A. Infection by spirilla in the stomach of the rhesus monkey. *Vet. Pathol.* 1982;**19**(suppl 7):17–25.

133 Curry, A, Jones, D, & Eldridge, J. Spiral organisms in the baboon (letter). *Lancet* 1987; **ii**:634–5.

134 Penfold, SS, Lastovica, AJ, & Elisha, BG. Demonstration of plasmids in *Campylobacter pylori* (letter). *J. Infect. Dis.* 1988;**157**:850–1.

135 Majewski, SIH, & Goodwin, CS. Restriction endonuclease analysis of the genome of *Campylobacter pylori* with a rapid extraction method: evidence for considerable genomic variation. *J. Infect. Dis.* 1988;**157**:465–71.

136 Langenberg, W, Rauws, EAJ, Widjojokusumo, A, Tytgat, GNJ, & Zanen, HC. Identification of *Campylobacter pyloridis* isolates by restriction endonuclease DNA analysis. *J. Clin. Microbiol.* 1986,**24**:414–7.

137 Perez-Perez, GI, & Blaser, MJ. Conservation and diversity of *Campylobacter pyloridis* major antigens. *Infect. Immun.* 1987;**55**:1256–63.

3: Non-ulcer dyspepsia — epidemiology, natural history, and association with Helicobacter pylori

N.J. TALLEY

Introduction

To effectively study and understand any disease requires that its relative rates and natural history are known. For non-ulcer dyspepsia, these basic issues are still unsettled, this being a major reason why knowledge about its etiology is so limited. This chapter will review the frequency of non-ulcer dyspepsia, its natural history and possible relationship with *Helicobacter pylori.*

Definition of dyspepsia and non-ulcer dyspepsia

Over 20 definitions of dyspepsia have been proposed, but the term has been used very loosely to encompass many gastrointestinal symptoms arising from almost anywhere in the gut [1–3]. Gastroenterologists generally tend to associate gastroduodenal disease, and particularly chronic peptic ulceration, with the term "dyspepsia" [1, 3, 4]. One of the key features of non-ulcer dyspepsia is pain, which is frequently described as "ulcer-like" [1, 3–5]. Yet, even patients with chronic peptic ulceration may have pain that is "atypical."

Classical ulcer pain or discomfort has been defined as two or more of the following symptoms: epigastric pain relieved by food or antacids; periodic epigastric pain; postprandial epigastric pain; and epigastric pain waking the patient from sleep at night [4, 6]. "Ulcer-like" pain, as so defined, occurs in only 60% of patients with chronic peptic ulceration, but is present in half of patients with non-ulcer dyspepsia [7].

Heartburn with or without acid regurgitation is also a very common complaint [5, 8]; while this on its own is often termed "dyspepsia," heartburn is a strong indicator of esophageal reflux disease, and so should be considered separately [1, 5, 9]. Other patients who present with upper gastrointestinal discomfort may have symptoms such as belching, bloating, visible distention, nausea, or early satiety that predominate [1, 5]; such "flatulent dyspepsia" may be more prevalent in patients who have the irritable bowel syndrome or aerophagia, and may reflect an underlying gastroduodenal motility disorder in some cases [4, 10–12].

The following definition of dyspepsia has therefore been recommended in an international working team report [4].

Dyspepsia

"Dyspepsia" should specifically refer to episodic or persistent upper abdominal pain or discomfort, which may or may not be related to meals; to be termed "chronic," symptoms should have been present for 3 months or longer [4]. This definition has the advantages of describing location, duration and exclusions, and will be used here.

Non-ulcer dyspepsia

Non-ulcer dyspepsia has been variably known as "functional dyspepsia," "X-ray-negative dyspepsia," "nervous dyspepsia," the "epigastric distress syndrome," or the "pseudo-ulcer syndrome" [1, 13]. When dyspepsia is present with a negative endoscopy (to exclude peptic ulceration, macroscopic esophagitis, and cancer), and when the physical examination and simple laboratory tests are non-contributory, the term "non-ulcer dyspepsia" has been applied [1, 11].

Non-ulcer dyspepsia is a heterogeneous syndrome clinically. Patients may have symptoms that strongly suggest peptic ulcer disease (termed "ulcer-like" dyspepsia). On the other hand, some may have pain and associated symptoms that suggest a gastric or small intestinal motility disorder ("motility-like" or "flatulent" dyspepsia) [4, 14, 15]. Others may have additional symptoms that suggest reflux of acid into the esophagus (termed "reflux-like" dyspepsia). Over and above these symptom subgroups, the complaints may be explained by a distinct functional bowel disorder such as the irritable bowel syndrome [4, 11].

If gastric biopsies are obtained from patients with non-ulcer dyspepsia, approximately 50% will have *H. pylori*-associated gastritis [14, 16]; whether the prevalence of *H. pylori* is different in the various symptom subgroups is unknown. Indeed, the relationship between gastritis and dyspepsia is unclear [16–18]; this important issue will be discussed later.

While the term "non-ulcer dyspepsia" is widely used, it is clearly inadequate because it groups together a number of disparate diseases and disorders. It would be just as logical to use vague terms like "non-gallstone" or "non-pancreatic" pain to describe a patient's symptoms, which are clearly nonsense [19]. For this reason the term "idiopathic dyspepsia" may be preferable. However, "non-ulcer dyspepsia" remains firmly entrenched in the medical literature.

Epidemiology of dyspepsia and non-ulcer dyspepsia

Measures of clinical frequency: prevalence and incidence

Determining the frequency of a disorder such as non-ulcer dyspepsia in any population entails measuring the prevalence and incidence. *Prevalence* is defined as the proportion of a group possessing a clinical outcome at a given point in time, and is measured by a single examination or survey of a group [20]. *Incidence* is defined as the proportion of a group initially free of the clinical outcome, but who develop the outcome over a given period of time [20].

Establishing the prevalence and incidence of non-ulcer dyspepsia remains more difficult than establishing these parameters in peptic ulcer disease [21, 22]. There are several reasons for these problems. The diagnosis of the disorder can cause difficulties. Peptic ulceration, for example, has been diagnosed in different studies at post mortem, by pan-endoscopy or barium meal, or, least reliably, on the basis of symptoms alone. Non-ulcer dyspepsia, on the other hand, can only be diagnosed if an accurate history is known and investigations or post mortem reveal no peptic ulceration or other significant organic disease. Non-ulcer dyspepsia is a diagnosis of exclusion, yet many of the data in the literature are unsatisfactory because they relied upon barium meal examinations, which are inaccurate; a significant number of cases of duodenal ulceration are missed, while a scarred duodenum may be misdiagnosed as active chronic duodenal ulceration [23, 24].

Estimating the prevalence and incidence is also difficult because non-ulcer dyspepsia and peptic ulcer are usually chronic recurrent disorders; indeed, sometimes patients with dyspepsia may have an ulcer crater, yet at other times with similar symptoms no crater is demonstrable [25, 26]. Therefore, assessments of the rates of non-ulcer dyspepsia and peptic ulcer are hampered by the lack of universally accepted criteria for determining whether or not the population has the disorder. Finally, to compound the problems, information in the literature can be misleading, because prevalence and incidence rates are often not clearly distinguished, and the measures used to determine these rates are often not described [21].

As the majority of dyspepsia sufferers have non-ulcer dyspepsia, rather than peptic ulceration (Table 3.1), data on the prevalence and incidence of dyspepsia will be presented before the frequency of non-ulcer dyspepsia is addressed.

Prevalence of dyspepsia

The magnitude of the disorder is very impressive, based on the figures available. In the United Kingdom, Doll and associates reported that 31% of the adult population over a 5-year period complained of indigestion or pains in the stomach [27]. Tibblin, in a cross-sectional

Table 3.1 Studies (conducted between 1943 and 1985) of the proportion of patients with dyspepsia without peptic ulceration, based on barium meal or endoscopic diagnostic testing

Investigators	Year of report	Number of patients	Proportion without peptic ulcer, gastric cancer, or esophagitis (%)
Edwards & Copeman [44]	1943	436	50
Avery Jones & Pollak [45]	1945	1522	37
Friedmann (male only) [46]	1948	138	67
Lipetz [47]	1955	463	30
Williams *et al.* [48]	1957	775	60
Krag [49]	1969	532	42
Edwards & Coghill [50]	1968	424	52
Davis & Williams [51]	1968	1663	47
Bonnevie *et al.* [52]	1971	114	26
Gregory *et al.* [53]	1972	276	37
Barnes *et al.* [54]	1974	50	40*
Mollman *et al.* [55]	1975	197	55
Mollman *et al.* [56]	1976	209	52
Mead *et al.* (all patients less than 50 years of age) [57]	1977	100	90
Oddsson *et al.* [58]	1977	181	47 (38*)
Bonnevie [40]	1976	2101	75
Horrocks & de Dombal [59]	1978	360	14
Beavis *et al.* [60]	1979	110	91*
Gear & Barnes [39]	1980	346	62*
Gear *et al.* [61]	1980	968	67*
Priebe *et al.* [62]	1982	88	42*
Becker *et al.* (all patients less than 40 years of age) [63]	1983	150	95
Watt *et al.* [64]	1984	1444	84
Lance *et al.* [65]	1985	100	71*
Edenholm *et al.* [66]	1985	165	51*
Sircus & Prescott [67]	1985	291	29*

* Endoscopy diagnosis.
Data on gastric cancer and esophagitis were not available in every study.
Adapted from Thompson, WG *Can. Med. Assoc. J.* 1984;**130**:565.

study, found that dyspepsia (which was not defined) peaked at age 50 and was reported by 26% of the men surveyed [28]. A Danish study of 1839 persons, sampled by opinion poll, indicated that the point prevalence of abdominal discomfort in the week of asking was 27% in those aged 15–70 years, and was almost constant at 30% in those aged 25–70 years [29]. In one-third of these cases, the symptoms were predominantly in the upper abdomen. Johnsen *et al.*, in a cross-sectional survey of 14 390 middle-aged persons in Norway, reported that 13% of men and 12% of women often had a gnawing pain in the pit of the stomach [30]. Other Danish studies have reported similar results [31]. An even higher prevalence of dyspepsia has been reported in the United Kingdom, but the vague (and undefined) term "indigestion" was used in their questionnaire [32]. Talley *et al.* randomly sampled a representative United States caucasian population of 835 persons, aged 30–64 years, using a previously validated symptom questionnaire. The overall age- and sex-adjusted prevalence rate of abdominal pain more than six times in the previous year was 26 per 100; the prevalence rates of upper abdominal pain and nausea were 16 and 7 per 100, respectively [33].

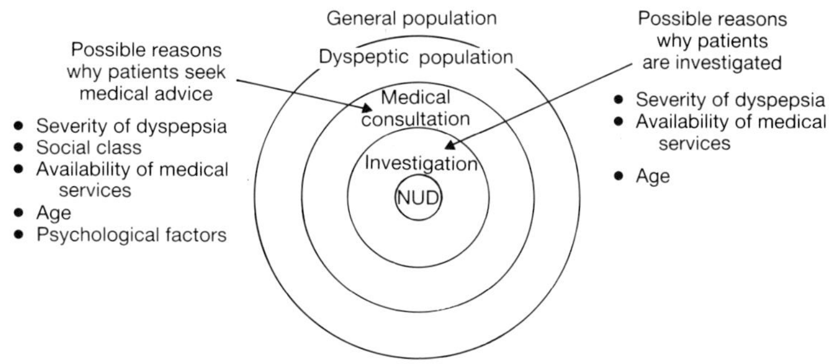

Fig. 3.1 Potential factors that influence health care seeking by persons with dyspepsia in the community. NUD, non-ulcer dyspepsia. (From Nyrén *et al.* [37].)

Wadsworth *et al.* were the first to report that only some patients with digestive complaints sought medical advice; 23% of their sample had been to see a doctor at some time for indigestion [34]. Of those who had seen a doctor, most were aged in the 30–39, or 60 years and above age groups, and this was more common among the unemployed. Other evidence supports the notion that most patients with dyspepsia do not see doctors [32–35]. Of those who take antacids, 90% do not obtain them by prescription [34].

In a study of 301 apparently healthy adults, abdominal pain occurred more than six times per year in 21%, with 7% having ulcer-like pain [35]. Importantly, in the year prior to interview, not more than 23% of these subjects had seen a doctor about the abdominal pain. Whether health care-seeking behavior is related to symptom severity, increased anxiety, neurosis, anticancer propaganda, free health care availability, or other factors, remains unknown [36, 37] (Fig. 3.1).

Incidence of dyspepsia

There have been very few studies of the incidence of dyspepsia. Over 20 years ago, Weir & Backett investigated a stable rural population in north-east Scotland [38]. A questionnaire was sent to 1500 men over the age of 15 years. After a 3-year period a second questionnaire was sent to the same men. "Ulcer-like" dyspepsia was reported by 15% of the population. A comparison of the results at the beginning and end of the study suggested that the rate of new dyspeptics was 1.6% per year, but this was balanced by a substantial recovery rate of 1.7% per year. Thus, the number of patients who become symptom-free or die may be balanced by a similar number who develop dyspepsia for the first time.

Gear & Barnes investigated patients presenting to general practitioners; the annual incidence of "dyspepsia" (which was not defined) was 1%, and 60% of these patients had no organic gastrointestinal disease [39]. Similarly, in a Danish population study the incidence of patients referred for barium meal studies was nearly 2% annually for adults older than 15 years [40]. If the annual incidence of dyspepsia approaches 2%, the life-time incidence of dyspepsia may approach 100% [41]. These figures illustrate the potential enormous economic and social consequences of dyspepsia for the health-care system and the general population [42, 43].

Prevalence and incidence of non-ulcer dyspepsia

In the last 45 years, there have been over 20 studies of patients presenting to clinics complaining of dyspepsia (Table 3.1) [39, 40, 44–67]. The prevalence of non-ulcer dyspepsia has varied greatly, but the majority of patients who present with "dyspepsia", however defined, do not have a chronic peptic ulcer. Importantly, all these groups of patients were not identical, ranging from hospital inpatients to general practice outpatients. Moreover, all these studies assessed highly selected patients; as only a small proportion of the dyspeptic population seeks medical advice, the results of the studies on investigated patients may not be applicable to the general dyspeptic population who do not attend for treatment [37]. Unfortunately, there are no adequate population-based studies to determine how important this selection bias really is.

The magnitude of the problem of non-ulcer dyspepsia is further emphasized by hospital discharge statistics. It is likely that the majority of patients with non-ulcer dyspepsia are not hospitalized. Yet, in the United States in 1976, 37 000 hospital patients were labeled as having psychogenic gastrointestinal disorders, and 19 000 of these had this as their primary reason for hospitalization [22]. The problem may in fact be larger, as it is unknown how many patients labeled as having diseases such as gastritis or cholelithiasis really in fact had non-ulcer dyspepsia. Finally, no studies have addressed the incidence of non-ulcer dyspepsia in the community.

In summary, "dyspepsia", defined as episodic or persistent upper abdominal pain or discomfort, is a very common problem with a point prevalence of 10–20% and an incidence of approximately 1–2% per year. Patients with dyspepsia can be broadly classified into two groups: those who have chronic peptic ulcer disease and those who have non-ulcer dyspepsia. The majority of patients who present to physicians with dyspepsia do not have a peptic ulcer.

Natural history of non-ulcer dyspepsia

There are two important questions about the prognosis of non-ulcer dyspepsia. First, what is the natural history of symptoms? Second, is non-ulcer dyspepsia a precursor of peptic ulceration? Unfortunately, of the few prospective studies that have investigated the prognosis of patients with non-ulcer dyspepsia, all but one have been based on single-contrast barium meal examinations.

Natural history of symptoms

There is some evidence that non-ulcer dyspepsia, like *H. pylori*-associated gastritis, tends to be a lifelong disease. Bonnevie reviewed patients with duodenal ulcer, gastric ulcer, and non-ulcer dyspepsia 2.5 years after diagnosis [41]. No significant difference was found with regard to the number of days of abdominal pain between the non-ulcer dyspepsia and peptic ulcer groups, and also with regard to the number of days lost from work. Subsequently, 77 non-ulcer dyspepsia patients were prospectively followed up 1, 3, and 5 years later. At 5 years of follow-up, 68% continued to have pain, although less than half of these had pain which interfered with their working capacity. Age, gender, the length of dyspepsia history, peak acid output after pentagastrin stimulation, and smoking and alcohol were not predictors of clinical outcome. However, patients at the time of diagnosis with vomiting or abdominal pain that was provoked by a meal had more abdominal pain than those patients without these symptoms.

Others have also studied the course of non-ulcer dyspepsia in barium meal-negative cases. Gregory *et al.* found that 76% of X-ray-negative dyspeptics were symptomatically improved 6 years after diagnosis, with the remainder having persistent dyspepsia [53]. This study was based on a general practice population. Becker *et al.* studied younger non-ulcer dyspepsia patients (less than 40 years of age), and found that 3 months after examination 25% had symptomatically improved, and this was unrelated to the treatment received [63]. In the one study of prognosis following endoscopic diagnosis of non-ulcer dyspepsia, Talley *et al.* prospectively followed up 111 patients for up to 18 months [68]. While overall pain decreased after diagnosis, 70% of patients continued to be symptomatic during the follow-up. Age and gender, environmental exposures, and the length of dyspepsia history did not predict the disease course, as was found by Bonnevie [41].

Do dyspeptic symptoms in non-ulcer dyspepsia sufferers eventually disappear or "burn out" after a certain number of years? It has been claimed by some investigators that chronic peptic ulcer symptoms may in fact "burn out" after 7–15 years [69, 70]. There are no comparable long-term follow-up studies in patients with non-ulcer dyspepsia, but Talley *et al.* found that non-ulcer dyspepsia symptoms did not tend to diminish whether patients had very long or short dyspepsia histories [68].

Overall, the evidence suggests that non-ulcer dyspepsia is, in most patients, a chronic illness,

Table 3.2 Proportion of patients with non-ulcer dyspepsia in whom a peptic ulcer developed

Investigators	Year of report	Type of population studied	No. of patients	No. of years of follow-up	Proportion in whom a peptic ulcer diagnosed (%)
Barfred [71]	1959	Hospital (in- & out-patients)	235	9.5	31
Brummer & Hakkinen [73]	1959	Hospital	102	5–6.5	12
Krag [49]	1969	Hospital	223	7–27	41
Gregory *et al.* [53]	1972	General practice	102	6	3
Viskum [72]	1977	Hospital	1331	18–33	25
Talley *et al.** [68]	1987	Outpatient	111	1–2	3

* Endoscopic diagnosis of non-ulcer dyspepsia.
Adapted from Thompson, WG *Can. Med. Assoc. J.* 1984;**130**:567.

but the outlook for life expectancy is excellent. Whether the presence of *H. pylori* infection affects the prognosis of non-ulcer dyspepsia has not been studied.

Non-ulcer dyspepsia and chronic peptic ulceration

Early studies reported rather high rates of ulcers developing in X-ray-negative dyspeptics (Table 3.2). Krag, on reinvestigating his patients 7–27 years after diagnosis, found that 41% had developed radiological evidence of ulceration; the majority of these patients had duodenal ulceration (60%) with the remainder having pyloric canal ulcers (20%) or gastric ulcers (20%) [49]. Barfred reported similar results [71]. Viskum, in a large retrospective study of 1331 patients, also found that 25% had radiological evidence of peptic ulceration 18–33 years after diagnosis [72]. Other studies by Talley *et al.* [68], Gregory *et al.* [53], and Brummer & Hakkinen [73], found that few patients developed peptic ulcers on follow-up.

Although the studies all agree that some non-ulcer dyspepsia patients do appear to develop peptic ulceration, the incidence of peptic ulceration has varied from that expected in the general population to much greater. One of the major reasons for this may be that different definitions of dyspepsia were used and, therefore, different populations were studied. In some investigations [49, 71] only patients with classical ulcer pain were studied, while others [53, 73] chose patients with various types of "dyspeptic symptoms". More importantly, as the diagnosis was based on single-contrast barium meal examinations in all but one study, it is likely that a significant number of peptic ulcers were initially missed radiologically [24].

On the other hand, in none of these studies were patients systematically reinvestigated for peptic ulcer disease, so that the ulcer frequency may have been underestimated. Further investigations are therefore needed to determine if there is a true association between non-ulcer dyspepsia and peptic ulcer. As *H. pylori* infection is very strongly associated with chronic duodenal ulceration [74–77], perhaps those non-ulcer dyspepsia patients who also have *H. pylori* infection are indeed more likely to develop an ulcer.

H. pylori gastritis and non-ulcer dyspepsia: cause and effect?

There is convincing evidence that *H. pylori* is the major cause of chronic non-specific gastritis [17, 74–77]. Moreover, *H. pylori* is difficult to eradicate and is probably a lifelong infection in most untreated persons [78–80].

An association between *H. pylori* and non-

Table 3.3 *Helicobacter pylori* gastritis and non-ulcer dyspepsia: evidence for a cause-and-effect relationship

Evidence of causation	Chronic gastritis	Non-ulcer dyspepsia
Association precedes disease	++	?
Association is strong (a large relative risk)	+++	+
Consistent finding of an association in different populations	+++	+
Dose–response effect	0	?
Effect of intervention	+++	±
Biological plausibility	+++	?

+ to +++, positive association varying from mild to marked; ±, equivocal evidence of an association; 0, no association; ?, no data.
Adapted from Talley, NJ. *J. Clin. Gastroenterol.* 1988;**10**:10–12.

ulcer dyspepsia has also been reported. A number of studies suggest that the prevalence of *H. pylori*-associated gastritis in non-ulcer dyspepsia ranges between 30% and 70% [1, 14, 16, 17, 74, 75]. There is an understandable deep-rooted temptation to attribute dyspepsia to gastritis when they coexist, particularly if no other etiology such as the irritable bowel syndrome or gastroesophageal reflux is apparent. Yet *H. pylori*-associated gastritis is also very common in the general community; in Western nations the prevalence increases with age, so that by the fifth decade up to 50% of the population is infected [81]. In certain special populations, such as inmates of institutions for the mentally retarded [82], and in developing countries [83], the prevalence is strikingly greater. While well-characterized, population-based studies are lacking, the majority of infected persons appear to be asymptomatic.

An association of *H. pylori* with non-ulcer dyspepsia could be causal, but other explanations are possible, including the overlap of common diseases by chance alone or confounding by other associated factors. Koch's postulates for determining that an infectious agent is the cause of a disease were set forth in 1882, and have been fulfilled for *H. pylori*-associated gastritis [84–86]. However, a causal association with non-ulcer dyspepsia cannot be established using Koch's postulates, as only some of these patients have *H. pylori* infection and many infected persons never develop symptoms. Indeed, it is often impossible to prove beyond reasonable doubt the cause of many diseases; some have argued that one can only disprove a cause-and-effect relationship [87]. However, it is possible to increase one's conviction based on empirical evidence to the point where cause and effect are very likely; epidemiologists have defined several criteria which suggest an association is truly causal [88] (Table 3.3).

A cause must always precede the disease. While there are data which indicate that *H. pylori* infection precedes the development of chronic gastritis [85], no such data are available for non-ulcer dyspepsia and prospective cohort studies are needed to resolve this issue.

Strength of association, as expressed by a large relative risk, is also an important indicator of causality. The relative risk is a measure of how many times more likely exposed persons will become diseased, relative to those non-exposed [20]. At this time, there are no data on the incidence of non-ulcer dyspepsia in persons exposed to *H. pylori* and the incidence in those not exposed to calculate the relative risk. However, this relative risk is probably small, because *H. pylori* infection is so common in totally asymptomatic members of the community [81, 83]. If *H. pylori* is of causal importance in non-ulcer dyspepsia, then the high prevalence of infection in asymptomatic persons implies that other risk factors must be necessary before symptoms can occur [16]. No such factors have been identified.

Dose–response relationships occur when varying amounts of the purported cause are related to varying amounts of disease. No relationship between the density of *H. pylori* infection and symptoms has been reported, although one study suggested that the degree of active chronic gastritis associated with polymorphonuclear leukocyte infiltration did correlate with dyspepsia [89].

The effect of treatment is another important indicator of causality; if the association between *H. pylori* and symptoms is reversible, this suggests an etiologic relationship. A small number of randomized, double-blind, placebo-controlled treatment trials have been published [90–94]. Treatment of *H. pylori* with bismuth has been reported to reduce symptom scores [90–94], but, compared with placebo, the results have not reached statistical significance in some studies [90, 93]. Moreover, the absolute improvement over placebo has been small, pain has often been poorly responsive, symptom measurements have not employed validated methods, bismuth uncommonly eradicates the infection, and its other local effects may explain any benefit, heterogeneous populations including irritable bowel syndrome patients have often been studied, and trials have not always included *H. pylori*-negative controls with dyspepsia [17, 95].

Antibiotics alone have not produced significant symptom improvement in *H. pylori*-associated non-ulcer dyspepsia [90, 96, 97], although these disappointing results may be explained by the poor suppression rates obtained in same of the studies. At present, there is no convincing evidence that treatment of *H. pylori* is efficacious in non-ulcer dyspepsia [16–18, 98].

Biological plausibility is present when a purported cause-and-effect relationship is consistent with current knowledge about disease mechanisms. It is conceivable, for example, that an inflamed gastric mucosa is more sensitive to acid or bile than normal mucosa, so that pain results [99, 100]. While some data do not support this hypothesis [101], even a lack of biological plausibility does not negate a cause-and-effect relationship.

To establish beyond reasonable doubt that *H. pylori* causes non-ulcer dyspepsia, it therefore needs to be confirmed that: (1) the incidence of *H. pylori* infection is indeed more common in non-ulcer dyspepsia; (2) infection precedes the first onset of non-ulcer dyspepsia symptoms; and (3) eradication of infection of itself abolishes symptoms.

Conclusions

It is apparent that the prevalence and incidence of non-ulcer dyspepsia varies with the population assessed. Although there is a lack of firm data, it appears that the disorder is extremely common in the general population, and that only some of these sufferers seek medical care. It may be that patients who do present to the health care professional are quite different from those who do not present. Therefore, more reliable information needs to be obtained from random surveys of the population, and to do this will require an improvement in techniques for measuring each of the symptoms from which diagnostic categories are constructed [102].

The majority of patients with non-ulcer dyspepsia will probably have their complaints for life. Whether the development of chronic peptic ulceration is more common in non-ulcer dyspepsia than in the general population remains uncertain.

While it has been postulated that some patients with *H. pylori*-associated gastritis have symptoms related to this disease, this remains to be firmly established. If *H. pylori* is a cause of dyspepsia, the factors which predispose only some infected persons to develop symptoms, and the reason why symptoms are usually intermittent when infection is constant, will need to be identified.

References

1 Talley, NJ, & Phillips, SF. Non-ulcer dyspepsia: potential causes and pathophysiology. *Ann. Int. Med.* 1988;**108**:865–79.
2 de Dombal, FT. Analysis of foregut symptoms. In: Baron, JH, & Moody, FG (eds), *Butterworths International Medical Reviews. Gastroenterology I. Foregut.* London and Boston: Butterworths, 1981, pp. 49–66.
3 Kingham, JGC, Fairclough, PD, & Dawson, AM. What is indigestion? *J. Roy. Soc. Med.* 1983;**76**: 183–6.
4 Drossman, DA, Thompson, WG, Talley, NJ, Funch-Jensen, P, Janssens, J, & Whitehead, WE. Identification of subgroups of functional gastro-

intestinal disorders. *Gastroenterology International* 1990;**3**:159–72.
5 Colin-Jones, DG (Chairman). Management of dyspepsia: report of a working party. *Lancet* 1988;**i**:576–9.
6 Greenlaw, R, Sheahan, DG, De Luca, V, Miller, D, Myerson, D, & Myerson, P. Gastroduodenitis. A broader concept of peptic ulcer disease. *Dig. Dis. Sci.* 1980;**25**:660–72.
7 Talley, NJ, McNeil, D, & Piper, DW. Discriminant value of dyspeptic symptoms: a study of the clinical presentation of 221 patients with dyspepsia of unknown cause, peptic ulceration, and cholelithiasis. *Gut* 1987;**28**:40–6.
8 Nyrén, O, Adami, HO, Bates, S, *et al.* Absence of therapeutic benefit from antacids or cimetidine in non-ulcer dyspepsia. *N. Engl. J. Med.* 1986; **314**:339–43.
9 Joelsson, B. Gastro-esophageal reflux disease. *Scand. J. Gastroenterol.* 1988;**23**(suppl 155): 101–3.
10 Manning, AP, Thompson, WG, Heaton, KW, & Morris, AF. Towards positive diagnosis of irritable bowel. *Br. Med. J.* 1978;**2**:653–4.
11 Talley, NJ, & Piper, DW. The association between non-ulcer dyspepsia and other gastrointestinal disorders. *Scand. J. Gastroenterol.* 1985;**20**:896–900.
12 Talley, NJ, Phillips, SF, Melton, LJ, Mulvihill, C, Wiltgen, C, & Zinsmeister, AR. Diagnostic value of the Manning criteria in irritable bowel syndrome. *Gut* 1990,**31**:77–81.
13 Gustavsson, S, Bates, S, Adami, H-O, Loof, L, & Nyrén, O. Definition and discussion of nomenclature. *Scand. J. Gastroenterol.* 1985; **20**(suppl 109):11–13.
14 Wegener, M. Börsch, G, Schaffstein, J, Schulz-Flake, C, Mai, U, & Leverkus, F. Are dyspeptic symptoms in patients with *Campylobacter pylori*-associated type B gastritis linked to delayed gastric emptying? *Am. J. Gastroenterol.* 1988;**83**:737–40.
15 Wegener, M, Börsch, G, Schaffstein, J, Reuter, C, & Leverkus, F. Frequency of idiopathic gastric stasis and intestinal transit disorders in essential dyspepsia. *J. Clin. Gastroenterol.* 1989;**11**: 163–8.
16 Talley, NJ. Is *Helicobacter pylori* a cause of non-ulcer dyspepsia? In: Malfertheiner, P, & Ditschuneit, H. (eds), *Helicobacter pylori, Gastritis and Peptic Ulcer.* Berlin: Springer-Verlag, 1990, pp. 361–9.
17 Talley, NJ. *Campylobacter pylori*-associated gastritis. Is antibiotic therapy now justified? *J. Clin. Gastroenterol.* 1988;**10**:10–12.
18 Talley, NJ, & Ormand, JE. Is antibacterial therapy against *Campylobacter pylori* useful in the treatment of indigestion and chronic peptic ulceration? *Trends Pharm. Sci.* 1989;**10**:36–40.
19 Talley, NJ. The "epigastric distress syndrome": a misnomer? *J. Clin. Gastroenterol.* 1987;**9**:718.
20 Fletcher, RH, Fletcher, SW, & Wagner, EH. *Clinical Epidemiology — The Essentials*, 2nd edn. Baltimore: Williams and Wilkins, 1988.
21 Kurata, JH, & Haile, BM. Epidemiology of peptic ulcer disease. *Clin. Gastroenterol.* 1984;**13**: 289–307.
22 Mendeloff, AI. Epidemiology of functional gastrointestinal disorders. In: Chey, WY (ed), *Functional Disorders of the Digestive Tract.* New York: Raven Press, 1983, pp. 13–19.
23 Cotton, PB. Fibreoptic endoscopy and the barium meal — results and implications. *Br. Med. J.* 1973;**2**:161–5.
24 Cotton, PB. & Shorvon, PJ. Analysis of endoscopy and radiography in the diagnosis, follow-up and treatment of peptic ulcer disease. *Clin. Gastroenterol.* 1984; **13**:383–403.
25 Peterson, WL, Sturdevant, RAL, Frankl, HD, *et al.* Healing of duodenal ulcer with an antacid regimen. *N. Engl. J. Med.* 1977;**297**:341–5.
26 Bardhan, KD, Saul, DM, Edwards, JL, *et al.* Comparisons of two doses of cimetidine and placebo in the treatment of duodenal ulcer: a multicenter trial. *Gut* 1979;**20**:68–74.
27 Doll, R, Jones, FA, & Buckatzsch, MM. Occupational factors in the arbiology of gastric and duodenal ulcers, with an estimate of their incidence in the general population. Medical Research Council Special Report Series, 276: 1–9. London: H.M.S.O., 1951.
28 Tibblin, G. Introduction to the epidemiology of dyspepsia. *Scand. J. Gastroenterol.* 1985;**20**(suppl 109):29–33.
29 Banke, L. Ulcumygdommers epidemiologi Kobenhavn: F.A.D.L.'s Forlag, 1975. Thesis.
30 Johnsen, R, Straume, B, & Forde, OH. Peptic ulcer and non-ulcer dyspepsia — a disease and a disorder. *Scand. J. Prim. Health Care* 1988;**6**: 239–43.
31 Hollnagel, H, Norrelund, N, & Larsen, S. Mave-Tarmsymptomer blandt 40-arige i Glostrup. En epidemiologisk undersogelse. *Ugeskr. Laeger* 1982;**144**:267–73.
32 Jones, R, & Lydeard, S. Prevalence of symptoms of dyspepsia in the community. *Br. Med. J.* 1989; **298**:30–32.
33 Talley, NJ, Phillips, SF, Zinsmeister, AR, & Melton, LJ. Prevalence of functional bowel disease: a random community survey (abstract). *Gastroenterology* 1990;**98**:A396.
34 Wadsworth, MEJ, Butterfield, WJH, & Blaney, R. *Health and Sickness. The Choice of Treatment. Perception of Illness and Use of Services in an Urban Community.* Hampshire: Tavistock Publications, 1971, pp. 67–73.
35 Thompson, WG, & Heaton, KW. Functional bowel disorders in apparently healthy people.

Gastroenterology 1980;**79**:283–8.
36 Lennard-Jones, JE. Functional gastrointestinal disorders. *N. Engl. J. Med.* 1983;**308**:431–5.
37 Nyrén, O, Gustavsson, S, Adami, H-O, & Loof, L. Methodological aspects of clinical trials in non-ulcer dyspepsia with special reference to selectional factors. *Scand. J. Gastroenterol.* 1985;**20**(suppl 109):159–62.
38 Weir, RD, & Backett, EM. Studies of the epidemiology of peptic ulcer in a rural community: prevalence and natural history of dyspepsia and peptic ulcer. *Gut* 1968;**9**:75–83.
39 Gear, MWL, & Barnes, RJ. Endoscopic studies of dyspepsia in a general practice. *Br. Med. J.* 1980; **280**:1136–7.
40 Bonnevie, O. The incidence and result of radiological examination of the stomach using a barium meal. *Scand. J. Gastroenterol.* 1976;**11**: 839–47.
41 Bonnevie, O. Outcome of non-ulcer disease. *Scand. J. Gastroenterol.* 1982;**17**(suppl 79): 135–8.
42 Nyrén, O, Adami, HO, Gustavsson, S, & Loof, L. Excess sick-listing in non-ulcer dyspepsia. *J. Clin. Gastroenterol.* 1986;**8**:339–45.
43 Talley, NJ, & Piper, DW. A prospective study of social factors and major life event stress in patients with dyspepsia of unknown cause. *Scand. J. Gastroenterol.* 1987;**22**:268–72.
44 Edwards, H, & Copeman, WSC. Dyspepsia: an investigation. *Br. Med. J.* 1943;**2**:640–42.
45 Avery Jones, F, & Pollak, H. Civilian dyspepsia. *Br. Med. J.* 1945;**5**:499–515.
46 Friedmann, MH. Peptic ulcer and functional dyspepsia in the armed forces. *Gastroenterology* 1948;**10**:586–606.
47 Lipetz, S. Gastrointestinal ulceration and non-ulcerative dyspepsia in an urban general practice. *Br. Med. J.* 1955;**2**:172–7.
48 Williams, AW, Edwards, F, Lewis, THC, & Coghill, NF. Investigation of non-ulcer dyspepsia by gastric biopsy. *Br. Med. J.* 1957;**1**:372–7.
49 Krag, E. The pseudo-ulcer syndrome. A clinical, radiographic and statistical follow-up study of patients with ulcer symptoms but no demonstrable ulcer in the stomach or duodenum. *Dan. Med. Bull.* 1969;**16**:6–9.
50 Edwards, FC, & Coghill, NF. Clinical manifestations in patients with chronic atrophic gastritis, gastric ulcer and duodenal ulcer. *Q. J. Med.* 1968; **37**:337–60.
51 Davis, RH, & Williams, JE. X-ray unit for general practitioners. *Br. Med. J.* 1968;**1**:502–4.
52 Bonnevie, O, Kallehauge, HE, Wulff, HR, & Wulff, MR. Prognostic value of the augmented histamine test in ulcer disease and X-ray negative dyspepsia. *Scand. J. Gastroenterol.* 1971;**6**:723–9.
53 Gregory, DW, Davies, GT, Evans, KT, & Rhodes, J. Natural history of patients with X-ray negative dyspepsia in general practice. *Br. Med. J.* 1972;**4**: 519–20.
54 Barnes, RJ, Gear, MWL, Nicol, A, & Dew, AB. Study of dyspepsia in a general practice as assessed by endoscopy and radiology. *Br. Med. J.* 1974;**4**:214–16.
55 Möllman, KM, Bonnevie, O, Gudmand-Hoyer, E, & Wulff, HR. A diagnostic study of patients with upper abdominal pain. *Scand. J. Gastroenterol.* 1975;**10**:805–9.
56 Möllman, KM, Bonnevie, O, Gudmand-Hoyer, E, & Wulff, HR. Nosography of X-ray negative dyspepsia. *Scand. J. Gastroenterol.* 1976;**11**: 193–7.
57 Mead, GM, Morris, A, Webster, GK, & Langman, MJS. Uses of barium meal examination in dyspeptic patients under 50. *Br. Med. J.* 1977; **1**:1460–61.
58 Oddsson, E, Binder, V, Thorgeirsson, T, *et al.* Prospective comparative study of clinical and pathological characteristics in Icelandic and Danish patients with gastric ulcer, duodenal ulcer, and X-ray negative dyspepsia. II. Histologic results. *Scand. J. Gastroenterol.* 1978; **13**: 489–95.
59 Horrocks, JC, & de Dombal, FT. Clinical presentation of patients with 'dyspepsia.' Detailed symptomatic study of 360 patients. *Gut* 1978; **19**:19–26.
60 Beavis, AK, La Brooy, S, & Misiewicz, JJ. Evaluation of one-visit endoscopic clinic for patients with dyspepsia. *Br. Med. J.* 1979;**1**:1387–9.
61 Gear, MWL, Ormiston, MC, Barnes, RJ, Rocyn-Jones, J, & Voss, GC. Endoscopic studies of dyspepsia in the community: an "open-access" service. *Br. Med. J.* 1980;**280**:1135.
62 Priebe, WM, DaCosta, LR, & Beck, IT. Is epigastric tenderness a sign of peptic ulcer disease? *Gastroenterology* 1982;**82**:16–19.
63 Becker, U, Andersen, IB, Elsborg, L, Rygaard, H, & Oigard, A. Consequence analysis of barium meal in patients under 40 years (abstract). *Scand. J. Gastroenterol.* 1983;**18**(suppl 86):6.
64 Watt, PCH, Spence, RAJ, Campbell, RC, McGurk, JJ, & Whyte, DGC. Combined barium meal and cholecystogram — an analysis of 1444 patients. *Postgrad. Med. J.* 1984;**60**:518–22.
65 Lance, P, Gibson-Glubb, S, Gazzard, JA, & Gazzard, BG. Chronic dyspepsia pain in general practice — its causes and diagnosis. *Postgrad. Med. J.* 1985;**61**:411–13.
66 Edenholm, M, Gustavsson, R, Jansson, O, *et al.* Endoscopic findings in patients with ulcer-like dyspepsia. *Scand. J. Gastroenterol.* 1985;**20**(suppl 109):163–7.
67 Sircus, W, & Prescott, RJ. Relation between dentition and dyspeptic disorders. *Br. Med. J.* 1985;**290**:115.

68 Talley, NJ, McNeil, D, Hayden, A, Colreavy, C, & Piper, DW. Prognosis of chronic unexplained dyspepsia. A prospective study of potential predictor variables in patients with endoscopically diagnosed non-ulcer dyspepsia. *Gastroenterology* 1987;**92**:1060–66.
69 Fry, J. Peptic ulcer: a profile. *Br. Med. J.* 1964; **2**:809–12.
70 Griebe, J, Bugge, P, Gjrup, P, Lauritzen, T, Bonnevie, O, & Wulff, HR. Long-term prognosis of duodenal ulcer: follow-up study and survey of doctors' estimates. *Br. Med. J.* 1977;**2**:1572–4.
71 Barfred, A. Pseudo-ulcer and true peptic ulcer. Ten-year regional follow-up in Denmark of cases discovered by X-ray during a three-year period at Odense, Denmark; with particular consideration to behaviour patterns. *Proceedings of the World Congress of Gastroenterology*. Baltimore: Williams and Wilkins, 1959, pp. 352–9.
72 Viskum, K. Ulcer disease. A comparison of some clinical and genetic aspects in patients suffering from duodenal ulcer, gastric ulcer and the pseudo-ulcer syndrome. *Dan. Med. Bull.* 1977; **24**:213–35.
73 Brummer, P, & Hakkinen, J. X-ray negative dyspepsia: a follow-up study. *Acta. Med. Scand.* 1959;**165**:329–32.
74 Marshall, BJ, & Warren, JR. Unidentified curved bacilli in the stomach of patients with gastritis and peptic ulceration. *Lancet* 1984;**i**:1311–14.
75 Marshall, BJ, McGechie, DB, Rogers, PA, & Glancy, RJ. Pyloric *Campylobacter* infection and gastroduodenal disease. *Med. J. Aust.* 1985;**142**: 439–44.
76 Fong, T-L, Dooley, CP, Dehesa, M, *et al. Helicobacter pylori* infection in pernicious anemia: a prospective controlled study. *Gastroenterology* 1991;**100**:328–32.
77 Ormand, JE, Talley, NJ, Shorter, RG, *et al.* Prevalence of *Helicobacter pylori* in specific forms of gastritis. Further evidence supporting a pathogenic role for *H. pylori* in chronic non-specific gastritis. *Dig. Dis. Sci.* 1991;**36**:142–5.
78 Langenberg, W, Rauws, EAJ, Houthoff, JH, *et al.* Follow-up study of individuals with untreated *Campylobacter pylori*-associated gastritis and of non-infected persons with non-ulcer dyspepsia. *J. Infect. Dis.* 1988;**157**:1245–9.
79 Hirschl, AM, Hentschel, E, Schutze, K, *et al.* The efficacy of antimicrobial treatment in *Campylobacter pylori*-associated gastritis and duodenal ulcer. *Scand. J. Gastroenterol.* 1988; **23**(suppl 142): 76–81.
80 Rauws, EAJ, Langenberg, W, Houthoff, HJ, Zanen, HC, & Tytgat, GNJ. *Campylobacter pyloridis*-associated chronic active antral gastritis; a prospective study of its prevalence and the effects of antibacterial and anti-ulcer treatment. *Gastroenterology* 1988;**94**:33–40.
81 Dooley, CP, Cohen, H, Fitzgibbons, PL, *et al.* Prevalence of Helicobacter pylori and histologic gastritis in asymptomatic persons. *N. Engl. J. Med.* 1989;**321**:1562–6.
82 Berkowicz, J, & Lee, A. Person-to-person transmission of *Campylobacter pylori. Lancet* 1987;**ii**:680–81.
83 Mégraud, F, Brassens-Rabbé, MP, Denis, F, Belbouri, A, & Hoa, DQ. Seroepidemiology of *C. pylori* infection in various populations. *J. Clin. Microbiol.* 1989;**27**:1870–3.
84 Marshall, BJ, Armstrong, JA, McGechie, DB, & Glancy, RJ. Attempt to fulfil Koch's postulates for pyloric *Campylobacter. Med. J. Aust.* 1985; **142**:436–9.
85 Morris, A, & Nicholson, G. Ingestion of *Campylobacter pyloridis* causing gastritis and raised fasting gastric pH. *Am. J. Gastroenterol.* 1987; **82**:192–9.
86 Talley, NJ. Chronic (non-erosive) gastritis. Pathogenesis and management. *Dig. Dis.* 1989; **7**:61–75.
87 Rothman, KJ. Causal inference in epidemiology. *Modern Epidemiology*. Boston: Little, Brown and Co., 1986, pp. 7–21.
88 Hill, AB. The environment and disease: association or causation. *Proc. Roy. Soc. Med.* 1965;**58**: 295–300.
89 Toukan, AU, Kamal, MF, Amr, SS, Arnaout, MA, & Abu-Romiyeh, AS. Gastroduodenal inflammation in patients with non-ulcer dyspepsia. A controlled endoscopic and morphometric study. *Dig. Dis. Sci.* 1985;**30**:313–20.
90 McNulty, CAM, Gearty, JC, Crump, B, *et al. Campylobacter pyloridis* and associated gastritis: investigator-blind, placebo controlled trial of bismuth salicylate and erythromycin ethylsuccinate. *Br. Med. J.* 1986;**293**:675–9.
91 Rokkas, T, Pursey, C, Uzoechina, E, *et al.* Nonulcer dyspepsia and short term DeNol therapy: a placebo controlled trial with particular reference to the role of *Campylobacter pylori. Gut* 1988; **29**:1386–91.
92 Lambert, JR, Borromeo, M, Korman, MG, & Hansky, J. Role of *Campylobacter pyloridis* in non-ulcer dyspepsia — a randomized controlled trial (abstract). *Gastroenterology* 1987;**92**:1488.
93 Loffeld, RJLF, Potters, HVJP, Stobberingh, E, Flendrig, JA, van Spreeuwel, JP, & Arends, JW. *Campylobacter*-associated gastritis in patients with non-ulcer dyspepsia: a double-blind placebo-controlled trial with colloidal bismuth subcitrate. *Gut* 1989;**30**:1206–12.
94 Kang, JY, Tay, HH, Wee, A, Guan, R, Math, MV, & Yap, I. The effect of colloidal bismuth subcitrate on symptoms and gastric histology in non-ulcer dyspepsia — a double-blind placebo-controlled study. *Gut* 1990;**31**:476–80.
95 Talley, NJ. *Campylobacter pylori* and symp-

toms: is there a cause-and-effect relationship? *Gastroenterology* 1989;**96**:1228–9.
96 Glupczynski, Y, Burette, A, Labbe, M, *et al.* *Campylobacter pylori*-associated gastritis: a double-blind placebo-controlled trial with amoxycillin. *Am. J. Gastroenterol.* 1988;**83**:365–72.
97 Gastrointestinal Physiology Working Group of Cayetano Heredia and the John Hopkins Universities. Morgan, D, Kraft, W, Bender, M, & Pearson, A (eds) Nitrofurans in the treatment of gastritis associated with *Campylobacter pylori*. *Gastroenterology* 1988;**95**:1178–84.
98 Ormand, JE, & Talley, NJ. *Helicobacter pylori*: controversies and an approach to management. *Mayo Clin. Proc.* 1990;**65**:414–26.
99 de Moraes-Filho, JPP, & Bettarello, A. Lack of specificity of the acid perfusion test in duodenal ulcer patients. *Am. J. Dig. Dis.* 1974;**19**:785–90.
100 Joffe, SN, & Primrose, JN. Pain provocation test in peptic duodenitis. *Gastrointest. Endosc.* 1983; **29**:282–4.
101 Tschychiyose, M, George, A, & Dooley, CP. Sensitivity of the gastric mucosa to acid and duodenal contents in patients with non-ulcer dyspepsia. *Gastroenterology* 1991 (in press).
102 Talley, NJ, Phillips, SF, Melton, LJ, Wiltgen, C, & Zinsmeister, AR. A patient questionnaire to identify bowel disease. *Ann. Int. Med.* 1989; **111**:671–4.

4: The epidemiology of Helicobacter pylori infection

D.N. TAYLOR & M.J. BLASER

Introduction

Helicobacter pylori was first isolated in 1982 from a patient with gastritis [1]. In the short time since this first isolation, evidence for its causal role in the pathogenesis of gastritis and duodenal ulcer has been rapidly accumulating. Briefly stated, *H. pylori* has been isolated from essentially all of patients with chronic active type B gastritis or peptic ulcer, and is rarely isolated, if at all, from persons with normal gastric mucosa. *H. pylori* has been found to have a strong affinity for the mucus-producing cells of the gastric antrum. *H. pylori*-colonized mucosa shows a marked reduction of mucus that may possibly be mediated by the production of extracellular protease and cytotoxins. In response to the infection, the host produces specific local and systemic immune responses. Epidemics of *H. pylori* gastritis have been documented as well as experimental infections in humans and animals. Elimination of the organism leads to a distinct improvement of gastritis. Long-term elimination results in significantly lower ulcer recurrence rates.

Acute infection

There have been two well-documented self-inoculation experiments with *H. pylori* that serve to describe the acute infection and incubation period associated with *H. pylori* infection. The first experimenter was found to have a normal biopsy prior to ingestion of cimetidine, followed 3 hours later by 10^9 *H. pylori* organisms suspended in alkaline peptone water [2]. Seven days later he developed an illness characterized by epigastric fullness, a sensation of hunger, an episode of vomiting, headache, irritability, and halitosis. Gastroscopy on the 10th day showed a soft gastric mucosa, and a biopsy of the antrum revealed gastritis with polymorphonuclear cell infiltration and organisms on the surface. Repeat biopsy on the 14th day showed improvement, at which time he began treatment with tinidazole. He had no further symptoms and did not develop an antibody response to the organism.

A second self-inoculation experiment was done in New Zealand [3]. The investigator first ingested 4×10^7 organisms of the same strain that was used previously and failed to become infected. Forty days later he ingested 3×10^5 organisms of a fresh clinical *H. pylori* isolate from New Zealand. In 3 days he developed severe epigastric pain, stomach cramping, and occasional vomiting that lasted for 5 days; thereafter he continued to have mild abdominal symptoms until day 11, when his symptoms ceased. Biopsies of the stomach on day 5 showed acute antral gastritis. The gastric pH was 1.2 on day 5 and 7.6 on day 8, and remained high until treatment with doxycycline was begun on day 25. Biopsies continued to show gastritis, in every case of which *H. pylori* was present. Initial antimicrobial treatment appeared to clear the infection, but on follow-up the organisms were still present. The subject ultimately developed chronic gastritis in conjunction with his persistent infection.

An outbreak of hypochlorhydria occurred among healthy volunteers who underwent gastroscopy at a Texas university in 1976 and 1977 [4]. In retrospect, this outbreak appeared to be caused by *H. pylori*, apparently introduced into the stomachs of volunteers via a pH electrode [5]. Seventeen of the 37 volunteers developed hypochlorhydria. Prior to detection of hypochlorhydria, nine of the 17 subjects developed a clinical illness, consisting of epigastric pain, nausea, and vomiting lasting 1–4 days. The illness usually began 1 week after the first intubation studies were performed. An increased pH was detectable 7–49 days after the illness began (mean = 25 days), but also occurred in some of the subjects who did not develop symptoms. The duration of hypochlorhydria was 2–8 months (mean = 4 months). During periods of hypochlorhydria, all patients had severe fundal and antral gastritis.

These studies indicate that there is an initial symptomatic phase that begins 3–7 days after ingestion of *H. pylori* and lasts for several days. The symptoms are associated with histologic evidence of acute antral gastritis. Hypochlorhydria frequently occurs 3–4 weeks after ingestion and may last for 2–8 months.

Although not all persons from whom *H. pylori* has been isolated have symptoms, there is invariably histologic evidence of inflammation at the site where *H. pylori* is isolated, and there is also serologic evidence of immune response to infection. Studies from every region of the world have confirmed the association of *H. pylori* on the gastric mucosa and chronic antral gastritis [6–14]. The organism is specifically found in association with primary or otherwise unexplained gastritis, and is not present in cases of secondary gastritis [15]. Eradication of *H. pylori* results in a pronounced improvement or healing of gastritis in adults and children [16, 17]. Although *H. pylori* only colonizes gastric epithelium, it can be found in the duodenum and the esophagus at sites of gastric metaplasia. Within the stomach, the organism preferentially colonizes the antral mucosa.

Gastroscopic studies are similar for adults and children. For example, in a series of 67 consecutive children undergoing upper gastrointestinal tract endoscopy, antral gastritis was diagnosed histologically in 18 patients [16]. *H. pylori* was identified by both culture and histology on the antral mucosa in seven of 10 patients with unexplained gastritis (primary), and none of eight patients with gastritis associated with an identified underlying cause (secondary). *H. pylori* was not identified in any of 49 cases with normal histology. Five patients had duodenal ulcer; all five had *H. pylori* on the antral mucosa. How exactly *H. pylori* is involved in the pathogenesis of duodenal ulceration remains to be determined.

Perhaps equally as compelling are some of the epidemiologic questions. It is not known how *H. pylori* is transmitted to humans, or whether there is a non-human reservoir that might be important in transmission of the organism. The natural history of the infection is also not known. Infection is considerably more common than illness. What determines who becomes ill, why one person should have gastritis and another a duodenal ulcer, how the traditional risk factors of ulcer disease such as smoking, aspirin, and alcohol interact with *H. pylori* infection, and finally whether there are long-term consequences to infection?

Microbiologic methods

Taxonomy

Comparison of partial 16S rRNA sequences from representative *Campylobacter* species indicates that *Helicobacter pylori* species are distantly related to *Campylobacter* species [18]. It is because of these distinctions that, the new genus, *Helicobacter*, was proposed [19]. Studies have shown that *H. pylori* strains share almost identical protein profiles in whole cell, outer membrane, and acid-extracted preparations, and several of those proteins may be conserved as group antigens [20–25]. However, restriction endonuclease DNA studies indicate considerable chromosomal DNA diversity [26, 27]. This method of analysis has been used to type strains [27].

Diagnostic methods

Definitive diagnosis of *H. pylori* infection relies on isolation of the organism from the stomach. This requires endoscopy and methods to culture the organism. By endoscopy, infection can be defined by histologic examination, culture, and assessment of urease activity of the biopsies. These methods have good diagnostic accuracy, but they are invasive and time consuming. Endoscopy has the problem of sampling error; i.e. the area biopsied and cultured may not be the area of infection.

A diagnostic test that does not require endoscopy is the urea breath test. In this procedure patients ingest ^{13}C- or ^{14}C-labeled urea [28, 29]. Breath samples are subsequently analyzed for the incorporation of labeled carbon in exhaled CO_2. Based on both timing and quantity of labeled CO_2 exhalation, the presence of *H. pylori* within the gastric mucosa may be sensitively and specifically predicted. The breath test is non-invasive and correlates well with culture. However, it requires fasting and either exposure of patients to radioactivity or access to a referral laboratory.

Graham *et al.* found that the majority (>85%) of patients with duodenal or gastric ulcer had positive ^{13}C breath tests [29]. Among asymptomatic persons from the United States, they found that 24% of persons aged 20–39, 36% of persons aged 40–59, and 82% of persons over 60 years old had positive breath tests. In contrast, the breath test was positive in 60% of persons from the People's Republic of China who were between 20 and 39 years of age. These data suggest that people from developing countries have higher prevalence of infection than those from developed countries.

Serologic studies may be used to screen large numbers of persons rapidly and at low cost. The detection of antibodies to *H. pylori* indicate active infection but, as with the other diagnostic tests, there is no means to determine the length of time a person has been infected or the severity of infection. Certain serologic assays do not differentiate between *H. pylori* and cross-reacting organisms [30], whereas others have resolved this problem [31, 32].

Serologic tests that detect antibodies to *H. pylori* have proved to be highly sensitive and specific indicators of gastric colonization. Untreated infections are not eradicated by the natural immune response, and the antibody titer remains at relatively constant levels over long periods of time, reflecting the chronicity of the infection. Antibody titers may take several months to become elevated. In a description of acute gastritis that occurred in a 46-year-old man who was admitted with profuse vomiting, IgG levels began to rise at day 21 and full seroconversion was not apparent until the next specimen was obtained at 14 weeks [33]. IgG levels remained constantly elevated for nearly 2 years, whereas IgA and IgM levels were undetectable. Treatment is associated with a decrease in antibody level [34, 35].

Seroepidemiologic studies of *H. pylori* infection

Serologic assays are useful epidemiologic tools provided that sensitivity and specificity are high. Different antigens have been used for *H. pylori* serology: whole bacteria treated by formaldehyde or heated; sonic extract; acid glycine extract; and high-molecular-weight antigens. The exact preparation of *H. pylori* antigens and other variables of the serologic methodology is of critical importance in developing assays of optimal diagnostic value. Megraud *et al.* found that, with the sonically produced antigen, a threshold of 400 ELISA units gave a sensitivity of 89% and a specificity of 90% [36]. A threshold of 600 ELISA units gave a sensitivity of 84% and a specificity of 96%. Antibodies to a crude preparation of urease were very specific, but not as sensitive as acid extract [37, 38].

The high specificity of antiurease antibody may make it particularly useful in confirming high antibody levels in children in the developing world. The specificity of serology in the developing world, where most people have high levels of antibody to *Campylobacter* species, has come into question and may be related to the purity of the antigen preparation used to detect antibody response. Use of high-molecular-weight antigens appears to be specific for *H. pylori* infection [31]. With such antigens, *H. pylori* IgG antibody response can be detected at high dilutions (1:800). Absorption of these sera with *C. jejuni*, *C. coli*, or *E. coli* produced minimal decreases in antibody titer. When used in Thailand, where *C. jejuni* infection is endemic, the age-related antibody curve of *C. jejuni* (highest in young children) was different from that of *H. pylori* infection (highest in young adults) [39]. Patients in Thailand with

Table 4.1 *Helicobacter pylori* infection among asymptomatic populations in the developed world

Age of total reference population (years)	United States		France	Finland	Australia
	$n = 113$ Dooley[1]	$n = 53$ Graham[2]	$n = 1199$ Megraud[3]	$n = 500$ Kosunen[3]	$n = 785$ Mitchell[3]
0–9	ND	ND		ND	4
10–19	ND	ND	16	ND	5
20–29	20	24 (20–39)	22	10	18
30–39	27		23	31	14
40–49	33	36 (40–59)	31	39	27
50–59	42		38	40	37
>60	47	82	36	60	ND
All ages	32	45	ND	ND	20

ND, not done.
[1] Paid volunteers (Los Angeles); [2] Paid volunteers (Houston); [3] Blood donors.

culture-proven *H. pylori* gastritis have elevated *H. pylori* antibody titers. The titers are similar using antigen from strains isolated in the United States or in Thailand.

H. pylori typing schemes

Typing methods would be very useful for following the natural history of infection. Biotype and restriction endonuclease patterns have been used for this purpose. Langenberg *et al.* found that restriction endonuclease patterns were reproducible and were useful in transmission studies [27]. A serotyping scheme would also be useful and should be a research priority.

H. pylori prevalence by age

In England, Jones *et al.* found that 10% of healthy blood donors under 20 years old were seropositive for *H. pylori*, compared to 50% of persons over 50 [40]. Among 500 blood donors from Manitoba, the prevalence of antibodies to *H. pylori* rose to 60% in adult age groups. The rise was gradual, with an increase in seroprevalence of 1–2% per year [41]. Rates were equal among men and women in the Canadian blood donor survey. Among elderly persons in the United States (Denver), Canada (Manitoba), and Japan (Osaka), seroprevalence remains at the same high rate observed in persons who are 60 years old [41]. In Vietnam and Thailand there is also a slight decrease in seroprevalence in the elderly [36, 39].

The frequency of *H. pylori* colonization of the gastric mucosa increases progressively with age [8, 42, 43] (Tables 4.1, 4.2). In developed countries it is very uncommon for children to be colonized, whereas approximately 40% of adults are colonized by the age of 50 (Fig. 4.1A). In a small study, Graham *et al.* reported that prevalence of *H. pylori* approximately equaled the age of the subjects [43]. In developing countries colonization may occur during childhood [39]. In France few (<1%) children were infected before the age of 6 years; while 5% of children aged 6–12 years and 15% of children aged 15–18 years were infected. In Vietnam about 40% of teenagers were positive [36]. In Ivory Coast most children (55%) were infected between 3 and 6 years old. In Thailand 18% of children aged 5–9 were infected, a rate that reached 55% by age 30 and 75% by age 50 [39] (Fig. 4.1B).

Ethnic groups

In the United States, 76% of adult healthy hispanic and black populations were seropositive, compared to 26% in non-hispanic caucasian populations. Studies among Asians also showed higher seropositivity rates. In New Zealand, seropositivity ranged from 70% in adults of Tongan extraction, to 44% in

Table 4.2 *Helicobacter pylori* infection among asymptomatic populations in the developing world

Age of total reference population (years)	Algeria $n = 277$ Megraud[1]	Ivory Coast $n = 374$ Megraud[2]	Vietnam $n = 365$ Megraud[1]	Thailand $n = 161$ Perez-Perez[2]	Papua New Guinea $n = 157$ Mitchell[2]
0–9	44	53	12	10	36
10–19	70	71	42	50	59
20–29	83	70	70	61	66
30–39	85	80	75	70 (30–49)	58
40–49	92	74	83		75
50–59	85	68	50	65	64
>60	ND	74	52	60	ND

ND, not done.
[1] Blood donors; [2] Serum surveys.

Samoans, and 39% in Cook Islanders [44]. In contrast, 15% of caucasian New Zealanders were seropositive.

Dwyer *et al.* measured antibody response in adult refugees on entry into Australia, and found that 43% of Ethiopians, 40% of Salvadoreans, and 18% of Vietnamese were seropositive [45]. Among a population of Australian aborigines in whom duodenal ulcers were rarely diagnosed, only 0.5% had antibodies to *H. pylori* in contrast to 15% of caucasian Australians [46]. The lack of *H.*

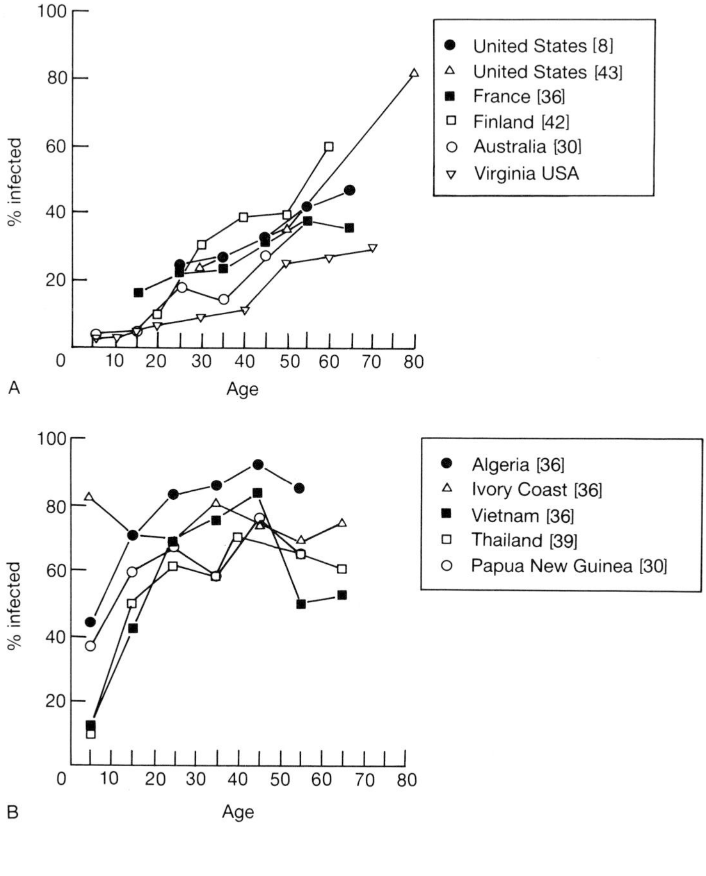

Fig. 4.1 Seroprevalence of *Helicobacter pylori* infection by age among healthy people in A, various developed countries; and B, various developing countries.

pylori infection in a population with a low incidence of duodenal ulcers further supports to the hypothesis that *H. pylori* is necessary for the development of duodenal ulcers.

Marshall has suggested that the age-related increase in *H. pylori* infection in developed countries could be explained by a cohort effect [47]. That is to say that *H. pylori* infections were more prevalent 20–30 years ago, so that a gradual age-related increase is observed as the cohort ages. In a study of young professionals working as Epidemic Intelligence Service (EIS) officers for the United States Public Health Service, paired sera were examined at average intervals of 8 years [48]. Among 37 people who were positive both times, the serum antibody titers were similar. This indicates that infection is chronic and not self-limited. In the years of the Centers for Disease Control study there was slight evidence for a cohort effect. In that study, most of the seroconverters had lived in New England or in the mid-Atlantic states.

Transmission

Perhaps the most compelling questions about the epidemiology of *H. pylori* infection center around transmission. Failure to understand the dynamics of transmission make it difficult to recommend methods of prevention.

Person-to-person transmission

In a Belgian study, clustering of cases in families and institutions was frequent, suggesting person-to-person transmission. Several studies have found an increased seroprevalence in populations where crowding and low sanitary levels might increase person-to-person transmission. At a Thai orphanage where enteric infections are hyperendemic, *H. pylori* seropositivity was 75% in children aged 1–3 years [39]. Further, the age-related acquisition of antibodies in rural Thailand was similar to that of hepatitis A. Berkowitz & Lee found that at all ages inmates of mental institutions were much more frequently seropositive than were healthy blood donors [49].

Marshall *et al.* performed 1 year follow-up studies after treatment with bismuth subsalicylate (BSS) and antibiotics, and found that none of the patients were reinfected [17]. They concluded that reinfection was uncommon in Australia.

Drumm *et al.* found that among children with *H. pylori* infection, 74% of 34 fathers, 83% of 18 mothers, and 55% of siblings were also infected. This was significantly more frequent than in children who were *H. pylori*-negative, where 26% of 27 fathers, 13% of 15 mothers, and 6% of a control group representing siblings were infected [50]. In particular, a seropositive mother was associated with infection in children.

Despite evidence that person-to-person transmission occurs, *H. pylori* has rarely been isolated from the mouth, dental plaque, or gingival scrapings [51, 52]. Furthermore, *H. pylori* appears to be quite sensitive to normal gastric pH, so it is not clear how small numbers of organisms could survive to reach the submucosa.

Sexual transmission

There is no evidence that *H. pylori* is sexually transmitted. In a survey among men attending a Denver sexually transmitted diseases (STD) clinic, heterosexual men were more likely to be seropositive than were homosexual men, but the difference could be explained by ethnic differences among the group [53]. There was also no difference in lifetime sexual partners or human immunodeficiency virus (HIV) status among men infected with *H. pylori*, compared to those who were not infected. Among men with *H. pylori* infection, the average number of sexual partners was 20 in the heterosexual men and 37 in homosexual men. Among men not infected with *H. pylori* the number of partners was 26 and 44, respectively.

Animal-to-human transmission

In one study, seropositivity rates were higher in persons who worked with animals, such as veterinarians and farmers, and lower among workers who had desk jobs [54]. Whether this indicates higher rates of infection with human strains of *H. pylori* is not yet known, and if so, whether socioeconomic differences might not be important.

Natural history of infection

Siurala *et al.* found that in longitudinal studies the prevalence of gastritis increases with age [55]. On average it took 18 years to develop mild atrophic gastritis, and 18 more years to develop severe atrophic gastritis. People with type B gastritis are more likely to develop gastric carcinoma. A hypothetical course of events is that *H. pylori* infection leads to type B gastritis, which may in some cases lead to atrophic gastritis and eventually to gastric carcinoma over a span of more than 40 years. In the United States and other developed countries the rates of gastric cancer have decreased, while rates of other cancers have increased. It is possible that as *H. pylori* infection is acquired at increasingly older ages in developed countries, there is not time enough for gastritis to progress to cancer.

The question of the natural history of long-term infections can best be answered in developing countries, where *H. pylori* is acquired at an early age. Another possible sequela of *H. pylori* infection is malabsorption. Hill *et al.* reported three cases of transient protein-losing enteropathy associated with acute gastritis in whom *H. pylori* was identified on the gastric mucosa [56]. With eradication of *H. pylori* infection with erythromycin, the gastric mucosa returned to normal and the protein loss ceased.

Conclusions

H. pylori infection is common and has a worldwide distribution. Present evidence indicates that it is more common in developing than in developed countries. The prevalence of *H. pylori* infection increases with age in parallel with gastritis. *H. pylori* infection does not appear to have any seasonality, and is as common in men as in women. Without a significant animal or environmental reservoir for human strains of *H. pylori*, person-to-person transmission appears to be the most likely mode. Exactly how the organism is transmitted from the stomach of one person to the stomach of another is still far from clear. Further understanding of the natural history and consequences of *H. pylori* infection remains an important aim.

References

1 Marshall, BJ, & Warren, JR. Unidentified curved bacilli in the stomach of patients with gastritis and peptic ulceration. *Lancet* 1984;**i**:1311–15.

2 Marshall, BJ, Armstrong, JA, McGechie, DB, & Glancy, RJ. Attempt to fulfil Koch's postulates for pyloric campylobacter. *Med. J. Aust.* 1985; **142**:436–9.

3 Morris, A, & Nicholson, G. Ingestion of *Campylobacter pyloridis* causes gastritis and raised fasting gastric pH. *Am. J. Gastroenterol.* 1987;**82**:192–9.

4 Ramsey, EJ, Carey, KV, Peterson, WL, *et al.* Epidemic gastritis with hypochlorhydria. *Gastroenterology* 1979;**76**:1449–57.

5 Graham, DY, & Klein, PD. *Campylobacter pyloridis* gastritis: the past, the present, and speculations about the future. *Am. J. Gastroenterol.* 1987;**82**:283–6.

6 Drumm, B, Sherman, P, Cutz, E, & Karmali, M. Association of *Campylobacter pylori* on the gastric mucosa with antral gastritis in children. *N. Engl. J. Med.* 1987;**316**:1557–61.

7 Chodos, JE, Dworkin, BM, Smith, F, van Horn, K, Weiss, L, & Rosenthal, WS. *Campylobacter pylori* and gastroduodenal disease: a prospective endoscopic study and comparison of diagnostic tests. *Am. J. Gastroenterol.* 1988;**83**:1226–30.

8 Dooley, CP, Fitzgibbons, PL, Cohen, H, Appleman, M, Perez-Perez, GI, & Blaser, MJ. Prevalence of *Helicobacter pylori* infection and histologic gastritis in asymptomatic persons. *N. Engl. J. Med.* 1989;**321**:1562–6.

9 Fitzgibbons, PL, Dooley, CP, Cohen, H, & Appleman, MD. Prevalence of gastric metaplasia, inflammation, and *Campylobacter pylori* in the duodenum of members of a normal population. *Am. J. Clin. Pathol.* 1988;**90**:711–4.

10 Gilman, RH, Leon-Barua, R, Koch, J, *et al.* Rapid identification of pyloric *Campylobacter* in Peruvians with gastritis. *Dig. Dis. Sci.* 1986;**31**: 1089–94.

11 Jones, DM, Lessells, AM, & Eldridge, J. *Campylobacter*-like organisms on the gastric mucosa: culture, histological, and serological studies. *J. Clin. Pathol.* 1984;**37**:1002–6.

12 Kilbridge, PM, Dahms, BB, & Czinn, SJ. *Campylobacter pylori*-associated gastritis and peptic ulcer disease in children. *Am. J. Dis. Child.* 1988;**142**:1149–52.

13 Langenberg, W, Rauws, EA, Houthoff, HJ, *et al.* Follow-up study of individuals with untreated *Campylobacter pylori*-associated gastritis and of noninfected persons with non-ulcer dyspepsia. *J. Infect. Dis.* 1988;**157**:1245–9.

14 Coghlan, JG, Gilligan, D, Humphries, H, *et al. Campylobacter pylori* and recurrence of

duodenal ulcers — a 12-month follow-up study. *Lancet* 1987;**ii**:1109–11.
15 Dooley, CP, & Cohen, H. The clinical significance of *Campylobacter pylori. Ann. Int. Med.* 1988;**108**:70–79.
16 Drumm, B, Sherman, P, Chiasson, D, Karmali, M, & Cutz, E. Treatment of *Campylobacter pylori*-associated antral gastritis in children with bismuth subsalicylate and ampicillin. *J. Pediatr.* 1988;**113**:908–12.
17 Marshall, BJ, Goodwin, CS, Warren, JR, *et al.* Prospective double-blind trial of duodenal ulcer relapse after eradication of *Campylobacter pylori. Lancet* 1988;**ii**:1439–42.
18 Romaniuk, PJ, Zoltowska, B, Trust, TJ, *et al. Campylobacter pylori*, the spiral bacterium associated with human gastritis, is not a true *Campylobacter* sp. *J. Bacteriol.* 1987;**169**:2137–41.
19 Goodwin, CS, Armstrong, JA, Chilvers, T, *et al.* Transfer of *Campylobacter pylori* and *Campylobacter mustelae* to *Helicobacter* gen. nov. as *Helicobacter pylori* comb. nov. and *Helicobacter mustelae* comb. nov., respectively. *Int. J. System. Bacteriol.* 1989;**39**: 397–405.
20 Megraud, F, Bonnet, F, Garnier, M, & Lamouliatte, H. Characterization of "*Campylobacter pyloridis*" by culture, enzymatic profile, and protein content. *J. Clin. Microbiol.* 1985;**22**:1007–10.
21 Perez-Perez, GI, & Blaser, MJ. Conservation and diversity of *Campylobacter pyloridis* major antigens. *Infect. Immun.* 1987;**55**:1256–63.
22 Burnie, JP, Lee, W, Dent, JC, & McNulty, CA. Immunoblot fingerprinting of *Campylobacter pylori. J. Med. Microbiol.* 1988;**27**:153–9.
23 Hirschl, AM, Pletschette, M, Hirschl, MH, *et al.* Comparison of different antigen preparations in an evaluation of the immune response to *Campylobacter pylori. Eur. J. Clin. Microbiol. Infect. Dis.* 1988;**7**:570–5.
24 Hook, J, Blomberg, B, Danielsson, D, & Kosunen, TU. Detection of antibody responses in rabbits hyperimmunized with *Campylobacter pylori* enzyme immunoassay indicates extensive antigenic similarities. *APMIS* 1989;**97**:56–60.
25 Kaldor, J, Tee, W, Nicolacopolous, C, Demirtzoglou, K, Noonan, D, & Dwyer, B. Immunoblot confirmation of immune response to *Campylobacter pyloridis* in patients with duodenal ulcers. *Med. J. Aust.* 1986;**145**:133–5.
26 Majewski, SI, & Goodwin, CS. Restriction endonuclease analysis of the genome of *Campylobacter pylori* with a rapid extraction method: evidence for considerable genomic variation. *J. Infect. Dis.* 1988;**157**:465–71.
27 Langenberg, W, Rauws, E, Widjojkusumo, A, Tygat, G, & Zanen, H. Identification of *Campylobacter pyloridis* isolates by restriction endonuclease DNA analysis. *J. Clin. Microbiol.* 1986;**24**:414–17.
28 Marshall, BJ, & Surveyor, I. Carbon-14 urea breath test for the diagnosis of *Campylobacter pylori*-associated gastritis. *J. Nucl. Med.* 1988;**29**: 11–16.
29 Graham, DY, Klein, PD, Evans, DJ Jr, *et al. Campylobacter pylori* detected noninvasively by the ^{13}C-urea breath test. *Lancet* 1987;**i**:1174–7.
30 Mitchell, HM, Lee, A, Berkowicz, J, & Borody, T. The use of serology to diagnose active *Campylobacter pylori* infection. *Med. J. Aust.* 1988;**149**:604–9.
31 Perez-Perez, GI, Dworkin, BM, Chodos, JE, & Blaser, MJ. *Campylobacter pylori* antibodies in humans. *Ann. Intern. Med.* 1988;**109**:11–17.
32 Evans, DJ Jr, Evans, DG, Graham, DY, & Klein, PD. A sensitive and specific serologic test for detection of *Campylobacter pylori* infection. *Gastroenterology* 1989;**96**:1004–8.
33 Frommer, DJ, Carrick, J, Lee, A, & Hazell, SL. Acute presentation of *Campylobacter pylori* gastritis. *Am. J. Gastroenterol.* 1988;**83**:1168–71.
34 Oderda, G, Ansaldi, N, Boero, M, Ponzetto, A, & Bellis, D. *Campylobacter pylori* in families of children with relapsing gastroduodenal disease due to *C. pylori* infection (letter). *Am. J. Gastroenterol.* 1988;**83**:1437–8.
35 Vaira, D, Holton, J, Cairns, SR, *et al.* Decreased antibody titres to *Campylobacter pylori* after treatment of gastritis. *Br. Med. J.* 1988;**297**:397.
36 Megraud, F, Brassens-Rabbe, M-P, Denis, F, Belbouri, A, & Hoa, DQ. Seroepidemiology of *Campylobacter pylori* infection in various populations. *J. Clin. Microbiol.* 1989;**27**:1870–3.
37 Dent, JC, McNulty, CAM, Uff, JS, Gear, MWL, & Wilkinson, SP. *Campylobacter pylori* urease: a new serological test. *Lancet* 1988;**i**:1002.
38 Newell, DG. Human serum antibody responses to the surface protein antigens of *Campylobacter pyloridis. Serodiagn. Immunother.* 1987; **1**:209–17.
39 Perez-Perez, GI, Bodhidatta, L, Wongsrichanalai, J, *et al.* Seroprevalence of *Campylobacter pylori* infections in Thailand. *J. Infect. Dis.* 1990;**161**: 1237–41.
40 Jones, DM, Eldridge, J, Fox, AJ, Sethe, P, & Whorwell, PJ. Antibody to the gastric campylobacter-like organism (*Campylobacter pyloridis*): clinical correlations and distribution in the normal population. *J. Med. Microbiol.* 1986;**22**:57–62.
41 Perez-Perez, GI, Marrie, T, Inouye, H, Shimoyama, T, Meiklejohn, G, & Blaser, MJ. The effect of age on seroprevalence of *Campylobacter pylori* infections (abstract 1015). In: *Proceedings of the 29th Interscience Conference on Antimicrobial Agents and Chemotherapy.*

Washington, DC: American Society for Microbiology, 1989.

42 Kosunen, TU, Hook, J, Rautelin, HI, & Myllyla, G. Age-dependent increase of *Campylobacter pylori* antibodies in blood donors. *Scand. J. Gastroenterol.* 1989;**24**:110–14.

43 Graham, DY, Klein, PD, Opekun, AR, & Boutton, TW. Effect of age on the frequency of active *Campylobacter pylori* infection diagnosed by the ^{13}C-urea breath test on normal subjects and patients with peptic ulcer disease. *J. Infect. Dis.* 1988;**157**:777–80.

44 Morris, A, Nicholson, G, Lloyd, G, Haines, D, Rogers, A, & Taylor, D. Seroepidemiology of *Campylobacter pyloridis. N. Z. Med. J.* 1986;**99**: 657–9.

45 Dwyer, B, Kaldor, J, Tee, W, Marakowski, E, & Raios, K. Antibody response to *Campylobacter pylori* in diverse ethnic groups. *Scand. J. Infect. Dis.* 1988;**20**:349–50.

46 Dwyer, B, Sun, NX, Kaldor, J, *et al.* Antibody response to *Campylobacter pylori* in an ethnic group lacking peptic ulceration. *Scand. J. Infect. Dis.* 1988;**20**:63–8.

47 Marshall, BJ. *Campylobacter pylori*: its link to gastritis and peptic ulcer disease. *J. Infect. Dis.* 1990;**12**(suppl 1):587–93.

48 Parsonnet, J, Blaser, MJ, Perez-Perez, GI, Hangnett-Bean, N, & Tauxe, R. Symptoms and risk factors of Helicobacter pylori infection in a cohort of epidemiologists. *Gastroenterology* 1991 (in press).

49 Berkowicz, J, & Lee, A. Person-to-person transmission of *Campylobacter pylori* (letter). *Lancet* 1987;**ii**:680–1.

50 Drumm, B, Perez-Perez, GI, Blaser, MJ, & Sherman, P. Intrafamilial clustering of *Campylobacter pylori* infection. *Gastroenterology* 1989;**96**:130.

51 Rosenthal, LE, Smoot, D, Mobley, HL, & Guisbert, W. *Campylobacter pylori* gastritis not related to periodontal disease (letter). *Am. J. Gastroenterol.* 1988;**83**:202.

52 Krajden, S, Fuksa, M, Anderson, J, *et al.* Examination of human stomach biopsies, saliva, and dental plaque for *Campylobacter pylori. J. Clin. Microbiol.* 1989;**27**:1397–8.

53 Polish, LB, Douglas, JM, Davidson, AJ, Le, YK, Perez-Perez, GI, & Blaser, MJ. Effect of ethnicity, sexual preference and HIV antibody status on *Campylobacter pylori* seroprevalence (abstract 1014). In: *Programmed Abstracts of the 29th Interscience Conference on Antimicrobial Agents and Chemotherapy*. Washington D.C.: American Society for Microbiology, 1989.

54 Vaira, D, D'Anastasio, C, Holton, J, *et al. Campylobacter pylori* in abattoir workers: is it a zoonosis? *Lancet* 1988;**ii**:725–6.

55 Siurala, M, Sipponen, P, & Kekki, M. Chronic gastritis: dynamic and clinical aspects. *Scand. J. Gastroenterol.* 1985;**20**(suppl):69–76.

56 Hill, ID, Sinclair-Smith, C, Lastovica, AJ, Bowie, MD, & Emms, M. Transient protein-losing enteropathy associated with acute gastritis and *Campylobacter pylori. Arch. Dis. Child.* 1987; **62**:1215–19.

5: Gastric Campylobacter-like organisms, ulcer disease and gastritis in animals and animal models of Helicobacter pylori gastritis

L. ENGSTRAND & S. GUSTAVSSON

Introduction

Since the initial report from Marshall & Warren in 1983, a large number of investigators have agreed that *Helicobacter pylori* is an emerging candidate agent for the genesis of gastritis and peptic ulcers. As with many human diseases, progress in the understanding of *H. pylori* gastritis would be increased if there was an animal model of the infection for experimental use.

Gastric ulcer and gastritis are recognized disorders in cats, dogs, and pigs. Endoscopic investigation of the esophagus, stomach, and duodenum in dogs and even cats with symptoms are routine in some veterinary hospitals. Ulceration in pigs causes economic consequences to animal breeders worldwide but, because of difficulties of diagnosis, the early stages of ulceration are usually undetected. In rhesus monkeys chronic gastritis has been observed in combination with *H. pylori*, and in ferrets gastritis has been observed in combination with gastric spiral bacteria, but the association with gastritis is inconsistent.

Pigs, dogs, and cats are all well-known laboratory animals, and there are reports describing naturally-occurring gastric ulcers and gastritis in these animals. The rhesus monkey is less common as a laboratory animal so far, because of the cost and the difficulties of breeding. The ferret is more or less unknown, but might be more practical than either monkeys or pigs. A few recent reports initiated by *H. pylori* research have described gastritis but no ulcers in ferrets.

In order to assess the susceptibility of an animal to *H. pylori* infection, several points should be considered. Are there similarities to the human gastrointestinal system (anatomic, histologic, physiologic, hormones, acid, etc.)? Is naturally-occurring gastritis or ulcer present in the animal? Does the animal harbor gastric *Campylobacter*-like organisms (CLO) in the stomach, and how does the normal gastric flora appear? Cost, size, age, and ease of breeding are other factors that might determine whether or not an animal is suitable, and if the model will be convenient.

Anatomy of different animal stomachs

Simple and compound stomachs in some animals are shown in Fig. 5.1. Obviously there are similarities and dissimilarities to the human stomach. The ruminant stomach differs a lot from the others. Cats, dogs, and pigs all have a fundic and pyloric gland region. The fundic region corresponds to the corpus of the stomach in humans and the pyloric region to the antrum. Pigs, horses, and ruminants have a non-glandular region lined by stratified squamous epithelium, the pars esophagea, which has no equivalent in the human stomach. In ruminants several outpouchings of the lower esophagus and gastric cardia form the three components of the fermentation system, i.e. the rumen, reticulum, and omasum.

Naturally-occurring ulcers/gastritis in dogs and pigs

As pigs and dogs are well-known laboratory animals, and several reports describe gastritis and ulcers in these animals, this review will concentrate on these animals with respect to inflammatory changes in the gastric mucosa. It is the opinion of the authors that the dog and

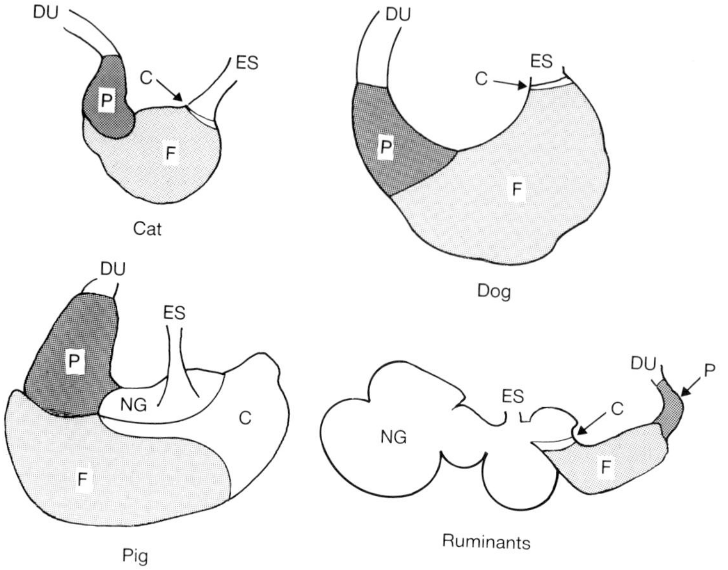

Fig. 5.1 Illustrations of simple and compound stomachs. C, cardiac region; DU, duodenum; ES, esophagus; F, fundic gland region; NG, non-glandular region (squamous epithelium); P, pyloric gland region.

the pig today are the most promising animals as models for *H. pylori* infection.

A gastric biopsy technique in dogs has been described [1–3], and the findings of biopsy examination have been presented [4, 5]. Gastritis has been observed in combination with pyloric stenosis [6], and duodenogastric reflux has been studied [4]. In a recent paper, van der Gaag describes the histopathologic appearance of endoscopic gastric biopsies in dogs with or without symptoms like vomiting, weight loss, and poor appetite [7]. As in humans, histopathologic examination of biopsies does not always correlate with the clinical symptoms. In the van der Gaag study, 35% of the dogs showed slight to severe gastritis, but gastric erosions and ulcers were rarely found. The classification of dog gastritis is nearly identical to the conventional human classification of gastritis. Chronic hyperplastic gastritis of the pyloric mucosa, and diffuse chronic gastritis of the body mucosa in dogs, are shown in Figs. 5.2A and 5.2B, respectively.

In pigs there is a difference between ulcers occurring in the glandular and non-glandular areas of the stomach [8]. The stomach is not a common site of infectious disease, but its mucosa is prone to damage due to acid–peptic autodigestion, ingested irritating agents, etc. The non-glandular area surrounds the cardia and is frequently the site of ulceration (Fig. 5.1). In the literature describing gastric ulceration in pigs, authors have only quite recently made the important distinction between ulcers of the pars esophagea (non-glandular region) and ulcers of the glandular gastric mucosa. The peptic ulcer of the glandular area is primarily seen in the fundic region, but on rare occasions is accompanied by ulceration of the non-glandular esophageal area. Symptoms like anemia, anorexia, and weight loss may occur in the chronic form of the disease, but often few if any clinical signs may be seen [9]. These ulcers are often noted in the slaughterhouse. The etiology of the esophageal ulceration still needs clarification, but some causative agents like infections, gastric acidity, dietary factors, and food processing are established [10–12].

Experimental models for gastric ulcer production have been reported. Increase of gastric acid and pepsin, secretion stimulators like histamine [13], and ulcerogenic drugs [14] all lead to ulceration in the stomach. Inoculation of *Ascaris suum* eggs produced ulcers in the pars esophagea, but these findings are inconsistent [15].

Gastritis of the glandular region is most pronounced on the greater curvature. The pathogenesis is poorly understood. Physiologic hyperemia, hemorrhage, infarction, and erosion

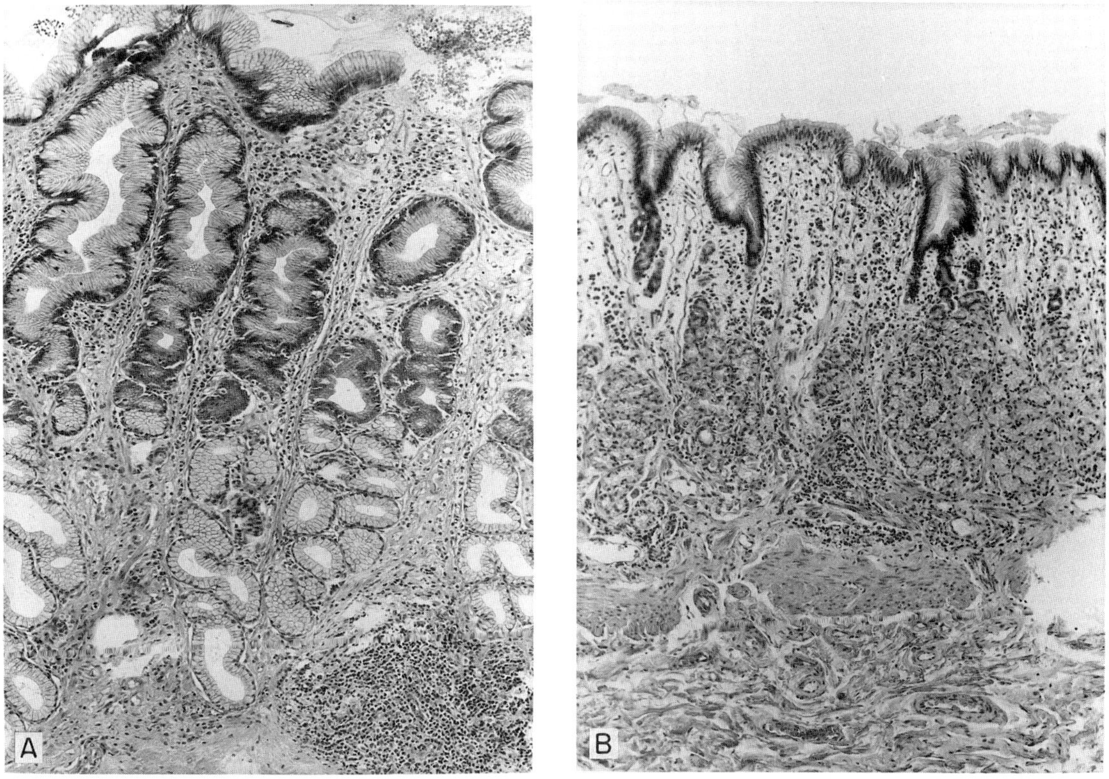

Fig. 5.2 Examples of histologic chronic gastritis in dogs. A, hyperplastic gastritis of the pyloric mucosa; B, chronic diffuse gastritis of the body mucosa. (Courtesy of R. Lindberg, Department of Pathology, Faculty of Veterinary Medicine, Uppsala, Sweden.)

may be observed but are non-specific. The lesion merely reflects an enteric disease or septicemic process [16].

Commensal spiral bacteria in animals and their relevance for *H. pylori* infection in man

Several types of spiral-shaped bacteria are found in the gastric mucosa of many animals like cats, dogs, baboons, and ferrets. These bacteria, often called gastric *Campylobacter*-like organisms (GCLO), are usually commensals and do not cause gastritis or ulcer. Several types may be cultured or detected histologically in the one animal.

Cat

Lee *et al.* describe the isolation of GCLO from the cat stomach [17] (see also Chapter 2). The organism is strongly urease- , catalase- and oxidase-positive with double axial filaments. This organism has also been observed in human gastric biopsies, and serologic studies suggest that spiral bacteria from animals may colonize the human stomach. This organism is supposed to be adapted to the gastric mucosa in the same manner as has been reported for *H. pylori* in the human gastric mucosa. The cat GCLO could be an alternative model of bacterial colonization of the stomach and would add important information to the association of *H. pylori* with the human gastric mucosa. Culture of this organism will allow biochemical studies and determination of minimal inhibitory concentrations (MICs) of anti-*H. pylori* drugs. Colonization studies by *in vivo* culture in mice might also be a useful experimental model [18].

Dog

Spiral-shaped bacteria have been described in the gastric mucosa of dogs [19, 20]. These

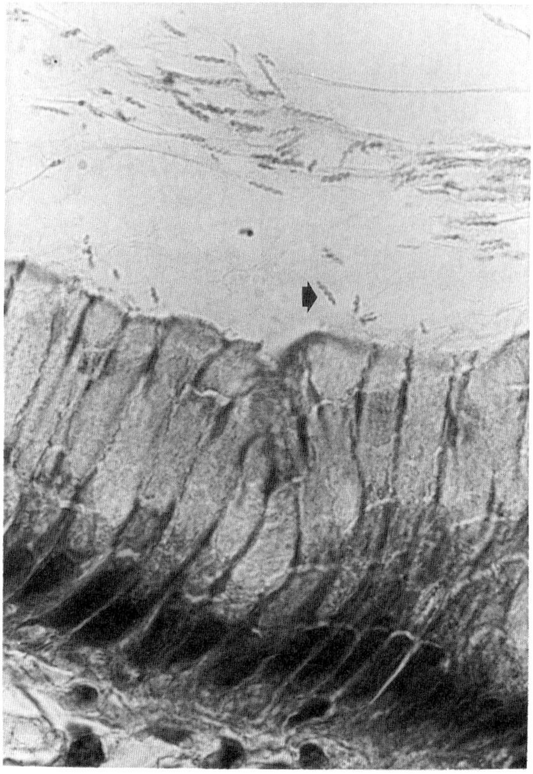

Fig. 5.3 Spiral-shaped bacteria overlying the surface epithelium in a dog with chronic gastritis of the pyloric mucosa. (Courtesy of R. Lindberg, Department of Pathology, Faculty of Veterinary Medicine, Uppsala, Sweden.)

bacteria are probably identical to the bacteria present in cats. Observation of similar bacteria in a dog with histologic gastritis of the pyloric mucosa is shown in Fig. 5.3 (R. Lindberg, personal communication).

Baboon

Spiral organisms in the baboon stomach have been reported by Curry *et al.* [21]. This organism is probably similar to the GCLO of cats and dogs, but recently an observation of baboon GCLO describes similarities to *H. pylori* with respect to DNA homology and cellular fatty acid profile [22]. The bacteria live at the base of crypts close to the epithelial cells.

Ferret

In ferrets, the spiral-shaped bacterium is unlike the GCLO in cats, dogs, and baboons. It is urease-, catalase-, and oxidase-positive but has no axial filaments. Tasman-Jones found that the organism was not present in all ferrets, and the association with gastritis was unclear [23]. DNA-hybridization indicates that ferret GCLO are of the same genus as *H. pylori* [24].

Primates

Observation of GCLO in the stomach of macaques has been reported by Euler *et al.* [25]. This tightly-spiraled organism was found in all animals, but culture attempts were unsuccessful. *H. pylori* was not observed in this study. Newell *et al.* describe the isolation of GCLO from the stomach of rhesus monkeys, identified as *H. pylori* [26]. In these animals the finding of *H. pylori* was associated with chronic gastritis (see below).

H. pylori infection in animals

When *H. pylori* has been observed in animals it has been associated with gastritis. *Macaca mulatta, M. nemestrina* [27], and probably baboons seem to be the only animals so far that naturally harbor *H. pylori*. Baskerville & Newell found histologically-confirmed gastritis in combination with *H. pylori* infection [28]. Antibodies to *H. pylori* were detected in serum by ELISA, and immunoperoxidase staining, using an *H. pylori*-specific monoclonal antibody, confirmed these findings. The organism was compared with *Campylobacter jejuni* and *H. pylori* isolated from humans. They were similar to *H. pylori* by light microscopy, in enzymic, fatty-acid-methyl ester, and protein profile analysis. Unlike the GCLO in animals described above, *H. pylori* in monkeys is not commensal and seems to be most prevalent in the antrum.

Recently, Rivera *et al.* [29] reported the presence of naturally occurring *H. pylori* infection in approximately 30% of swine being slaughtered in Mexico City. The infection was associated with gastritis in the animals, and may have been transmitted to slaughterhouse workers.

Experimental animal models of *H. pylori* infection

Oral challenge with *H. pylori* of numerous small laboratory animals like mice, rats, rabbits, guinea pigs, and germ-free rats have, so far, all been unsuccessful [30]. The gastrointestinal systems of these animals are all different from the human, and examination of biopsy samples cannot be performed without difficulty because of the size of the animals. However, attempts to infect small laboratory animals will continue, since there is a necessity for a convenient animal model, easily reproduced by other investigators. To this end, oral challenge of only a few animals has been successful, i.e. gnotobiotic and barrier-reared pigs, and recently even germ-free dogs [31].

Establishment of *H. pylori* in neonatal gnotobiotic piglets

Krakowka *et al.* and Lambert *et al.* have described the successful colonization of *H. pylori* in gnotobiotic piglets [32, 33]. After pretreatment with cimetidine, *H. pylori* was given orally and the pigs were examined up to 4 weeks after challenge. Bacteria colonized only the gastric and proximal duodenal mucosa, development of gastritis was observed (infiltration of mononuclear leukocytes), and *H. pylori* antibodies were found in serum samples collected at necropsy. The disadvantages with this model are the short observation period permitted, and difficulties with endoscopic examination, treatment regimens, and breeding (because of the need to keep the pigs in separated isolation units).

H. pylori in barrier-born pigs

As a few recent studies indicate that pigs might be suitable animals to study the characteristics and pathologic mechanisms of *H. pylori*, the authors decided to use barrier-born pigs in an animal model for *H. pylori* infection. These pigs could also be used to assess the therapeutic possibilities once an *H. pylori* infection is established. The aims of the study were to establish growth, to elucidate local inflammatory and systemic immune response, and to try to eradicate the organism from infected mucosa.

The barrier-born pig (specific pathogen-free) is of Swedish land race, not delivered by caesarian section, but kept isolated from common infectious agents in pigs. At 8 weeks of age (bodyweight 20 kg) the pigs were transferred to ordinary experimental stables. The pigs were kept isolated from other pigs and given ordinary pig feed.

Preparation of bacteria

A human strain of *H. pylori* was isolated 4 weeks before the inoculation started and subcultivated four times. The bacteria were grown on blood agar plates without antibiotics in anaerobic jars, and the colonies were harvested after 4 days and suspended in sterile saline at room temperature. The suspension was administered within 45 minutes after harvesting and part of it was cultured on blood agar plates to check living bacteria.

Experimental design

Seven pigs were inoculated and two served as controls. Before inoculation, acid secretion in all pigs was suppressed by oral omeprazole therapy (40 mg daily) for 1 week. The pigs were fasted for 14 hours before challenge. Four pigs from one litter received a suspension of 5×10^7 colony-forming units (CFU) in 5 ml sterile saline repeated twice during 2 weeks. After 3 weeks, 3×10^8 CFU were adminstered with gruel before and after bacterial suspension, and fat was injected into the duodenum to achieve prolonged gastric emptying. Three pigs from a second litter were inoculated once with a suspension of 10^9 CFU with fat and gruel as described above. All inoculated pigs were given 40 mg intravenous papaverin 5 minutes after inoculation. Con-

Table 5.1 Growth of *Helicobacter pylori* in antral biopsies from pigs inoculated with *H. pylori* and from uninfected controls. Treatment was performed in all pigs in litter 1 after 10 weeks' observation

		Week									
Litter no.	Pig no.	0	1	2	3	4	6	8	10	12	
1	1	—	—	+	+	+	+	+	+	—	
	2	—	—	+	+	+	+	+	+	—	
	3	—	—	—	+	+	+	+	+	—	
	4	—	—	+	+	+	+	+	+	—	Treatment
2	5	—	—	—	—	—	—	—			
	6	—	—	—	—	—	—	—			
	7	—	+	+	+	+	+	+	+	+	
	8	—	—	—	—	—	—	—			Controls, not inoculated
	9	—	—	—	—	—	—	—			

trols were maintained separately from the infected pigs. All infected pigs were observed for 12 weeks, the uninfected controls and the inoculated-but-not-infected pigs for 8 weeks. Endoscopy with biopsy was repeated weekly for the first 3 weeks and then every second week. Serum samples were taken at the same intervals. After 10 weeks, all infected pigs in litter one were treated with a combination of bismuth, metronidazole, and ampicillin for 2 weeks.

Endoscopy and biopsy specimens

Endoscopy (Olympus GIF-Q) was performed under Stressnil–Hypnodil anesthesia for inoculation of *H. pylori* and for observation and biopsy of the gastric mucosa. Two biopsy specimens were taken from the prepyloric area within 2–5 cm from the pylorus, and two biopsy specimens from the corpus. One biopsy from each site was frozen in isopentane and stored at −70 °C for subsequent immunohistochemical staining using an *H. pylori*-specific mouse monoclonal antibody [34]. Frozen sections were also stained by Mayer's hematoxylin and the presence and intensity of gastritis were observed. The other specimen was homogenized and cultured for *H. pylori*.

Serum immune response

Serum samples were taken as described above and tested for the development of *H. pylori* antibodies using an enzyme immunoassay (EIA). As antigen, the same bacterial strain as was used for inoculation was added to 96-well PVC trays. After blocking of uncoated sites and washing, peroxidase-conjugated rabbit anti-swine immunoglobulins (Dakopatts, Copenhagen, Denmark) were added. Antibody binding was estimated by reactivity with 1,2-phenylenediamine, and the EIA was measured in a Titerec multiscan photometer at 495 nm. Control sera from uninfected pigs were included in each assay.

Results

Detection of H. pylori. Culture and immunohistochemical staining were performed in all pigs. *H. pylori* could be detected by growth in antral biopsy specimens from all inoculated pigs in the first litter (Table 5.1). In litter 2 (including two controls), only one out of three pigs proved to be *H. pylori*-positive (HP+) after challenge. Once infected, the pigs remained HP+ during the observation period and the *H. pylori*-negative (HP−) pigs remained HP− in spite of close contacts with HP+ pigs. After therapy the bacteria disappeared from the gastric mucosa (Table 5.1). A stained cryostat section with *H. pylori* is shown in Fig. 5.4.

Histopathology. Mononuclear cells were present in the submucosa and in the epithelial regions in all pigs before the inoculation started. These cells appeared occasionally,

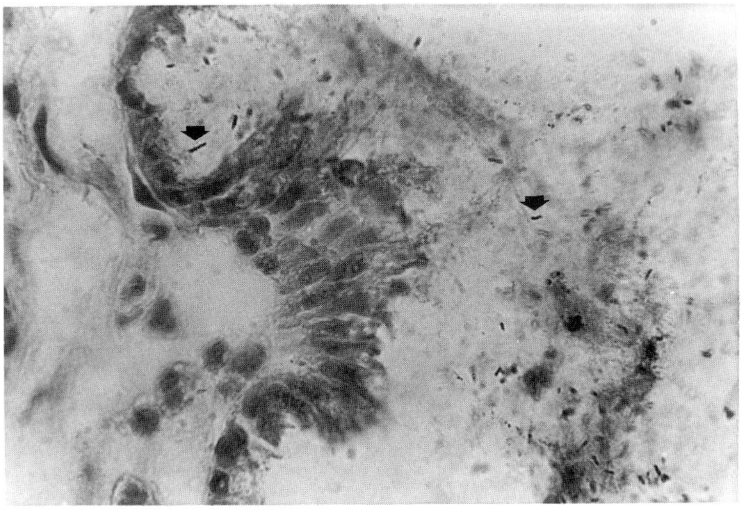

Fig. 5.4 Cryostat section of gastric pig mucosa stained with monoclonal antibodies and peroxidase–antiperoxidase. Bacteria are indicated. The section is counterstained with hematoxylin.

and no aggregates of inflammatory cells were observed (Fig. 5.5A). In the HP+ pigs, populations of these cells increased 4–6 weeks after inoculation, comparable with a superficial focal gastritis in man. The mononuclear cells were located in the submucosa and sometimes in aggregates (Fig. 5.5B). Intense infiltration deeply throughout the lamina propria was never observed. These findings in the HP+ pigs were varied, but with a clear difference from the uninfected pigs. The two controls, and the two inoculated-but-not-infected pigs, showed similar changes throughout the 8-week observation period, i.e. the same histopathologic findings as all pigs before inoculation.

Endoscopy observations. Technically, endoscopy was always easy to perform in anesthetized pigs, but sometimes the endoscopic view was obscured by gastric contents. Normally, the gastric mucosa of the corpus, i.e. below the evident squamous epithelial cell third proximal part (Fig. 5.1), is homogeneously reddened. This reddened area is sharply demarcated from the pale antrum. In HP+ pigs, the reddened area of the corpus was invading further distally and, typically, the red areas were encircling pale areas, giving the mucosa a characteristic appearance. These findings were observed in all HP+ pigs 2 weeks after inoculation of the bacteria, i.e. when *H. pylori* could be detected in these pigs, and remained throughout the observation period. In the immediate prepyloric area, or in the duodenum, no changes were ever observed, neither development of obvious erosive gastritis nor ulcer. No mucosal abnormality was observed in HP− pigs.

Serology. Raised antibody levels to *H. pylori* were detected in the serum from all infected pigs 2–4 weeks after challenge and remained at high levels throughout the observation period. Controls and inoculated-but-not-infected pigs had no antibody response specific to *H. pylori* (Fig. 5.6).

Discussion

It is possible to establish growth of *H. pylori* in the stomach of barrier-born pigs, and living bacteria are cultured for at least 9 weeks. These observations confirm the view that the bacteria actually colonize the gastric mucosa and do not merely remain in the stomach after inoculation (due to retarded gastric emptying, etc.). Raised antibody titers to *H. pylori* in the infected pigs further suggest that *H. pylori* survives in the pig stomach when the infection is established. Based on our observations, it seems that *H. pylori* is not commensal. Development of focal

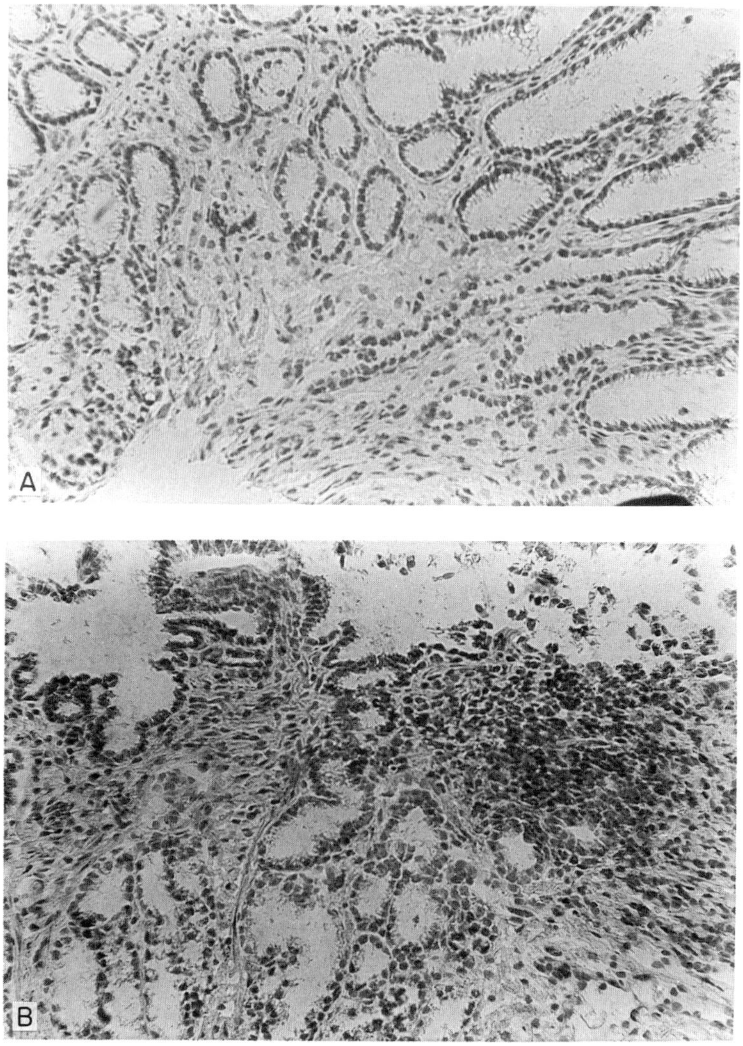

Fig. 5.5 Cryostat sections of gastric pig mucosa before (A) and after (B) inoculation with *H. pylori*. Note mononuclear cell infiltration in B. The sections are counterstained with hematoxylin.

superficial gastritis and endoscopic changes have been found in the infected pigs. In control or inoculated-but-not-infected pigs no such findings have been observed.

Our experiments indicate that a high inoculation dose and repeated inoculation enhance the infection rate. Hypochlorhydria and retarded gastric emptying seem to make the stomach more susceptible to colonization with *H. pylori*, but this hypothesis has to be further elucidated. As in humans, triple therapy eradicates the organisms from the gastric mucosa [35] but long-term observations have to confirm these results.

Future strategies in animal models of *H. pylori* infection

A non-expensive, easily reproducible and convenient animal model of *H. pylori* infection is urgently needed. Small animals like mice, rats, and rabbits were impossible to colonize by *H. pylori* [30]. Neither ordinary dogs nor ordinary pigs become colonized after oral challenge [36]. Rhesus monkeys naturally harbor the organism and could be presumptive candidates as *in vivo* experimental animals. Cost, and difficult breeding, make this animal less attractive. It seems that the animal fulfilling the criteria for

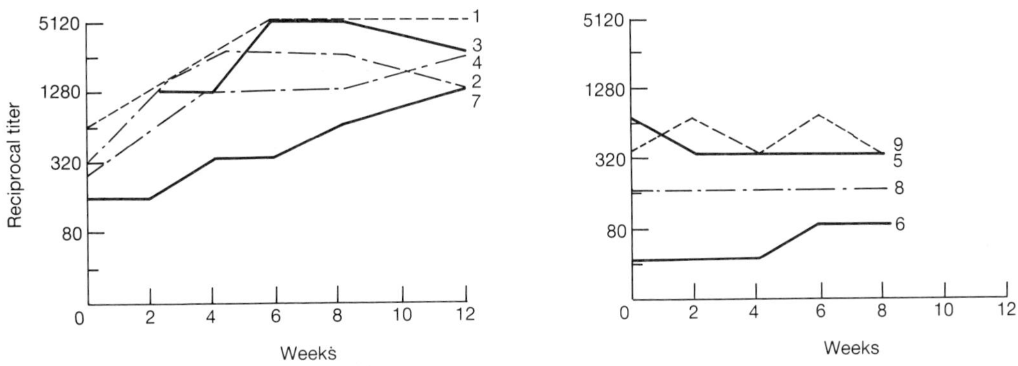

Fig. 5.6 Reciprocal antibody titers to *H. pylori* in sera of barrier-born pigs including controls (8 and 9) and inoculated-but-not-infected pigs (5 and 6). Reciprocal titer is the dilution factor of serum in the last well which produced a positive reaction defined as twice the background.

a good animal model has to be protected in some way against common infectious agents before challenge with *H. pylori*.

Gnotobiotic pigs and germ-free dogs are susceptible to *H. pylori*, and advances have been made with the barrier-born pig model. Dogs or pigs are well-known laboratory animals, and both have similarities to the human stomach concerning gastric physiology. *In vitro* experiments on the gastric mucosa from pigs have been performed, especially with regard to physiologic parameters like acid production in isolated parietal cells [37, 38]. Recently, an interesting study from Westblom *et al.* describes the gastric mucosa concentrations of antibiotics in a pig model [39]. This technique could be valuable in different pharmacokinetic studies of anti-*H. pylori* drugs.

Dogs and pigs are not ruminants or rodents, i.e. they have dietary characteristics similar to humans that can be studied. Dogs have been endoscoped for many years, and gastritis and ulcers have been observed whose classification is nearly identical to the human classification of gastritis. In pigs, ulceration of the pars esophagea is well known, and several etiologic factors have been established. Gastritis of the glandular region is less studied so far, perhaps because of its minimal diagnostic significance in pigs.

The pathogenesis of gastritis is poorly understood, and its relation to *H. pylori*-induced gastritis in man remains to be determined. Further investigations using monoclonal antibodies raised against *H. pylori* and swine B and T cell monoclonal antibodies will be performed to elucidate the inflammatory reaction.

Acknowledgments

The help of Olga Svensson is gratefully acknowledged. This study was supported by grants from the Swedish Medical Research Council, the Swedish Society of Medicine, and the Professor Nanna Suartz Foundation.

References

1 Bonneau, NH, & Reed, JH. Use of the gastrocamera in the dog. *J. Am. Vet. Med. Assoc.* 1972; **161**:185–9.
2 Happe, RP, & van der Gaag, I. Endoscopic examination of oesophagus, stomach and duodenum in the dog. *J. Am. Anim. Hosp. Assoc.* 1983;**19**: 197–206.
3 Sullivan, M, & Miller, A. Endoscopy (fibreoptic) of the oesophagus and stomach in the dog with persistent regurgitation or vomiting. *J. Small Anim. Pract.* 1985;**26**:369–79.
4 Happe, RP, van den Brom, WE, & van der Gaag, I. Duodenogastric reflux in the dog, a clinicopathological study. *Res. Vet. Sci.* 1982;**33**: 280–86.
5 van der Gaag, I, Happe, RP, & Wolvecamp, WthC. Investigation of the dog stomach. *Proc. Voorjaarsdagen Neth. Small Anim. Vet. Assoc.* PAO publication 1974;**5**:60–73.

6 Happe, RP, van der Gaag, I, & Wolvecamp, WC. Pyloric stenosis caused by hyperthropic gastritis in three dogs. *J. Small Anim. Pract.* 1981;**22**: 7–17.
7 van der Gaag, I. The histological appearance of peroral gastric biopsies in clinically healthy and vomiting dogs. *Can. J. Vet. Res.* 1988;**52**:67–74.
8 O'Brien, JJ. Gastric ulceration (of the pars oesophagea) in the pig. *Vet. Bull.* 1969;**39**:75–82.
9 Curtin, TM, Goetsch, GD, & Hollandbeck, R. Clinical and pathological characterization of esophagogastric ulcers in swine. *J. Am. Vet. Med. Assoc.* 1963;**143**:854–60.
10 Kowalczyk, T. Gastric ulcers. In: Dunne, HW, & Leman, AD (eds), *Diseases of Swine*, 4th edn. Iowa: Iowa State University Press, 1975, pp. 978–1010.
11 Qureshi, SR, Olander, HJ, & Gaafar, SM. Oesophagogastric ulcers associated with *Ascaris suum* infestation in swine. *Vet. Pathol.* 1978;**15**: 353–7.
12 Arnot, RS, Terblanche, J, Hickman, R, van H. Barbezat, GO, & Louw, JH. Acid secretion in the bile duct ligated pig. *S. Afr. Med. J.* 1979;**56**:606.
13 Muggenburg, BA, Kowalczyk, T, Reese, NA, Hoekstra, WG, & Grummer, RH. Experimental production of gastric ulcers in swine by histamine in mineral oil–bees wax. *Am. J. Vet. Res.* 1966;**27**:292–9.
14 Hey, H, Wamberg, T, Rasmussen, M, & Jorgensen, F. Endoscopic evaluations of potentially ulcerogenic drugs. A new *in vivo* porcine test model. *Eur. Surg. Res.* 1987;**19**:312–17.
15 Gaafar, SM, & Keittevuti, B. Experimental induction of esophagogastric ulcers with inoculations of *Ascaris suum* eggs in swine. *Gastroenterology* 1972;**63**:423–6.
16 Jubb, KVF, & Kennedy, PC. *Pathology of Domestic Animals*, 2nd edn. New York: Academic Press, 1970, p. 67.
17 Lee, A, Hazel, SL, O'Rourke, J, & Kouprach, S. Isolation of a spiral-shaped bacterium from the cat stomach. *Infect. Immun.* 1988;**56**:2843–50.
18 Lee, A. *Campylobacter pylori* and CLO in animals: overview of mucus-colonizing organisms. In: Rathbone, BJ, & Heatly, RV (eds), *Campylobacter pylori and Gastroduodenal Disease*. Oxford: Blackwell Scientific Publications, 1989, pp. 246–60.
19 Lockart, VG, & Boler, RK. Ultrastructure of a spiralled microorganism in the gastric mucosa of dogs. *Am. J. Vet. Res.* 1970;**31**:1453–62.
20 Weber, AF, & Schmittdiel, EF. Electron microscopic and bacteriologic studies of spirilla isolated from the fundic stomach of cats and dogs. *Am. J. Vet. Res.* 1962;**23**:422–7.
21 Curry, A, Jones, DM, & Eldridge, J. Spiral organisms in the baboon stomach. *Lancet* 1987; **ii**:634–5.
22 Newell, DG. *Campylobacter pylori* infections in non-human primates. In: Rathbone, BJ, & Heatly, RV (eds), *Campylobacter pylori and Gastroduodenal Disease*. Oxford: Blackwell Scientific Publications, 1989, pp. 265–73.
23 Tasman-Jones, C. Failure to detect gastric *Campylobacter*-like organisms in a group of ferrets in New Zealand. *N.Z. Med. J.* 1988;**101**: 275.
24 Fox, JG, Edmonds, P, Taylor, NS, Paster, B, & Dewhirst, F. Comparison of the phylogenetic, biochemical, phenotypic and morphological characteristics of gastric campylobacters from humans and ferrets. In: Kaijser, B, & Falsen, E (eds), *Campylobacter IV. Proceedings of the Fourth International Workshop on Campylobacter Infection*. Göteborg: University of Göteborg, 1987, pp. 50–53.
25 Euler, A, Moe, J, Zurenko, R, Schaadt, R, & Ulrich, R. Documentation of a "spiral organism" not *Campylobacter pylori* (CP) in the stomach of *Macaca fascicularis* (MF) and *Macaca mulatta*. In: Megraud, F, & Lamouliatte, H (eds), *Proceedings of Workshop on Gastroduodenal Pathology and Campylobacter pylori*. Amsterdam: Elsevier, 1989.
26 Newell, DG, Hudson, MJ, & Baskerville, A. Isolation of a gastric *Campylobacter*-like organism from the stomach of four rhesus monkeys, and identification as *Campylobacter pylori*. *J. Med. Microbiol.* 1988;**27**:41–4.
27 Bronsdon, MA, & Schoenknecht, FD. *Campylobacter pylori* isolated from the stomach of the monkey *Macaca nemestrina*. *J. Clin. Microbiol.* 1988;**26**:1725–8.
28 Baskerville, A, & Newell, DG. Naturally occurring chronic gastritis and *Campylobacter pylori* infection in the rhesus monkey: a potential model for gastritis in man. *Gut* 1988;**29**:465–72.
29 Rivera, E, Luqueno, V, Calva, JJ, & Ruiz-Palacios, GM. Exposure to swine, a risk factor for human *Campylobacter pylori* infection. *The Vth International Workshop on Campylobacter Infections. Puerto Vallarta, Mexico, 25 Feb–1 March, 1989*, p. 45 (abstract).
30 Ehlers, S, Warrelmann, M, & Hahn, H. In search of an animal model for experimental *Campylobacter pylori* infection: administration of *Campylobacter pylori* to rodents. *Zentralb. Bacteriol. Microbiol. Hyg.* 1988;**268**:341–6.
31 Radm, MJ, Eaton, KA, Krakowka, S, *et al. Helicobacter pylori* gastric infections in gnotobiotic beagle dogs. *Infect. Immun.* 1990;**58**:2606–12.
32 Krakowka, S, Morgan, DR, Kraft, WG, & Leund, RD. Establishment of gastric *Campylobacter pylori* infection in the neonatal gnotobiotic piglet. *Infect. Immun.* 1987;**55**:2789–96.

33 Lambert, JR, Borromeo, M, Pinkard, KJ, Turner, H, Chapman, CB, & Smith, ML. Colonization of gnotobiotic piglets with *Campylobacter pyloridis* — an animal model? *J. Infect. Dis.* 1987;**155**:1344.
34 Engstrand, L, Påhlson, C, Schwan, A, & Gustavsson, S. Monoclonal antibodies for detection of *Campylobacter pylori* in biopsy smears and frozen sections. *Scand. J. Gastroenterol.* 1988;**23**(142):50–52.
35 Börsch, G, Wegener, M, Mai, U, & Opferkuch, W. Efficiency of oral triple therapy to eradicate *Campylobacter pylori*. In: Megraud, F, & Lamouliatte, H (eds), *Proceedings of Workshop on Gastroduodenal Pathology and Campylobacter pylori*. Amsterdam: Elsevier, 1989.
36 Zinner, MJ, Couse, NF, Yeo, CJ, Dick, JD, & Antiohus, C. The effect of acute and chronic *Campylobacter pyloridis* exposure in 2 animal models. Proc Keystone Colorado, 1987.
37 Mårdh, S, Norberg, L, Ljungström, M, Humble, L, Borg, T, & Carlsson, C. Preparation of cells from pig gastric mucosa. Isolation of parietal cells by isopyknic centrifugation on linear density gradients of Percoll. *Acta Physiol. Scand.* 1985;**123**:349–54.
38 Gustavsson, S, & Lundqvist, G. Participation of antral somatostatin in the local regulation of gastrin release. *Acta Endocrinol.* 1978;339–46.
39 Westblom, TU, Duriex, DE, Madan, E, & Belshe, RB. Guinea pig model for antibiotic transport across gastric mucosa: Inhibitory tissue concentrations of clindamycin against *Helicobacter pylori* (*Campylobacter pylori*) following two separate dose regimens. *Automicrob. Agents Chemotherapy* 1990;**34**:25–8.

6: Interactions of microbial adhesins and toxins with the gastrointestinal mucosa

R.L. GUERRANT & C.A. LINGWOOD

Introduction

The pathogenesis of diseases caused by viral, bacterial, parasitic, and fungal pathogens in the gastrointestinal tract involves two characteristic steps. An understanding of these steps is critical to determining how different microorganisms specifically alter gastrointestinal function to cause disease, as well as to finding ways of interrupting the disease process by immunologic, pharmacologic, epidemiologic, or biochemical means.

The first step is the ability of the microorganism to colonize the relevant portion of the gastrointestinal tract where the disease is being caused (Table 6.1). Effective pathogens may attach to either specific mucosal cell receptors or the overlying mucus coat. The second step is the disruption of intestinal cell function by the microorganism through either direct or indirect functional derangement. Direct effects may occur by a cytotoxic or enterotoxic product; whereas indirect effects may involve other cells or mediators, such as local neurons or recruited inflammatory neutrophils or macrophages. Numerous lessons are already being learned from other enteric pathogens that appear to have relevance to *Helicobacter pylori* disease. It is the purpose of this chapter to review some of these lessons from enteric pathogens, with particular focus on the interactions of adhesins and toxins with receptors in host tissues.

Mechanisms of target cell disruption: the examples of *Escherichia coli*

To a remarkable degree, the wide array of mechanisms by which enteric pathogens can derange gut function can be examined in a single species, *Escherichia coli*. Because the traits that enable an organism to colonize or cause disease are often encoded by transmissible genetic elements, such as plasmids or phages, *E. coli* can be harmless normal bowel flora or can produce a cholera-like enterotoxin hemorrhagic cytotoxin, may destructively colonize the bowel, or be locally invasive like *Shigella* (Table 6.2).

Although certain serotypes of *E. coli* were recognized to be associated with infantile diarrhea in the 1940s, it was the early 1970s before *E. coli* was found to produce a secretory enterotoxin, using ligated rabbit ileal loops as used to study cholera toxin [1]. Like cholera toxin, the heat-labile enterotoxin of *E. coli*, LT, was found to activate adenylate cyclase, following binding to a ganglioside receptor, GM1 [2, 3], an effect that has been used to develop highly sensitive tissue culture assays for these enterotoxins [4–6]. Further studies distinguished an entirely different heat-stable enterotoxin, STa, that contains only 18–19 amino acids and activates guanylate rather than adenylate cyclase [7–11]. Still another, unrelated heat-stable enterotoxin, STb, causes intestinal bicarbonate secretion via a cyclic nucleotide independent mechanism [12, 13]. Another heat-labile enterotoxin, LT-II, has been isolated from a water buffalo in Thailand; LT-II also activates adenylate cyclase via ADP-ribosylation of Gs (like LT and cholera toxin) [14, 15]. The roles of STb and LT-II in human disease remain unclear [16].

While investigating alternative methods for detecting *E. coli* LT, Konowalchuk *et al.* [17] discovered yet another *E. coli* toxin particularly cytotoxic to vero cells in culture. This vero

Table 6.1 Pathogenesis of enteric infections

1	Colonization (mucus or epithelium)
2	Target cell disruption (direct or indirect)

cytotoxin was later found to be closely related to shiga toxin, and was therefore also termed shiga-like toxin (SLT) [18]. *E. coli* producing this toxin were isolated in low frequency from the stool of patients with bloody diarrhea in early clinical studies [19, 20].

The beginnings of an appreciation of the true clinical significance of this toxin occurred in 1983, when studies were published linking these infections, originating from contaminated food products, with hemorrhagic colitis (HC) [21], and in Karmali *et al.*'s landmark study, with hemolytic uremic syndrome (HUS) [22]. (Both syndromes were of previously unknown etiology, but are related, since HC follows a prodromal diarrheal illness which may be followed by HUS.) Since that time many studies have confirmed this association (reviewed in [23]), such that vero toxin is now the major common feature in the clinical epidemiology of HUS patients. Similar gastrointestinal lesions are observed in rabbits following administration of the purified toxin [24]. Shiga toxin has also been proposed as the primary cause of colonic vascular damage which may be associated with shigella dysentery [25].

Initially a single rare serotype, O157:H7, was isolated, but many serotypes have now been shown to elaborate this toxin. Variants of this toxin (VT2, SLTII [26, 27]), originally detected immunologically, have now been described. All these toxins, including shiga toxin itself, comprise an A cytotoxic subunit in association with a B subunit pentamer which binds specifically to the glycolipid globotriosyl ceramide (Gb_3) [28–31] to effect entry into susceptible cells. The A subunit acts intracellularly by cleaving adenosine from an *N*-glycoside bond at position 4324 in the 28S RNA from the 60S ribosomal subunit, to block protein synthesis by inhibiting elongation factor-1 (EF-1) dependent aminoacyl tRNA binding, much like the active subunit of ricin [32–34]. Recent studies have indicated that endothelial cells are particularly sensitive to vero toxin *in vitro* [35], and this is consistent with the site of lesions in HC and HUS, i.e. in the capillary bed of the gastrointestinal mucosa and the renal glomerulus [36]. Moreover Gb_3 has been found to be the major glycolipid of human kidney [37].

Table 6.2 Mechanisms of diarrhea

E. coli	Mechanism	Analogy
ETEC	Enterotoxin	*Vibrio cholerae*
LT-I, LT-II		
STa, STb		
EHEC	Cytotoxin	*Clostridium difficile*
VT (SLT) I, II		
EIEC	Invasion	*Shigella*
EPEC	Effacement	? *Cryptosporidium*
Class I, II		
EAEC	Colonization	? *Giardia*

See Glossary for explanation of abbreviations.

A further variant of vero toxin, the pig edema toxin, has been isolated from *E. coli* and causes a hemolytic gastrointestinal disease in pigs [38]. Edema and neurological disorder are also observed. Although this toxin (termed VTE or SLTIIv) is highly homologous to other members of the vero toxin family [39, 40], it has recently been shown to bind to a different glycolipid receptor, globotetraosyl ceramide (Gb_4) [41], which may explain its different cell susceptibility and pathogenesis *in vivo*.

About 10% of *E. coli* from human stool express Galα1-4Gal-specific adhesins and therefore also bind to Gb_4 [42], but the mannose-specific type 1 fimbriae may mediate the majority of binding of commensal *E. coli* to gastrointestinal colonic cells [43].

Still other *E. coli* have a large 140 MDa plasmid that seems partly responsible for certain serotypes to be invasive, much like *Shigella*. The capacity to invade colonic mucosa, like that to cause conjunctivitis in the guinea pig "Sereny" test, also appears to be dependent at least in part on chromosomally encoded lipopolysaccharide structure [44].

The classically recognized "enteropathogenic" serotypes of *E. coli* (EPEC) have the capacity to both adhere to and efface the intestinal mucosal epithelium, effects that appear to be encoded by a plasmid (for a fimbriate adhesin) as well as chromosomal elements (for "actin condensation factor (acf)", the effacement trait) [45, 46]. The two "classes" of EPEC both have acf (effacement) trait; however, they differ in that the class II EPEC lack the pMAR2 attachment plasmid, responsible for the characteristic focal human epithelial cell line (HEp-2) cell adherence [47, 48].

Finally, the capacity to colonize alone may derange intestinal function. Not only do the colonizing vaccine strains cause diarrhea in human volunteers, much as they had in studies by Smith & Linggood in piglets reported in 1971 [49], but these strains impair water and electrolyte absorption and disaccharidase activity, and cause prolonged diarrhea in the reversible ileal tie rabbit (RITARD) model [50, 51]. Whether the diarrhea associated with the enteroadherent, aggregating *E. coli*, recently described by Vial *et al.* [52], and by Bhan *et al.* [53], occurs by this type of functional derangement remains to be determined.

Microbial traits critical to colonization

The initial encounter of microorganisms with any mucosal surface necessitates an interaction with the overlying mucus. With increasing resolution, several specific microbial virulence traits are now being dissected, including motility, chemotaxis, production of mucolytic enzymes and lectin-like fimbriate surface adhesins, and hydrophobicity, all to enable the organism to deliver its enterotoxin or cytotoxin, or the organism itself, to the relevant site to cause disease.

Motility

Although the motility of the pathogen is probably important with several bacterial and parasitic pathogens, the specific contribution it makes to pathogenesis is probably best studied with *Vibrio cholerae*. In 1975, Guentzel & Berry showed that non-motile derivatives of *Vibrio cholerae* had strikingly reduced ability to cause fatal diarrhea in suckling mice [54]. They further showed that ^{14}C radiolabeled non-motile *V. cholerae* strains had a reduced capacity to adsorb to the surface of washed mouse small intestinal segments *in vitro*. Similar studies by Schrank & Verwey showed that mucus prevented the penetration of inert carbon particles, while motile *Vibrio cholerae* rapidly and effectively penetrated the mucus overlying the rabbit intestinal mucosa [55]. Either active or passive antibody against cell wall antigen clumped the vibrios in the lumen and prevented their penetration of mucus. However, whether this apparent role for *Vibrio* flagella and motility in contributing to virulence was independent of other pilus-like filamentous projections of a slime envelope, and the potential roles for motility with other enteric pathogens, are currently unclear. Analogous to motile virulent vibrios, the intense motility of *Helicobacter pylori* probably contributes to its pathogenicity in penetrating gastric mucus. However, other non-motile organisms such as *Shigella* species are fully capable of causing bowel infection by other means.

Chemotaxis

The ability of enteric pathogens such as *Vibrio cholerae, E. coli* and *Salmonella typhimurium* to respond chemotactically to mucosal surface-attractive substances or "taxins" has been suggested by several workers, including Adler [56], Allweiss *et al.* [57], and Freter & O'Brien [58]. Although recognized for over a century in capillaries or in soft agar (in 1881 by Engelmann, and in 1884 by Pfeffer), the ability of bacteria to move toward attractants or away from repellants has sparked renewed interest in recent years. Meticulous studies have suggested that attractants result in counterclockwise rotation of flagella, which causes smooth swimming, while repellants cause clockwise flagellar rotation, flagellar bundle disruption and aimless bacterial tumbling [56].

Allweiss *et al.* showed that only chemotactic and not non-chemotactic mutants of *V. cholerae, E. coli* and *S. typhimurium* rapidly associated with slices of mouse or rabbit small intestine immersed in bacterial suspensions [57]. They also showed that a pepsin digest of rabbit intestinal mucosa inhibited the chemotactic response, and that this mucosal digest could also be placed in agar blocks or in capillary tubes and provide the chemotactic attractant. Further work by Freter & O'Brien has shown that the non-chemotactic mutants of *V. cholerae* were unable to penetrate deep into the intervillus spaces, even though their motility, growth, and adherence to intestinal brush border membranes were normal [58]. Therefore, only the motile, chemotactic strains were fully virulent and able to penetrate the mucus gel to the deep intervillus spaces.

Microbial products

The role of bacterial products, such as neuraminidase and mucolytic enzymes, has been demonstrated by Schneider & Parker, who have shown that protease-deficient mutants of *Vibrio cholerae* are strikingly less virulent in infant mice, despite their normal motility and toxigenicity [59, 60]. They have further shown that the protease they studied is associated with a mucinase, and that antiserum to the mucinase passively protects mice from *V. cholerae* diarrhea. The ability of microbes to produce glycosidases, goblet cell secretagogues, or proteases, that may alter the structure or function of the mucosa, has also been suggested. Certainly the potential role of the capacity of *H. pylori* to degrade gastric mucin probably contributes to its pathogenicity [61].

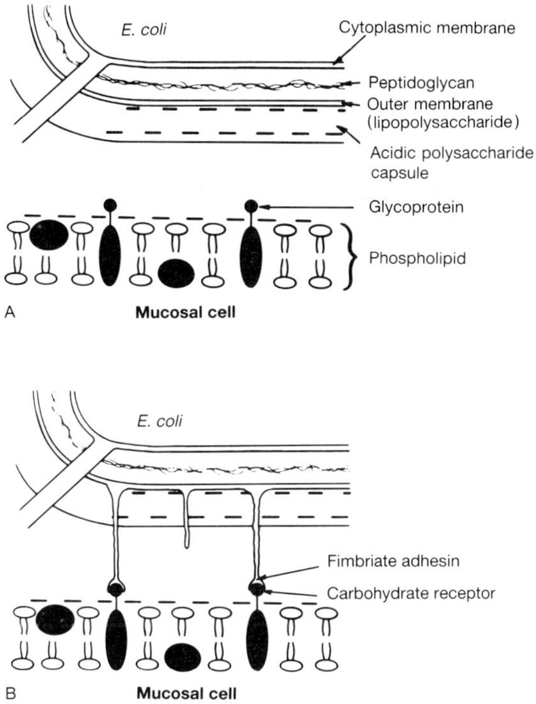

Fig. 6.1 Diagram of the means by which surface fimbriae overcome the normally repulsive surfaces of bacterial and host cells. A, repulsion of negatively charged bacterial and mucosal cell surfaces. B, attachment of bacterial ligand to complementary receptors.

Microbial adhesins

The role of lectin-like protein bacterial surface fimbriate structures, which are responsible for adherence to mucosal surfaces, has been the subject of great interest in the gastrointestinal as in the genitourinary and respiratory tracts [62–64]. As shown in Fig. 6.1, these fimbriate structures overcome the repelling negative charges on the surfaces of the organism as well as the host cell. In group A streptococci, for example, the lipoteichoic acid adhesin on surface bacterial M protein fibrils interacts through its lipid moiety with fatty acid binding sites in the amino-terminal region of fibronectin molecules on the host cell surface [63]. In type 1 fimbriated *E. coli*, a specific 29 kDa protein at the fimbriate tip interacts with D-mannose on glycoprotein receptors on host cells and in mucus [64].

In enterotoxigenic *E. coli*, when organisms adhere to transmembrane, cytoskeleton-anchored proteins (like integrins), instead of extracellular matrix, they may invade instead of colonizing the surface [65], because these fimbriate adhesins are under the control of transmissible plasmids, some very elegant studies that defined their role in the pathogenesis of enterotoxigenic *E. coli* diarrhea were made possible. From veterinary work in the early 1970s, it became clear that the ability of an organism to colonize the upper small bowel was a prerequisite for an enterotoxigenic *E. coli* to cause disease [49]. A major attachment adhesin in *E. coli* that causes diarrhea in piglets is the protein, fimbriate K88 antigen. The ability to produce enterotoxin (Ent+) alone was insufficient to cause diarrhea. Only when the K88 colonizing antigen was present did the Ent+ strains cause diarrhea. Indeed, mild diarrhea also resulted from the ability to colonize in the upper small bowel, even without enterotoxin production. It is the receptor for this K88 adhesin that Sellwood found was the autosomal dominant trait necessary for disease suscepti-

Table 6.3 *Escherichia coli* adhesins

Adhesin	Receptor		HA
UTI			
Type 1 pili (7 nm)	M–	D-Mannosides	MSHA guinea pig
S-fimbriae	S–		
P-fimbriae	Gn–G–L–Cer	Globoside	
ETEC (animal)			
K88 (2 nm)	G–	D-Galactoside	MRHA guinea pig RBC
K99 (4.8 nm)	NeuGc–L–Cer	*N*-Glycolyl-neuraminyl	MRHA sheep RBC
987 P		L–C	—
F41		Glycophorin A^m	—
ETEC (human)			
CFA/I (7 nm)	Gn–L–Cer (S on L)	GM_2	MRHA human-A RBC
CFA/II			
CS-1 (7 nm)			MRHA bovine RBC
2 (7 nm)	S–		
3 (2 nm)			—
CFA/III (7 nm, Honda)	?		Non-HA
CFA/IV (E8775)			
CS-4 (7 nm)			
5 (7 nm)	? like CFA/I		MRHA bovine + human RBC
6 (2 nm)			Non-HA
CFA/V (PCF 159) (7 nm)	?		Non-HA

See Glossary for explanation of abbreviations.

bility in piglets [66].

Similar findings have been reported for *E. coli* with the human colonization factor antigen (CFA/I) given to human volunteers [67]. Six of seven individuals who ingested 10^8 CFA/I+ enterotoxigenic *E. coli* developed diarrhea and excreted the organism for 7 days, while none of six volunteers who ingested 10^8 CFA/I– enterotoxigenic *E. coli* (LT+, although this organism may have become ST–) developed diarrhea or shed the organism for more than 4 days. In addition, none who ingested the CFA– derivative strain developed antibody titer rises, while four and six of the seven who ingested the CFA+ strain developed serum antibody responses to the toxin and somatic antigens, respectively.

The best recognized and relatively species-specific fimbriate adhesins among *E. coli* are K88 (pig), K99 (calf, pig, lamb), 987P (pig), F41 (calf) and CFA/I, CFA/II (CS1-3), CFA/III, CFA/IV (E8775, with CS4-6), and PCF 159 (?CFA/V) (see Glossary) (Table 6.3) [68]. These varied bacterial surface adhesins are antigenically distinct and are often detected by a characteristic hemagglutination pattern, as shown in Table 6.3. However, the actual receptors on the red blood cells and the intestinal epithelial cells or glycocalyx may be quite different. Consequently, the carbohydrate blockers of hemagglutination may not necessarily inhibit adhesion of these organisms to the intestinal epithelium [69].

The K99 fimbriae have been recently shown to bind to *N*-glycolylsialic acid residues of glycoconjugates, particularly *N*-glycolyl-GM_3 and *N*-glycolylsialoparagloboside [70]. Sialic acid is found only as the *N*-acetyl derivative in humans, which may explain the lack of human colonization of *E. coli* expressing this hemagglutinin.

Although the degree of mannose resistance

with CFA/I attachment to epithelial cells is variable, and *N*-acetyl-neuraminic acid (NANA) may non-specifically inhibit adherence by increasing negative surface charges [69], a ganglioside (GM_2)-like glycoconjugate has been postulated as the possible erythrocyte receptor for CFA/I and K99 hemagglutinins [71, 72]. Extensive studies of the hemagglutination and porcine epithelial cell brush border binding by K88 suggest that its binding may involve galactosyl residues on the host cell [73]. The degree of hydrophobicity, particularly with these fimbriate surface adhesins, has been correlated with adhesiveness [74]. Freter & Jones have shown that L-fucose inhibited the adherence of *V. cholerae* to intestinal brush border membranes, although *V. cholerae* motility and chemotaxis were more important in the association with slices of intact ileal mucosa [75]. Whether the control of expression of these surface fimbriae is under catabolite repression, or is altered by the reduced oxygen tension in the intestinal tract or other factors, is under current active study.

These fimbriate adhesins provide promising antigens for the development of protective immunity, locally in the mucosa, or for passive transfer via colostrum or milk [76]. Indeed, animal vaccines are already being used. However, protective immunity appears to be adhesin type specific, and the number of types of human *E. coli* surface adhesins remains unknown [69, 77]. Likewise, the host species and age specificities of the receptors for these adhesins remain poorly understood [78].

Capsular adhesins

The roles for glycans and lipoteichoic acids of streptococci and K1 polysaccharide antigen of *E. coli* are well established. The bacterial capsule may be involved in the close adherence of the rabbit diarrhea *E. coli* strain (RDEC-I) and possibly in the classical enteropathogenic *E. coli* serotypes to intestinal cells [79, 80]. This close adherence appears to disrupt the brush border and is probably important in the pathogenesis of diarrhea associated with these *E. coli* [80]. The degree of species and bowel regional specificity reported with RDEC [81] remains unclear with the human pathogens.

Glycoconjugate receptors for toxins and adhesins

The carbohydrate receptors for microbial protein toxins and adhesins may be linked to glycolipids or to glycoproteins. Glycolipids are strictly membrane-bound, while glycoproteins may be membrane-bound or secreted [82]. The location of the glycoconjugate receptor is a critical determinant of the location of adhesin-specific binding; for example of CFA/I and II to brush borders vs type 1 fimbriae to basolateral surfaces of enterocytes [83]. Furthermore, tissue adherence may enhance the nutrition and growth of the microorganism, as well as the delivery of toxin(s) to the host cell [84]. Conversely, the adherence of organisms may be primarily to glycoproteins in the overlying mucus coat, rather than to the mucosal cell surface itself [85–87]. Indeed, the mucus gel may provide a competitive barrier to microbial adhesion to the cell surface, especially when combined with synergistically cooperative antibody [88]. The distribution and nature of carbohydrate receptors on the mucosal surface or in mucus may also be influenced significantly by age, which probably determines the window of age susceptibility characteristically seen in many enteric infections [89–91].

The membrane glycolipid receptors for several bacterial toxins are shown in Table 6.4. One of the best characterized is the monosialoganglioside receptor for cholera toxin, GM_1 [92]. As shown in Fig. 6.2, this structure is composed of galactosyl-galactosamine and sialic acid groups attached to a lactosyl-ceramide core. Although the heat-labile toxin (LT) of *E. coli* binds to GM_1 receptors like cholera toxin, LT appears to bind less specifically to other ganglioside and galactoprotein receptors as well [6, 93]. Building on a remarkably common theme, the receptors for tetanus, botulinum, shiga, and *Clostridium difficile* toxins appear to have glycolipid receptors [28, 29, 94–96].

Analogous to glycoconjugate receptors for microbial toxins, many microbial adhesins for target host cell attachment or entry also appear to involve remarkably similar glycoconjugate receptors (Table 6.4). From early work with the neuraminidase "receptor destroying enzyme"

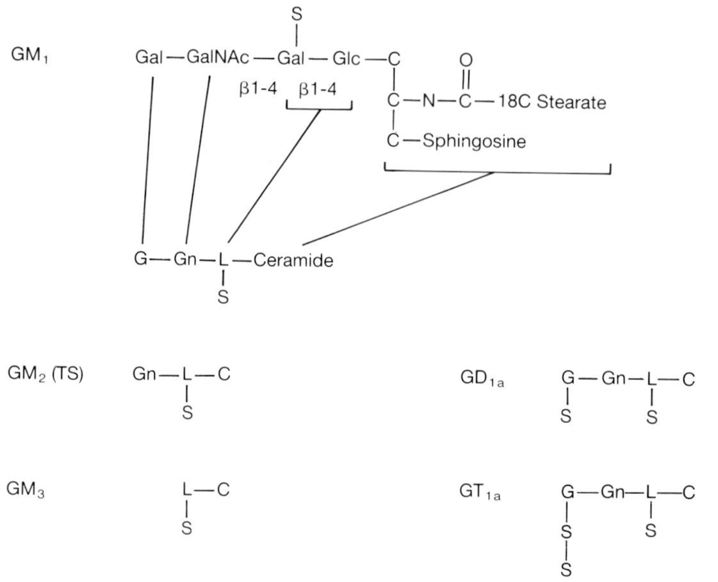

Fig. 6.2 Structures of key gangliosides, GM_1, GM_2 (Tay–Sachs ganglioside), GM_3, GD_{1a}, and GT_{1a}.

(from *V. cholerae*) dating back to 1947, the receptor for influenza virus involves a critical sialic acid moiety [97, 98]. Similarly, Sendai virus interacts with ganglioside-containing liposomes [99]. More recent data demonstrate the binding of *Propionobacterium*, *Bordetella pertussis*, and several colonic bacteria to lactosyl or lactosylceramide residues [82, 100, 101]. Interestingly, certain normal strains of human fecal bacteria produce exoglycosidases capable of digesting gastrointestinal blood group glycolipids down to lactosyl ceramide [102], and thus provide receptors for these microorganisms. Still other carbohydrate receptors for gonococci have been postulated [103]. Among protozoan parasites, a Gal–GalNAc adherence lectin of *Entamoeba histolytica* provides virulent amoebae with their capacity to adhere to target cells, which enables their subsequent characteristic lysis of target tissue [104]. In addition, the Duffey blood group is the key to the ability of the malarial parasite, *Plasmodium vivax*, to invade host erythrocytes [105, 106].

A major determinant of surface carbohydrates on epithelial cells and in mucus glycoproteins, as well as on red blood cells, is the genetically-determined blood type (Fig. 6.3). Such specificities may determine susceptibilities to certain infections or toxins, such as the repeatedly demonstrated association of symptomatic cholera and LT *E. coli* infections with individuals with blood group O (whether by fucose adhesins or by competing A blood group glycoconjugates that sequester active toxin [107]). Blood group specificities may also determine adhesin susceptibilities [108], indeed glycolipids containing both cholera toxin binding specificity and blood group activity have been detected [109]. Such "chimeric" receptors might result in a genetic predisposition to pathogenesis. The mechanisms of association of peptic ulcer disease, gastric ulcers, and achlorhydria with blood type or secretor status, remain to be elucidated.

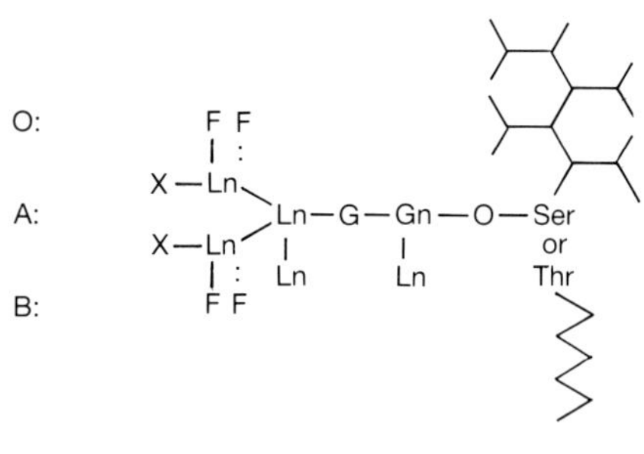

Fig. 6.3 Glycoconjugate structures in mucus glycoproteins and membrane glycolipids in individuals with A, B and O blood types. Gn, GalNAc; Ln, Gal–GlcNAc. For blood group A, X = Gn; B, X = G; O, X = no residue.

Table 6.4 Glycoconjugate receptors for microbial toxins and adhesins

Receptor	Molecular structure	Chemical name
Cholera toxin/LT	S G–Gn–L–Cer–	GM_1
Colonic *Propionobacterium* *Bacteriodes, Clostridium,* *Fusobacterium* *Lactobacillus* ?*Bordetella pertussis* *Neisseria gonorrhoea*	L–C–	Lactosyl ceramide
Shiga toxin, vero toxins	G–L–Cer–	Globotriosyl ceramide (Gb_3)
Pig edema toxin	Gn–G–L–Cer–	Globoside
Tetanus toxin	S–S (S)–G–Gn–L–Cer–	GD_{1b} (or GT_{1b})
Botulinum toxin	S S–S–G–Gn–L–Cer–	? GT_{1a}
C. difficile toxin A	G–G–GlcNAc–L–Cer–	Ceramide pentahexoside (type B blood group)
P-fimbriae	Gn–G–L–Cer– Gn–Gn–G–L–Cer–	Globoside (Forssman glycolipid)
S-fimbriae	S–G---O–S/T	Glycophorin A
Neisseria gonorrhoeae	G–Gn–L–Cer–	Gangliotetraosylceramide
Mycoplasma	SO_4–L–Cer–	Sulfatides
Escherichia coli CFA/I	S Gn–L–Cer–	Ganglioside GM_2
Influenza virus	S–	Glycophorin
Plasmodium vivax	? S–	Duffey Fy^b/Fy^a
Entamoeba histolytica	G–Gn–M–M–O–S/T (N) (R)	Glycoproteins
Pseudomonas cepacia *Pseudomonas aeruginosa* *Haemophilus influenzae* *Staphylococcus aureus* *Streptococcus pneumoniae*	Gn–L–Cer–	Gangliotriosyl ceramide
Helicobacter pylori	S L–Cer–	*N*-Acetylneuraminyllactose Ganglioside GM_3 Alkylacylglycerolipid

See Glossary for explanation of abbreviations.

H. pylori adhesins

Several groups have noted the capacity of *H. pylori* to agglutinate many different types of red blood cells. Emody *et al.* demonstrated mannose-resistant, monosialoganglioside-sensitive hemagglutination of rabbit, human, or sheep erythrocytes [110]. Evans *et al.* have demonstrated a fibrillar *N*-acetylneuraminyllactose-binding hemagglutinin on all 10 *H. pylori* isolates, which was sensitive to heat, pronase, and papain, but resistant to pepsin and trypsin [111]. This hemagglutinin was solubilized with *N*-octylglucoside, and was inhibited by the sialoproteins fetuin, α_2-macroglobulin, and glycophorin A.

Neuraminidase specificity and preferential binding suggest that the NeuAc(2–3)Gal isomer of NeuAc-lactose is critical to the receptor. Furthermore, they were able to demonstrate serum IgG antibody to this neuraminyllactose binding hemagglutinin in 82% of ulcer patients, 68% of asymptomatic *H. pylori*-infected individuals, and 2% of uninfected individuals [112]. However, treatment of the red cells with trypsin or pronase did not reduce the hemagglutination. In addition, the receptor for binding *H. pylori* to erythrocytes may not be the same as that for gastric epithelium. Leunk *et al.* reported that the inhibition of binding HEp-2 cells was quite different from that of hemagglutination [113]. Furthermore, Dunn *et al.* noted that binding of *H. pylori* to KATO (human gastric carcinoma) cells was only slightly reduced by neuraminidase or by sialo- or asialo-glycoproteins [114].

Using a different approach, extraction of lipids from cells known to bind *H. pylori* (red blood cells, gastric mucosa, and HEp-2 cells), Lingwood *et al.* have detected a common *H. pylori*-binding lipid in these tissues. Binding was detected by thin layer chromatogram overlay using a specific antibody–peroxidase conjugate system [115]. The charged *H. pylori*-binding lipid was isolated from A, B, and O red blood cells, pig and human gastric mucosa, and recently from KATO cells also. The receptor lipid was acid- and base-labile. Acid treatment of the *H. pylori*-binding lipid resulted in the complete loss of binding, while base treatment resulted in a reduction in thin layer chromatography mobility (indicating loss of a single fatty acid ester) but binding was maintained. The authors suggested that this represented a novel gastric alkylacylglycerolipid (see Fig. 6.4). The presence of carbohydrate was suspected since sulfated glyceroglucolipids are common components of the gastric mucosa. The receptor species has since been found to contain phosphate and not sulfate, and the presence of sugar has not yet been structurally confirmed. The lipid has been partially characterized (CA, Lingwood, in progress), and is being studied for ability to inhibit *H. pylori* adhesion *in vitro*. The lipid was found in the adult human gastric antrum, at reduced levels in the fundus, and barely detectable in infant antrum, and thus correlates with the known incidence of *H. pylori* colonization *in vivo*. Only viable organisms were found to bind, and binding was found to be lost following prolonged *in vitro* passage. Since these properties also correlate with the pathogenesis of *H. pylori*, it is likely that such glycerolipid binding is involved in the mechanism of pathogenesis of this organism. Similar binding specificity has been reported for exoenzyme-5 from *Pseudomonas aeruginosa* [116].

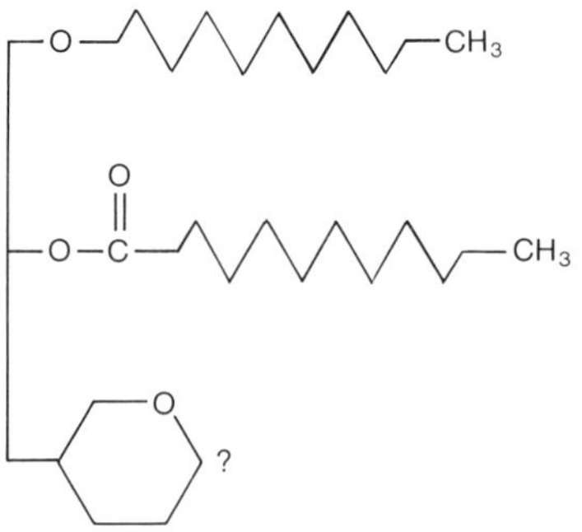

Fig. 6.4 Novel gastric alkylacylglycerolipid postulated as a receptor for *H. pylori.*

H. pylori cytotoxin(s)

As shown in Table 6.5, several invasive or inflammatory pathogens have been recognized to produce characteristic cytotoxins that may contribute to their virulence in causing inflammatory enteritis. These include *Shigella* species, enterohemorrhagic *E. coli* (EHEC), *Clostridium difficile, Campylobacter jejuni,* and *H. pylori.*

These organisms produce, respectively, shiga toxin, shiga-like toxins I and II (also called "vero cytotoxins I and II"), *C. difficile* toxins A and B, a polymyxin-released cytotoxin, and two *H. pylori* cytotoxins. Analogous to a polymyxin-

Table 6.5 Cytotoxins produced by inflammatory pathogens

Inflammatory pathogens	Cytotoxin
Shigella dysenteriae	Shiga toxin
Enterohemorrhagic *Escherichia coli* (EHEC) (e.g. O157:H7, O26, etc.)	Vero cytotoxins I & II (SLT-I, SLT-II)
Clostridium difficile	Toxins A (hemorrhagic enterotoxin) B (cytotoxin)
Campylobacter jejuni	*C. jejuni* cytotoxin (e.g. C-31 cytotoxin)
Helicobacter pylori	Vacuolating and cytolethal toxins Phospholipases Urease and ammonia

releasable cytotoxin from *C. jejuni* (and shiga toxin) [117], 57% of 66 clinical isolates of *H. pylori* produce reasonably high titers ($\geq$ 1:16) of a Chinese hamster ovary (CHO) cell cytotoxin that is non-dialyzable, heat- and trypsin-labile, and distinct from SLT-I, SLT-II, *C. difficile* toxins A or B, and from the vacuolating cytotoxin described by Guerrant *et al.* and Leunk *et al.* [118, 119]. The distinct vacuolating cytotoxin is usually produced (or released) in relatively low titers (usually $\leq$ 1:4) of unconcentrated *H. pylori* culture filtrates of up to 42% of isolates [119, 120]. Figura *et al.* noted that 67% of *H. pylori* isolated from patients with peptic ulcer disease, but only 30% of strains from patients with only gastritis ($P <$ 0.01) [118], had this activity. This vacuolating cytotoxin is maximal at 7–11 days in *Brucella* broth with 5% fetal bovine serum, and cytotoxigenic strains produce immunogenic proteins of 82, 95 or 132 kDa [121]. The role, if any, of these cytotoxins in contributing to the diseases that may be caused by *H. pylori*, remains to be determined.

Summary

The pathogenesis of a wide range of types of enteric infections shares an instructive number of principles. Those that are not simply preformed toxins (like staphylococcal or botulinal food poisoning) require a colonization step, followed by a step of target cell functional disruption (in order to qualify as a "pathogen" from the perspective of the human host). These steps involve target cell or mucus receptors that often share a set of specific carbohydrate moieties on membrane glycoproteins. An improved understanding of these key steps in pathogenesis will probably enlighten the varied range of clinical and pathological manifestations, as well as potential means to treat or prevent disease, caused by these common enteric pathogens.

Glossary of abbreviations

A^m	A type of glycophorin
Cer	Ceramide
CFA	Colonization factor antigen
CS	*E. coli* surface antigen
E8775	*E. coli* strain
EAEC	Enteroadherent *E. coli*
EF	Elongation factor
EHEC	Enterohemorrhagic *E. coli*
EIEC	Enteroinvasive *E. coli*
EPEC	Enteropathic *E. coli*
ETEC	Enterotoxigenic *E. coli*
F41	A type of fimbriae in calf diarrhea *E. coli*
Gal (G)	Galactose
GalNAc (Gn)	*N*-Acetyl-D-galactosamine
Gb	Globoside
GD	Disialoganglioside
Glc	Glucose
GM	Monosialoganglioside
Gn	Galactosamine
G_s	G (GTP binding) protein that is stimulatory for adenylate cyclase
GT	Trisialoganglioside
HA	Hemagglutinin
HC	Hemorrhagic colitis

HUS	Hemolytic uremic syndrome
L	Lactose (Gal–Glc)
Ln	Gal–GlcNAc
LT	Heat-labile toxin
M	D-Mannosides
MRHA	Mannose-resistant hemagglutination
MSHA	Mannose-sensitive hemagglutination
NANA	*N*-Acetyl-neuraminic acid
NeuGe	*N*-Glycolyl-neuraminyl
PCF	Putative colonization factor
R	Asparagine
S	Sialic acid (NANA)
SLT	Shiga-like toxin
S/T	Serine/theronine linked glycolipid
ST	Heat-stable toxin
UTI	Urinary tract infection
VT	Verotoxin

References

1 Gorbach, SL, Banwell, JG, Chatterjee, BD, *et al.* Acute undifferentiated human diarrhea in the tropics. I. Alterations in intestinal microflora. *J. Clin. Invest.* 1971;**50**:881.

2 Evans, DJ Jr, Chen, LC, & Curlin, GT. Stimulation of adenyl cyclase by *Escherichia coli* enterotoxin. *Nature (New Biol.)* 1972;**236**:137.

3 Guerrant, RL, Ganguly, U, Casper, AGT, *et al.* Effect of *Escherichia coli* on fluid transport across canine small bowel: mechanism and time course with interotoxin and whole bacterial cells. *J. Clin. Invest.* 1973;**52**:1707.

4 Donta, ST, Moon, HW, & Whipp, SC. Detection of heat-labile *Escherichia coli* enterotoxin with the use of adrenal cells in tissue culture. *Science* 1974;**183**:334.

5 Guerrant, RL, Brunton, LL, Schnaitman, TC, *et al.* Cyclic adenosine monophosphate and alteration of Chinese hamster ovary cell morphology: a rapid, sensitive *in vitro* assay for the enterotoxins of *Vibrio cholerae* and *Escherichia coli*. *Infect. Immun.* 1974;**10**:320.

6 Guerrant, RL, & Brunton, LL. Characterization of the Chinese hamster ovary cell assay for the enterotoxins of *Vibrio cholerae* and *Escherichia coli* and for antitoxins: differential inhibition by gangliosides, specific antisera and toxoid. *J. Infect. Dis.* 1977;**135**:720–28.

7 Evans, DG, Evans, DJ Jr, & Pierce, NF. Differences in the response of rabbit small intestine to heat-labile and heat-stable enterotoxins of *Escherichia coli*. *Infect. Immun.* 1973; **7**:873.

8 Greenberg, RN, & Guerrant, RL. *E. coli* heat stable enterotoxin. In: Dorner, F & Drews, J (eds), *Pharmacology of Bacterial Toxins*. New York: Pergamon Press, 1986, pp. 115–52.

9 Hughes, JM, Murad, F, Chang, B, *et al.* Role of cyclic GMP in the action of heat-stable enterotoxin of *Escherichia coli*. *Nature* 1978;**271**:755.

10 Field, M, Graf, LH Jr, Laird, WJ, *et al.* Heat stable enterotoxin of *E. coli*. *In vitro* effects on guanylate cyclase activity, cyclic GMP concentration, and ion transport in small intestine. *Proc. Natl. Acad. Sci. USA*. 1978;**75**:2800.

11 Guerrant, RL, Hughes, JM, Chang, B, *et al.* Activation of intestinal guanylate cyclase by heat-stable enterotoxin of *E. coli*: studies of tissue specificity, potential receptors and intermediates. *J. Infect. Dis.* 1980;**142**:220.

12 Kennedy, DJ, Greenberg, RN, Dunn, JA, Abernathy, R, Ryerse, JS, & Guerrant, RL. Effects of *Escherichia coli* heat-stable enterotoxin STb on intestines of mice, rats, rabbits, and piglets. *Infect. Immun.* 1984;**46**:639–43.

13 Weikel, CS, Nellans, HN, & Guerrant, RL. The *in vivo* and *in vitro* effects of a novel enterotoxin, STb, produced by *Escherichia coli*. *J. Infect. Dis.* 1986;**153**:893–901.

14 Seriwatana, J, Echeverria, P, Taylor, DN, *et al.* Type II heat-labile enterotoxin-producing *Escherichia coli* isolated from animals and humans. *Infect. Immun.* 1988;**56**:1158–61.

15 Holmes, RK, Twiddy, EM, & Pickett, CL. Purification and characterization of type II heat labile enterotoxin of *Escherichia coli*. *Infect. Immun.* 1986;**53**:464–73.

16 Weikel, CS, Tiemens, K, Moseley, S, & Guerrant, RL. Species specificity and lack of production of STb enterotoxin by *Escherichia coli* strains isolated from humans with diarrheal illness. *Infect. Immun.* 1986;**52**:323–5.

17 Konowalchuk, J, Speirs, JI & Stavric, S. Vero response to a cytotoxin of *Escherichia coli*. *Infect. Immun.* 1977;**18**:775–9.

18 O'Brien, AD, LaVeck, GD, Thompson, MR & Formal, SB. Production of *Shigella dysenteriae* type 1-like cytotoxin by *Escherichia Coli*. *J. Infect. Dis.* 1982;**1446**:763–9.

19 Hardas, UD, Jalgaonkar, SV & Kulkarni, VK. Cytotoxic effect of culture filtrate of enteropathogenic *Escherichia coli* from diarrhea in children on vero cell culture. *Indian J. Med. Res.* 1982;**76**:86–88.

20 Wade, WG, Thom, BT & Evans, N. *Lancet* 1979; **ii**:1235.

21 Riley, LW, *et al.* Hemorrhagic colitis associated with a rare *Escherichia coli* serotype. *N. Engl. J. Med.* 1983;**308**:681–5.

22 Karmali, MA, Steele, T, Petric, M & Lim, C. Sporadic cases of hemolytic uremic syndrome

associated with fecal cytotoxin and cytotoxin-producing *Escherichia coli*. *Lancet* 1983;**i**: 619–20.
23 Karmali, MAB. Infection by verocytotoxin-producing *Escherichia coli*. *Clin. Microbiol. Rev.* 1989;**2**:15–38.
24 Barrett, TJ, Potter, ME & Wachsmuth, IK. Continuous infusion of Shiga-like-toxin II as a model for SLTII-induced diseases. *J. Infect. Dis.* 1989;**159**:774–7.
25 Fontain, A, Arondel, J & Sansonetti, PJ. The role of shiga toxin in the pathogenesis of bacilliary dysentery studied by using a tox⁻ mutant of *Shigella dysenteriae* 1. *Infect. Immun.* 1988;**56**: 3099–109.
26 Head, SC, Petric, M, Richardson, SE, Roscoe, ME, & Karmali, MA. Purification and characterization of vero cytotoxin 2. *FEMS Microbiol. Lett.* 1988;**51**:211–16.
27 Strockbine, NA, Marques, LRM, Newland, JW, Smith, HW, Holmes, RK & O'Brien, AD. Two toxin-converting phages from *Escherichia coli* O157:H7 strain 933 encode antigenically distinct toxins with similar biological activities. *Infect. Immun.* 1986;**53**:135–40.
28 Jacewicz, J, Clausen, H, Nudelman, E, Donohue-Rolfe, A, & Keusch, GT. Pathogenesis of *Shigella* diarrhea. XI. Isolation of a *Shigella* toxin-binding glycolipid from rabbit jejunum and HeLa cells and its identification as globotriosylceramide. *J. Exp. Med.* 1986;**163**: 1391–1404.
29 Lindberg, AA, Brown, JE, Stromberg, N, Westling-Ryd, M, Schultz, JE, & Karlsson, K-A. Identification of the carbohydrate receptor for shiga toxin produced by *Shigella dysenteriae* type 1. *J. Biol. Chem.* 1987;**262**:1779–85.
30 Lingwood, CA, Law, H, Richardson, SE, *et al.* Glycolipid binding of natural and recombinant *Escherichia coli* produced vero toxin *in vitro*. *J. Biol. Chem.* 1987;**262**:8834–9.
31 Waddell, T, Head, S, Petric, M, Cohen, A, & Lingwood, C. Globotriosyl ceramide is specifically recognized by the *Escherichia coli* vero cytotoxin 2. *Biochem. Biophys. Res. Commun.* 1988;**152**:674–9.
32 Obrig, TG, Moran, TP, & Brown, JE. The mode of action of shiga toxin on peptide elongation of eukaryotic protein synthesis. *Biochem. J.* 1987; **244**:287–94.
33 Endo, Y, Tsurugi, K, Yuksudo, T, Takeda, Y, Ogasawara, K, & Egarashi, K. Site of action of a vero toxin (VT2) from *Escherichia coli* O157:H7 and of shiga toxin on eukaryotic ribosomes RNA *N*-glycosidase activity of the toxin. *Eur. J. Biochem.* 1988;**171**:45–50.
34 Sakena, SK, O'Brien, AD, & Ackerman, EJ. Shiga toxin, shiga-like toxin II variant and ricin are all single-site RNA *N*-glycosidases of 28S RNA when injected into *Xenopus* oocytes. *J. Biol. Chem.* 1989;**264**:596–601.
35 Obrig, TG, Del Vecchio, PJ, Brown, JE, *et al.* Direct cytotoxic action of shiga toxin on human vascular endothelial cells. *Infect. Immun.* 1988; **56**(9):2373–8.
36 Richardson, SE, Karmali, MA, Becker, LE, & Smith, CR. The histopathology of the hemolytic uremic syndrome associated with vero cytotoxin-producing *Escherichia coli* infections. *Hum. Pathol.* 1988;**19**:1102–8.
37 Boyd, B, & Lingwood, C. Vero toxin glycolipid in human renal tissue. *Nephron* 1989;**51**: 207–210.
38 Linggood, MA, & Thompson, JM. Vero toxin production among porcine strains of *Escherichia coli* and its association with oedema disease. *J. Med. Microbiol.* 1987;**25**:359–62.
39 Marques, LRM, Peirris, JSM, Cryz, SJ, & O'Brien, AD. *Escherichia coli* strains isolated from pigs with edema disease produce a variant of shiga-like toxin II. *FEMS Microbiol. Lett.* 1987;**44**:33–8.
40 Gyles, CL, DeGrandis, SA, MacKenzie, C, & Brunton, JL. Cloning a nucleotide sequence analysis of the genes determining verocytotoxin production in a porcine edema disease isolate of *Escherichia coli*. *Microbial Pathog.* 1988;**5**: 419–26.
41 DeGrandis, S, Law, H, Brunton, J, Gyles, C, & Lingwood, CA. Globotetraosyl ceramide is recognized by the pig edema disease toxin *J. Biol. Chem.* 1989;**264**(21):12520–25.
42 Svanborg-Eden, C, Erikssen, B, Hansen, SLA, *et al.* Adhesion to normal human uroepithelial cells of *Escherichia coli* from children with various forms of urinary tract infection. *J. Pediatr.* 1978;**93**:398–403.
43 Wold, AE, Thorsson, M, Hold, S, & Svanborg-Eden, C. Attachment of *Escherichia coli* via mannose or Galα1-4Galβ-containing receptors to human colonic epithelial cells. *Infect. Immun.* 1988;**56**:2531–7.
44 Sasonetti, PJ, Hale, TL, & Oaks, EV. Genetics of virulence in enteroinvasive *Escherichia coli*. In: *Microbiology 1985*, pp. 74–7.
45 Knutton, S, Baldini, MM, Kaper, JB, & McNeish, AS. Role of plasmid-encoded adherence factors in adhesion of enteropathogenic *Escherichia coli* to HEp-2 cells. *Infect. Immun.* 1987;**55**:78–85.
46 Knutton, S, Baldwin, T, Williams, PH, & American Society of Microbiology, Washington DC. McNeish, AS. Actin accumulation at sites of bacterial adhesion to tissue culture cells: basis of a new diagnostic test for enteropathogenic and enterohemorrhagic *Escherichia coli*. *Infect. Immun.* 1989;**57**:1290–8.

47 Baldini, MM, Kaper, JB, Levine, MM, *et al.* Plasmid mediated adhesion of enterophogenetic *Escherichia coli*. *J. Pediatr. Gastroenterol. Nutr.* 1983;**2**:534–8.
48 Nataro, JP, Kaper, JB, Robins-Browne, R, *et al.* Patterns of adherence of diarrheagenic *Escherichia coli* to HEp-2 cells. *Pediatr. Infect. Dis. J.* 1987;**6**:829–31.
49 Smith, HW, & Linggood, MA. Observations of the pathogenic properties of the K88, Hly and Ent plasmids of *Escherichia coli* with particular reference to porcine diarrhea. *J. Med. Microbiol.* 1971;**4**:467.
50 Wanke, C, & Guerrant, RL. Small-bowel colonization alone is a cause of diarrhea. *Infect. Immun.* 1987;**55**:1924–6.
51 Schlager, TA, & Guerrant, RL. Net fluid secretion and impaired villous function induced by small intestinal colonization by non-toxigenic, colonizing *E. coli* (abstract 1133). *28th Interscience Conference on Antimicrobial Agents and Chemotherapy* Los Angeles, 1988, p. 310.
52 Vial, PA, Robins-Browne, R, Lior, H, *et al.* Characterization of enteroadherent aggregative *E. coli*, a putative agent of diarrheal disease. *J. Infect. Dis.* 1988;**158**:70–79.
53 Bhan, MK, Raj, P, Levine, MM, Kaper, JB, Bhandain, N, Kumar, R, & Sazawal, S. Enteroadherent aggregative *E. coli*: a cause of persistent diarrhea in a cohort of rural Indian children. *J. Infect. Dis.* 1989 (in press).
54 Guentzel, MN, & Berry, LJ. Mortality as a virulence factor for *Vibrio cholerae*. *Infect. Immun.* 1975;**11**:890–97.
55 Schrank, GD, & Verwey, WF. Distribution of cholera organisms in experimental *Vibrio cholerae* infections: proposed mechanisms of pathogenesis and antibacterial immunity. *Infect. Immun.* 1976;**13**:195–203.
56 Adler, J. Chemotaxis in bacteria. *Rev. Biochem.* 1976;**44**:341–56.
57 Allweiss, B, Dostal, J, Carey, KE, Edwards, TF, & Freter, R. The role of chemotaxis in the ecology of bacterial pathogens of mucosal surfaces. *Nature* 1977;**266**:448–50.
58 Freter, R, & O'Brien, PCM. Role of chemotaxis in the association of motile bacteria with intestinal mucosa: chemotactic responses of *Vibrio cholerae* and description of motile nonchemotactic mutants. *Infect. Immun.* 1981;**34**:214–49.
59 Schneider, DR, & Parker, CD. Isolation and characterization of protease-deficient mutants of *Vibrio cholerae*. *J. Infect. Dis.* 1978;**138**:143–51.
60 Schneider, DR, & Parker, CD. Purification and characterization of the ucinose of *Vibrio cholerae*. *J. Infect. Dis.* 1982;**145**:474–82.
61 Slomiany, BL, Bilski, J, Sarosiek, J, Murty, VLN, JDworkin, B, van Horn, K, Zielenski, J, & Slomiany, A. *Campylobacter pyloridis* degrades mucin and undermines gastric mucosal integrity. *Biochem. Biophys. Res. Commun.* 1987;**144**: 307–14.
62 Jones, GW. The attachment of bacteria to the surfaces of animal cells. In: Reissig, JL (ed), *Microbial Interactions; Receptors and Recognition*, Series B, Vol. 3. London: Chapman & Hall, 1977, pp. 139–76.
63 Beachey, EH, Giampapa, CS, & Abraham, SN. Adhesin receptor-mediated attachment of pathogenic bacteria to mucosal surfaces. *Am. Rev. Resp. Dis.* 1988;**138**:45–8.
64 Svandborg-Eden, C, Hansson, S, Jodal, U, *et al.* Host–parasite interaction in the urinary tract. *J. Infect. Dis.* 1988;**157**:421–6.
65 Isberg, RR. Discrimination between intracellular uptake and surface adhesion of bacterial pathogens. *Science* 1991;**252**:934–8.
66 Sellwood, R. The interaction of the K88 antigen with porcine intestinal epithelial cell brush borders. *Biochim. Biophys. Acta* 1980;**632**: 326–35.
67 Satterwhite, TK, Evans, DG, DuPont, HL, *et al.* Role of *Escherichia coli* colonization factor antigen in acute diarrhea. *Lancet* 1978;**ii**:181–4.
68 McConnell, MM, Thomas, LV, Willshaw, GA, Smith, HA, & Rowe, B. Genetic control and properties of coli surface antigens of colonization factor antigen IV (PCF8775) of enterotoxigenic *Escherichia coli*. *Infect. Immun.* 1988;**56**: 1974–80.
69 Bergman, MJ, Updike, SJ, Wood, SE, Brown, III, & Guerrant, RL. Attachment factors among enterotoxigenic *Escherichia coli* from patients with acute diarrhea from diverse geographic areas. *Infect. Immun.* 1981;**32**:881–8.
70 Kyogashima, M, Ginsburg, V, & Krivan, HC. *Escherichia coli* K99 binds to *N*-glycolylsialoparagloboside and glycolyl-GM_3 found in piglet small intestine. *Arch. Biochem. Biophys.* 1989;**270**:391–7.
71 Faris, A, Lindahl, M, & Wadstrom, TI. Gm2-like glycoconjugate as possible erythrocyte receptor for the CFA/I and K99 haemagglutinins of enterotoxigenic *Escherichia coli*. *FEMS Microbiol. Lett.* 1980;**7**:265–9.
72 Ono, E, Abe, K, Nakazawa, M, & Naiki, M. Ganglioside epitope recognized by K99 fimbriae from enterotoxigenic *Escherichia coli*. *Infect. Immun.* 1989;**57**:907–11.
73 Sellwood, R. The interaction of the K88 antigen with porcine intestinal epithelial cell brush borders. *Biochim. Biophys. Acta* 1980;**632**: 326–35.
74 Faris, A, Wadstrom, T, & Freer, JH. Hydrophobic adsorptive and hemagglutinating properties of *Escherichia coli* possessing colonization factor antigens (CFA/I or CFA/II), Type I pili, or other pili. *Current Microbiol.* 1981;**5**:67–72.

75 Freter, R, & Jones, GW. Adhesive properties of *Vibrio cholerae*: nature of the interaction with intact mucosal surfaces. *Infect. Immun.* 1976; **14**:246–56.

76 Marx, JL. Vaccinating with bacterial pili. *Science* 1980;**209**:1103–6.

77 Deneke, CF, Thorne, GM, & Gorbach, SL. Serotypes of attachment pili of enterotoxigenic *Escherichia coli* isolated from humans. *Infect. Immun.* 1981;**32**:1254–60.

78 Runnels, PL, Moon, HW, & Schneider, RA. Development of resistance with host age to adhesion of K99+ *Escherichia coli* to isolated intestinal epithelial cells. *Infect. Immun.* 1980; **28**:298–300.

79 Cantey, JR, & Inman, LR. Diarrhea due to *Escherichia coli* strain RDEC-1 in the rabbit: the Peyer's patch as the initial site of attachment and colonization. *J. Infect. Dis.*1981;**143**:440–46.

80 Ulshen, MH, & Rollo, JL. Pathogenesis of *Escherichia coli* gastroenteritis in man: another mechanism. *N. Engl. J. Med.* 1980;**302**:99, with accompanying editorial by Guerrant, RL, pp. 113–15.

81 Cheny, CP, Schad, PA, Formal, SB, & Boedeker, EC. Species specificity of *in vitro Escherichia coli* adherence to host intestinal cell membranes and its correlation with *in vivo* colonization and infectivity. *Infect. Immun.* 1980;**28**:1019–27.

82 Karlsson, K. Animal glycolipids as attachment sites for microbes. *Chem. Phys. Lipids* 1986; **42**:153–72.

83 Knutton, S. *In vitro* adhesion of enterotoxigenic *Escherichia coli* to human intestinal epithelial cells from mucosal biopsies. *Infect. Immun.* 1984;**44**:514–18.

84 Zafriri, D. Growth advantage and enhanced toxicity of *Escherichia coli* adherent to tissue culture cells due to restricted diffusion of products secreted by the cells. *J. Clin. Invest.* 1987; **79**:1210–16.

85 Yamamoto, T. Electron microscopic study of *Vibrio cholerae* adherence to the mucus coat and villus surface in the human small intestine. *Infect. Immun.* 1988;**56**:2753–9.

86 Nevola, J. *In vivo* colonization of the mouse large intestine and *in vitro* penetration of intestinal mucus by an avirulent smooth strain of *Salmonella typhimurium* and its lipopolysaccharide-deficient mutant. *Infect. Immun.* 1987;**55**:2884–90.

87 Cohen, P. Adhesion of a human fecal *Escherichia coli* strain to mouse colonic mucus. *Infect. Immun.* 1985;**48**:139–45.

88 McSweegan, E. Intestinal mucus gel and secretory antibody are barriers to *Campylobacter jejuni* adherence to INT 407 cells. *Infect. Immun.* 1987;**55**:1431–5.

89 Dean, E. Age-specific colonization of porcine intestinal epithelium by 987P-piliated enterotoxigenic *Escherichia coli. Infect. Immun.* 1989; **57**:82–7.

90 Dean, E. Location and distribution of a receptor for the 987P pilus of *Escherichia coli* in small intestines. *Infect. Immun.* 1985;**47**:345–8.

91 Mobassaleh, M, Donohue-Rolfe, A, Jacewicz, M, Grand, RJ, & Keusch, GT. Pathogenesis of *Shigella* diarrhea: evidence for a developmentally regulated glycolipid receptor for *Shigella* toxin involved in the fluid secretory response of rabbit small intestine. *J. Infect. Dis.* 1988;**157**:1023–31.

92 Van Heyningen, W. Carpenter, CCJ, Pierce, NF, & Greenough W III. Deactivation of cholera toxin by ganglioside. *J. Infect. Dis.* 1971;**124**: 415–18.

93 Holmgren, J. Comparison of receptors for cholera and *Escherichia coli* enterotoxins in human intestine. *Gastroenterology* 1985;**89**:27–35.

94 Kamata, Y, Kozaki, S, Sakaguchi, G, Iwamori, M, & Nagai, Y. Evidence for direct binding of *Clostridium botulinum* type E derivative toxin and its fragments to gangliosides and free fatty acids. *Biochem. Biophys. Res. Commun.* 1986; **150**(3):1015–19.

95 Sakaguchi, G. *Clostridium botulinum* toxins. In: Dorner, F, & Drews, J (eds), *Pharmacology of Bacterial Toxins*. New York: Pergamon Press, 1986, pp. 519–48.

96 Krivan, HC, Clark, GF, Smith, DF, & Wilkins, TD. Cell surface binding site for *Clostridium difficile* enterotoxin: evidence for a glycoconjugate containing the sequence $Gal_{\alpha I\text{-}3}$ $Gal_{\beta I\text{-}4}$ GlcNAc. *Infect. Immun.* 1986;**53**:573–81.

97 Burnet, FM, & Stone, JD. *Aust. J. Exp. Biol. Med. Sci.* 1947;**25**:227–33.

98 Faillard, H. Uber die Abspaltung von *N*-acetylneuraminsaure aus mucine durch das "Receptor-destroying-enzyme" aus *Vibrio cholerae. Hoppe–Seyler's Zeitschrift für Physiologische Chemie* 1957;**307**:62–86.

99 Haywood, AM. Characteristics of sendai virus receptors in a model membrane. J. Mol. Biol. 1974, **83**:427–36.

100 Stromberg, N, Ryd, M, Lindberg, A, & Karlsson, K. Studies on the binding of bacteria to glycolipids. Two species of *Propionobacterium* apparently recognize separate epitopes on lactose of lactosylceramide. *FEBS Lett.* 1988;**232**:193–8.

101 Tuomanen, E, Towbin, H, Rosenfelder, G, Braun, D, Larson, G, Hansson, G, & Hill, R. Receptor analogs and monoclonal antibodies that inhibit adherence of *Bordetella pertussis* to human ciliated respiratory epithelial cells. *J. Exp. Med.* 1988;**168**:267–77.

102 Larson, G, Falk, P, & Lansing, CH. Degradation of human intestinal glycosphingolipids by extracellular glycosidases from mucin-degrading bacteria in the human fecal flora. *J. Biol. Chem.*

1988;**263**:10790–8.
103 Stromberg, N, Deal, C, Nyberg, G, Normark, S, So, M, & Karlsson, K. Identification of carbohydrate structures that are possible receptors for *Neisseria gonorrhoeae. Proc. Natl. Acad. Sci. USA* 1988;**85**:4902–6.
104 Ravdin, JI, & Guerrant, RL. The role of adherence in cytopathogenic mechanisms of *Entamoeba histolytica.* Study with mammalian tissue culture cells and human red blood cells. *J. Clin. Invest.* 1981;**68**:1305–13.
105 Miller, LH, Mason, SJ, & Dvorae, JA. Erythrocyte receptors for (*Plasmodium knowlesi*) malaria: Duffy blood group determinants. *Science* 1976; **189**:561–2.
106 Haynes, D, Dalton, JP, Klotz, FW, McGinniss, MH, Hadley, TJ, Hudson, DE, & Miller, LH. Receptor-like specificity of *Plasmodium knowlesi* malarial protein that binds to Duffy antigen ligands of erythrocytes. *J. Exp. Med.* 1988;**167**:1873–81.
107 Bennum, FR, Roth, GA, Monferran, CG, & Cumar, FA. Binding of cholera toxin to pig intestinal mucosa glycosphingolipids: relationship with the ABO blood group system. *Infect. Immun.* 1989;**57**:969–74.
108 Brooks, DE, Cavanagh, J, Jayroe, D, Janzen, J, Snoek, R, & Trust, T. Involvement of the MN blood group antigen in shear-enhanced hemagglutination induced by the *Escherichia coli* F41 adhesin. *Infect. Immun.* 1989;**57**: 377–83.
109 Bennum, FR, Roth, GA, Monferran, CG, & Cumar, FA. Binding of cholera toxin to pig intestinal mucosa glycosphingolipids; relationship with the ABO blood group system. *Infect. Immun.* 1989;**57**:969–74.
110 Emody, L, Carlsson, A, Ljungh, A, & Wadstrom, T. Mannose-resistant haemagglutination by *Campylobacter pylori. J. Infect. Dis.* 1988;**20**: 353–4.
111 Evans, DG, Evans, DJ, Moulds, JJ, & Graham, DY. *N*-Acetylneuraminyllactose-binding fibrillar hemagglutinin of *Campylobacter pylori*: a putative colonization factor antigen. *Infect. Immun.* 1988;**56**:2896–906.
112 Evans, DJ, Evans, DG, & Graham, DY. Serum antibody responses to the *N*-acetylneuraminyl-lactose-binding hemagglutinin of *Campylobacter pylori. Infect. Immun.* 1989;**57**:664–7.
113 Leunk, RD, Ferguson, M, & Morgan, D. *In vitro* adherence and hemagglutination by *Campylobacter pylori* (abstract 184). *Vth International Workshop on Campylobacter Infections. Puerto Vallarta, Mexico,* 1989.
114 Dunn, BE, Altmann, M, & Campbell, GP. Binding of *Campylobacter pylori,* to kato cells analyzed by flow cytometry. *Gastroduodenal Disease and Campylobacter pylori, Charlottesville, Va,* May 10–12, 1989.
115 Lingwood, CA, Law, H, Pellizzari, A, Sherman, P, & Drumm, B. A novel gastric glycolipid is a receptor for *Campylobacter pylori. Gastroduodenal Disease and Campylobacter pylori, Charlottesville Va.,* May 10–12, 1989.
116 Lingwood, CA, Cheng, M, Krivan, HC, & Woods, D. Glycolipid receptor binding specificity of exoenzyme-5 from *Pseudomanas aeniginosa. Biochem. Biop. Res. Com.* 1991;**175**:1076–81.
117 Guerrant, RL, Wanke, CA, Pennie, RA, Barrett, LJ, Lima, AAM, & O'Brien, AD. Production of a unique cytotoxin by *Campylobacter jejuni. Infect. Immun.* 1987;**55**:2526–30.
118 Guerrant, RL, Barrett, LJ, & Marshall, BJ. Cytotoxin production by *C. pylori* (abstract 188). *Vth International Workshop on Campylobacter Infections, Puerto Vallarta, Mexico,* 1989.
119 Leunk, RD, Johnson, PT, David, BC, Kraft, WG, & Morgan, DR. Cytotoxic activity in broth-culture filtrates of *Campylobacter pylori. J. Med. Microbiol.* 1988;**26**:93–99.
120 Figura, N, Gugliemetti, P, Rossolini, A, Barber, A, Cusi, G, Musmanno, RA, Russi, M, & Quaranta, S. Cytotoxin production by *Campylobacter pylori* strains isolated from patients with peptic ulcers and from patients with chronic gastritis only. *J. Clin. Microbiol.* 1989;**27**:225–6.
121 Cover, TL, Perez-Perez, Gl, & Blaser, JJ. Characterization of *C. pylori* cytotoxin (abstract 189). *International Workshop on Campylobacter Infections,* Puerto Vallarta, Mexico, 1989.

7: Laboratory diagnosis and handling of Helicobacter pylori

T.U. WESTBLOM

Introduction

In the days before the discovery of *Helicobacter pylori*, gastritis was commonly diagnosed by the endoscopist through visual inspection of the mucosa. With routine use of gastric biopsies, it became obvious that the naked eye was not able to distinguish between inflamed and non-inflamed mucosa the way histologic examination could. Seemingly normal tissue could be found to harbor great numbers of *H. pylori* under the microscope and to be accompanied by severe polymorphonuclear white cell infiltration. A good laboratory can therefore be of considerable assistance to the endoscopist, yet laboratory diagnosis of *H. pylori* can be intricate because of the fastidious nature of the organism and its peculiar biochemical characteristics.

Culture techniques for *H. pylori*

Even though culture is not the most sensitive way of diagnosing *H. pylori* infection it remains the most specific, and is essential for selecting therapy based on antimicrobial susceptibilities. With appropriate techniques, *H. pylori* can readily be cultured from endoscopic biopsies of the stomach and duodenum. It has also been recovered from esophageal biopsies [1, 2]; however, in this location it is usually a contaminant from concurrent *H. pylori* gastritis [3]. Even though it is reasonable to assume that the organism may be present in lower numbers in other parts of the gastrointestinal tract, as evidenced by histologic findings of *H. pylori*-like organisms in Meckel's diverticulum [4] and the rectum [5], so far it has not been possible to culture the organism from stool samples. Repeated attempts to culture *H. pylori* from the oral cavity have been unsuccessful [6, 7], except for a single isolate from dental plaque [6]. *H. pylori* does not grow in commercial blood culture systems [8].

Successful isolation of *H. pylori* therefore still requires gastric endoscopy. It is recommended that multiple biopsies be obtained for culture, since the organism can have a patchy distribution [9], and single biopsies can be subject to sampling error. *H. pylori* is most likely found in the antrum, which should always be biopsied, preferably with at least two biopsies. Depending on the clinical situation, biopsies from the fundus, duodenum, and esophagus may also be obtained. Before plating, biopsies are minced or ground. A regular small glass tissue grinder is used and a small volume (0.5–1.0 ml) of a nutrient broth is added, preferably the same broth used to transport the biopsy to the microbiology laboratory [10]. After grinding, 100 μl of the homogenate is spread onto each plate. If grinding cannot be performed, the fresh biopsy may be streaked across the agar, but the recovery rate is somewhat lower using this technique, especially if the number of organisms is low in the specimen.

Cultivation of *H. pylori* is best done at 37 °C and 100% humidity. Even though the organism has been recovered at both 35 °C and 42 °C, these temperatures are less than optimal [11, 12]. Below 28 °C it will not grow at all [11–13]. The critical point of humidity has been shown to be 98% [9] and for a suitable margin of safety 100% is recommended.

H. pylori is a microaerophilic organism and will not grow in normal atmospheric conditions. It grows best when the CO_2 content is 10% and the oxygen content is no more than 5% [9], but the organism is not strictly microaerophilic. It can be grown in a normal CO_2

incubator provided the CO_2 content is at least 10%, but the recovery rate in such an atmosphere, which contains about 19% oxygen, may be slightly lower. Anaerobic atmosphere has not been successful in promoting growth [9, 14, 15]. If a microaerophilic incubator is not available, a candle jar can be used [16], in which case it is recommended to include a small container of water to ensure a high humidity inside the jar. The best alternative to a microaerophilic incubator is the GasPak system using CampyPak envelopes (BBL Microbiology Systems, Cockeysville, Maryland). These will provide a humid atmosphere with 5% oxygen and 12% CO_2 when fully loaded. The CampyPak system provides excellent growth, but needs replacement of the gas envelopes every time the jar has been opened. This can be a disadvantage, compared to a microaerophilic incubator, if frequent handling of the specimens is needed in the laboratory.

H. pylori is a slow-growing organism on all media, and cultures take 2–5 days to become positive. Colonies are about 1 mm in diameter, pale to transparent in color, and can be either smooth or rough. Identification is made by typical morphology on Gram staining, as well as positive reactions for urease, catalase, and oxidase. Additional tests that can be used are alkaline phosphatase, γ-glutamyl aminopeptidase, leucine aminopeptidase, and DNase, which are positive in 100% of strains [17]. Overall, 31 enzymes have been identified [18], but the majority of these are not needed for routine identification.

Solid media

Given the right incubator environment, *H. pylori* will grow on several different agars, including commercially-available chocolate agars, blood agars, and Skirrow's medium [15, 17, 19–22]. Such agars may be used for subculturing and are usually economically attractive compared to home-made media. However, a lot of variation can be found between the formulas

Table 7.1 Solid agars used for *Helicobacter pylori* cultures

Author	Agar base	Supplements	Antibiotics
Goodwin *et al.* [9]	Brain–heart infusion	7% Horse blood 1% IsoVitalex	Nalidixic acid 20 mg l^{-1} Vancomycin 6 mg l^{-1} Amphotericin B 2 mg l^{-1}
Buck & Smith [23]	GC agar base	1% Hemin	None reported
Hirschl [24]	Mueller–Hinton	3% Sheep blood	Trimethoprim 5 mg l^{-1} Vancomycin 10 mg l^{-1} Polymyxin B 2500 IU l^{-1}
Queiroz *et al.* [25]	Brain–heart infusion	10% Sheep blood TTC 40 mg l^{-1}	Nalidixic acid 20 mg l^{-1} Vancomycin 6 mg l^{-1} Amphotericin B 2 mg l^{-1}
Glupczynski *et al.* [26]	Brain–heart infusion	10% Horse serum 0.2% Charcoal 1% Yeast extract TTC 40 mg l^{-1}	Cefsulodin 5 mg l^{-1} Trimethoprim 5 mg l^{-1} Vancomycin 10 mg l^{-1} Amphotericin B 10 mg l^{-1}
Dent & McNulty [27]	Columbia	7% Lysed horse blood	Cefsulodin 5 mg l^{-1} Trimethoprim 5 mg l^{-1} Vancomycin 10 mg l^{-1} Amphotericin B 5 mg l^{-1}
Westblom *et al.* [28]	Columbia	10% Egg yolk 1% IsoVitalex TTC 40 mg l^{-1}	Cefsulodin 5 mg l^{-1} Trimethoprim 5 mg l^{-1} Vancomycin 6 mg l^{-1} Amphotericin B 6 mg l^{-1}

TTC, 2,3,5-triphenyltetrazolium chloride.

used by different manufacturers, and each laboratory is recommended to test several of the available media before deciding which one best suits their local needs.

Even though commercially available media may be useful for subculturing, many of them are less suitable for primary isolation. For such cultures very rich media are needed, as well as antibiotic supplements to reduce overgrowth of faster growing contaminants. Several different formulas have been used successfully (Table 7.1). Most of them have in common a nutritious agar base supplemented with either blood or serum.

The original formula, reported by Goodwin *et al.* [9], used brain–heart infusion agar with 7% horse blood and 1% IsoVitalex. This is a rich medium that has proved to work very well. However, brain–heart infusion agar is costly if large quantities are used. *Brucella* agar has been shown to work just as well when supplemented with 10% bovine blood and 1% IsoVitalex. This medium also uses 40 mg l^{-1} TTC (2,3,5-triphenyltetrazolium chloride), an additive that was originally suggested by Queiroz *et al.* [25]. When *H. pylori* grows on media containing TTC it produces colonies with a golden hue, which is helpful in identification. A different type of medium has been reported by Glupczynski *et al.* [26], using 10% horse serum instead of blood, and supplemented with 0.2% charcoal and 1% yeast extract. Charcoal can bind toxic components in the medium and promote growth of *H. pylori*, which has also been shown earlier by Buck & Smith [23]. Unfortunately, charcoal may also bind some antibiotics, particularly the antifungal agents, and can therefore paradoxically lead to increased numbers of contaminants.

All agars for primary isolation need antibiotic supplementation to decrease contamination from the oral cavity. Since the endoscope passes through the oral cavity, it is hard to avoid contact with bacteria colonizing the mouth. Furthermore, patients who are taking H2-blockers or omeprazole may have a gastric pH above 4, which can lead to colonization of the stomach by both Gram-negative and Gram-positive bacteria. Several antibiotic combinations have been used in selective media (Table 7.1). Goodwin's original recipe called for nalidixic acid, vancomycin and amphotericin B. Some strains of *H. pylori* may, however, be sensitive to nalidixic acid, and trimethoprim can be used as an alternative. If fungal contamination is a particular problem, amphotericin B may not be enough to suppress the growth of contaminants. *Aspergillus* species can sometimes be resistant to amphotericin, in which case cycloheximide can be added to the medium in a concentration of 100 mgl^{-1}. Recently, Dent & McNulty [27] reported a modified Skirrow's medium which instead used cefsulodin, trimethoprim, vancomycin and amphotericin B. Cefsulodin is an antibiotic with good activity against *Pseudomonas*, but it is not yet available in many parts of the world, including the United States. When used in selective *H. pylori* media it effectively reduces the number of contaminants.

A completely different type of medium has recently been reported by Westblom *et al.* [28]. They developed a novel agar which contains egg yolk instead of serum or blood products. When this medium was compared to the traditional media by Goodwin [9], Glupczynski [26], and Dent & McNulty [27], it produced statistically significant higher growth at a faster rate. Colonies of *H. pylori* are easy to spot on the egg yolk medium since they stain bright red against a yellow background.

Liquid media

H. pylori does not grow well in regular nutrient broths, unless supplemented with serum. The serum should not be heat inactivated, but can be of either horse or bovine origin. Several different formulas have been used (Table 7.2).

When using a liquid medium it is important to facilitate the diffusion of CO_2 from the incubator atmosphere into the entire liquid phase. This can be accomplished by using an orbital shaker inside the incubator [29], but not all incubators can be equipped with such shakers. An alternative method is to use a very shallow body of liquid. This can be done using 100 ml tissue culture flasks instead of glass tubes. If such flasks are filled with no more than 10 ml of broth and left lying down flat in the incubator, the depth of the liquid will be only a few millimeters. This is sufficient for

Table 7.2 Liquid media used for *Helicobacter pylori* cultures

Author	Basic broth	Supplements
Buck & Smith [23]	*Brucella*	5% horse serum
Buck & Smith [23]	*Brucella*	1% corn starch
Morgan *et al.* [29]	*Brucella*	10% fetal calf serum
Armstrong *et al.* [30]	Brain–heart infusion	10% horse serum, 0.25% yeast extract
Hudson & Newell [31]	*Brucella*	1% fetal calf serum pyruvate
Westblom *et al.* [10]	*Brucella*	10% horse serum, 1% IsoVitalex

good diffusion of the CO_2, provided that the corks are not screwed in tightly. Best results are obtained with gas permeable corks. Most tissue culture flasks are grooved and can be stored on top of each other to give more space in the incubator. If traditional glass tubes are used instead, they should not be filled with more than 2–3 ml of liquid for optimal growth conditions.

If large volumes of bacteria need to be cultivated, 500 ml or 1000 ml tissue culture flasks with 50 ml or 100 ml of broth will provide the same favorable shallow depth. If an orbital shaker is used, it can be fitted with large flasks up to 2500 ml, giving an even larger capacity. When maximal production of bacteria is needed, one can use a continuous liquid culture medium. Such a system has been described by Hudson & Newell [31] and uses a chemostat with a constant 0.6 l culture volume. Fresh medium consisting of *Brucella* broth with 1% fetal calf serum is supplied at dilution rates varying between 0.05 and 0.2 per hour. This type of culture system may be particularly useful for large-scale production of antigen for serodiagnosis.

Transport media

For optimal culture results it is important to plate the biopsy as soon as possible while it is still fresh. However, plating the biopsy in the endoscopy suite, during ongoing endoscopy, is labor-consuming and merely increases the risk of contamination. In most instances, therefore, the biopsy has to be placed in a temporary transport medium. If the microbiology laboratory is located near the endoscopy suite, the composition of this transport medium is not crucial. If plating will be done within an hour, one can use sterile normal saline, provided it is free of bacteriostatic supplements. If longer time elapses, however, *H. pylori* will lose viability in saline [32]. Using a 20% glucose solution, Goodwin *et al.* showed that *H. pylori* can stay viable at 4 °C for at least 5 hours [9]. Freezing the biopsy for transportation is not recommended. The organism is vulnerable to freeze damage, and one study using this method failed to grow any isolates [33].

A biphasic medium has been used successfully for transportation and has the added advantage of functioning as a culture medium as well [10]. This medium contains a 20° slant of solid *Brucella* agar with 10% bovine blood and 1% IsoVitalex at the bottom of a 16 mm glass tube. Two milliliters of a liquid phase consisting of *Brucella* broth with 10% horse serum and 1% IsoVitalex covers the slant. Both the solid and liquid phase contain antibiotics to reduce growth of contaminants. In the microbiology laboratory the broth is poured off and used in the grinding of the biopsy. The remaining agar slant is not discarded but incubated along with the rest of the agars. In biopsies with low numbers of organisms, this method has sometimes resulted in positive cultures in the original transport tube when other plates have been without growth.

The distant microbiology laboratory, not located on the same premises as the endoscopy suite, poses a special problem. No transport medium suitable for mailing of the biopsies has been developed. However, a semi-solid medium has been used to ship pure cultures of *H. pylori* [34]. This medium consists of brain–heart infusion broth with 7% horse blood and 0.5% agar. In preliminary tests it could sustain

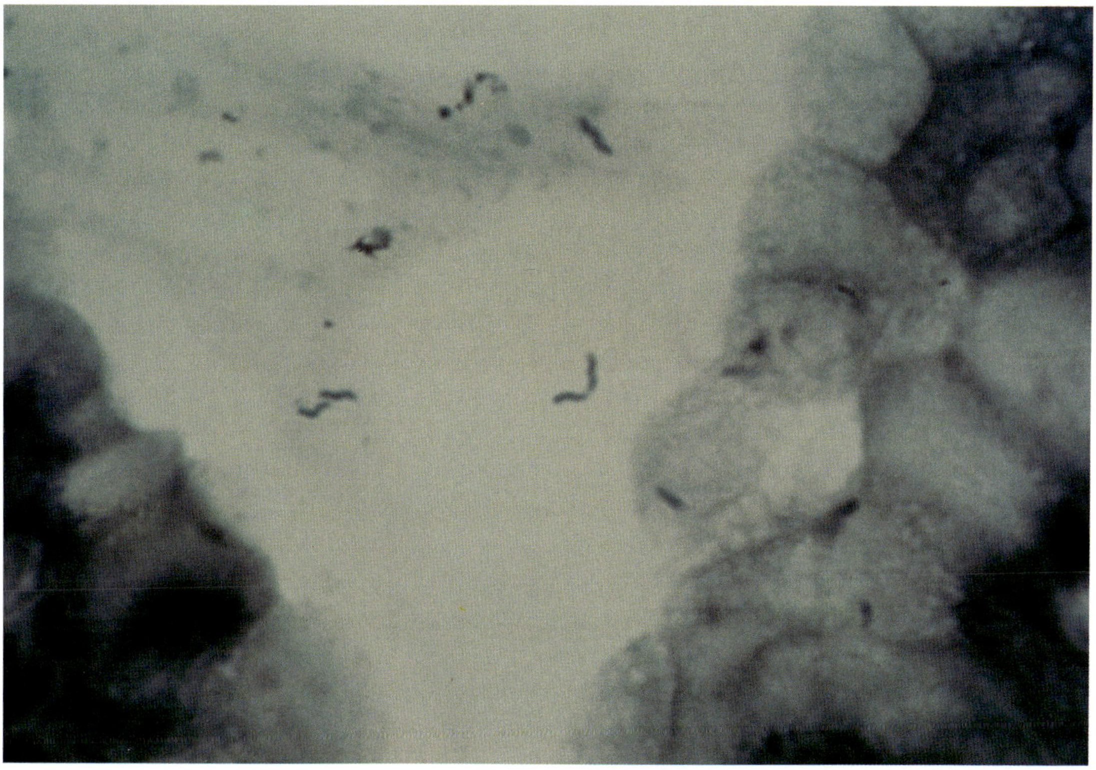

Plate 7.1 Modified Giemsa stain according to Madan *et al.* [39].

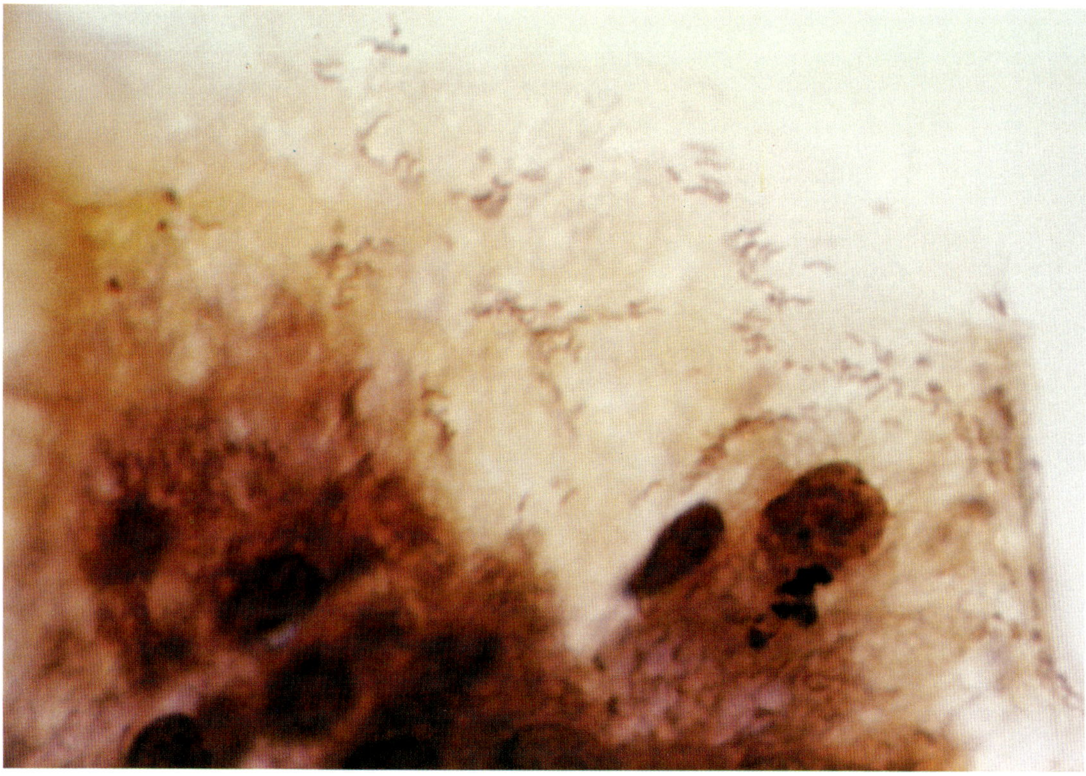

Plate 7.2 Brown–Hopps stain [41] showing *H. pylori* inside luminal mucus.

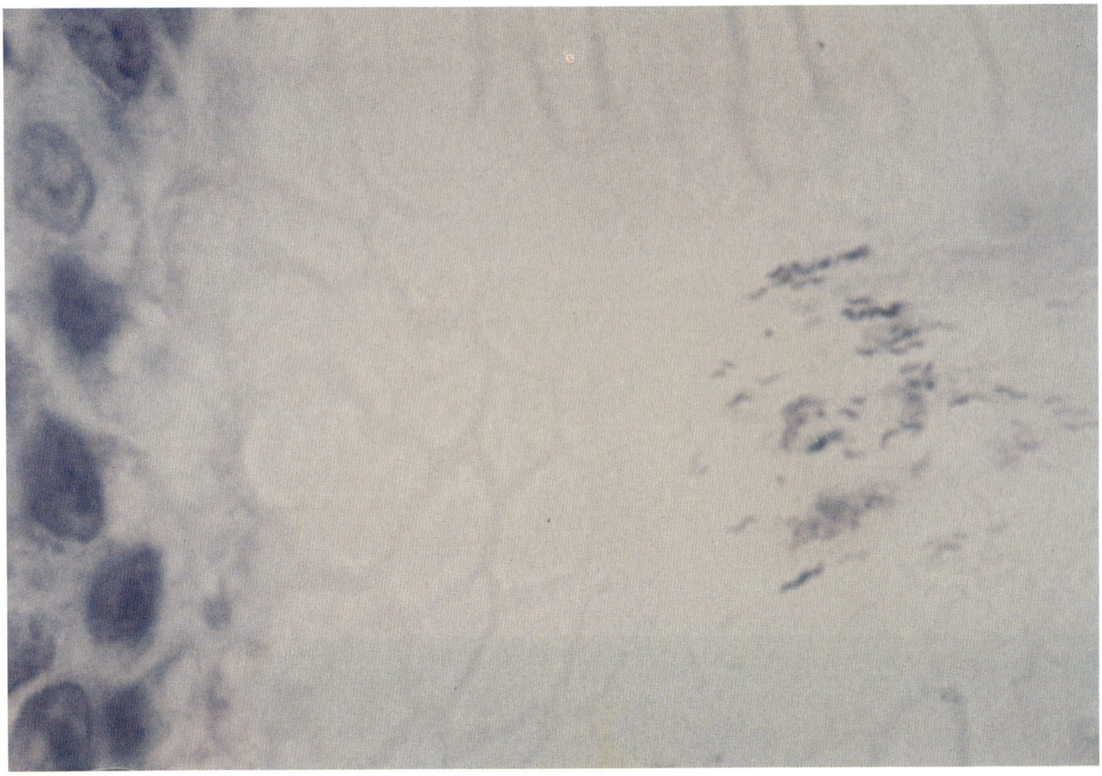

Plate 7.3 Cresyl fast violet stain according to Burnett *et al.* [42].

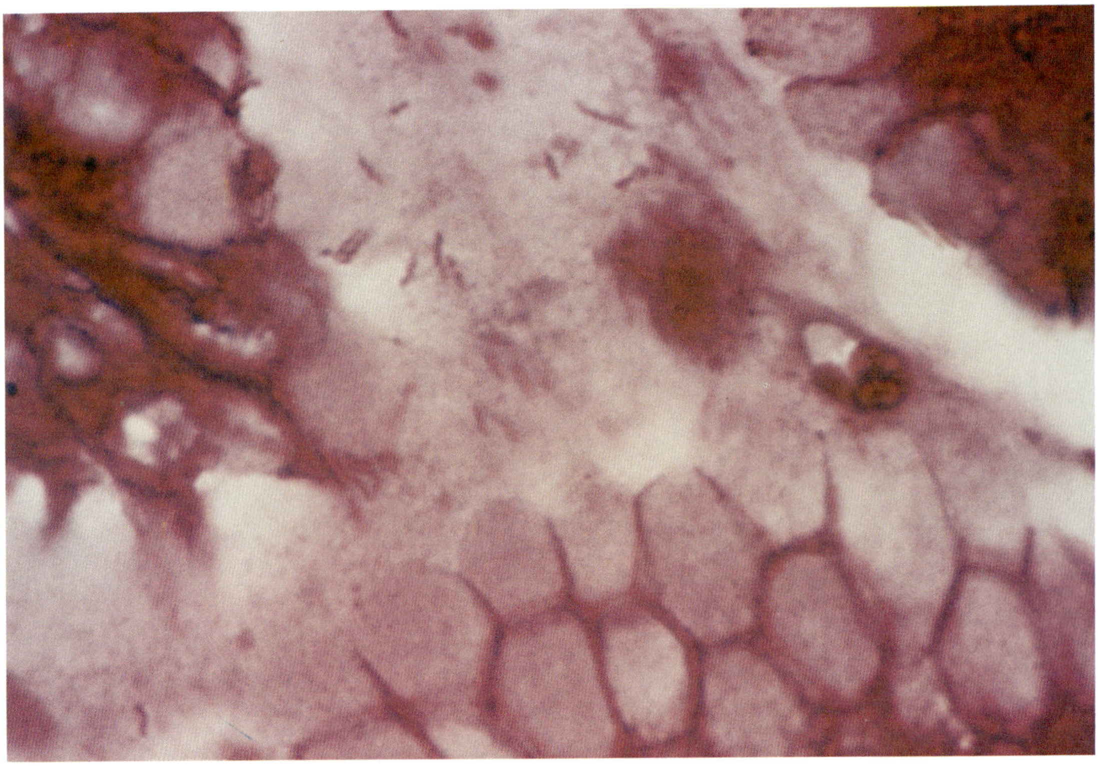

Plate 7.4 Carbol fuchsin stain according to Rocha *et al.* [45].

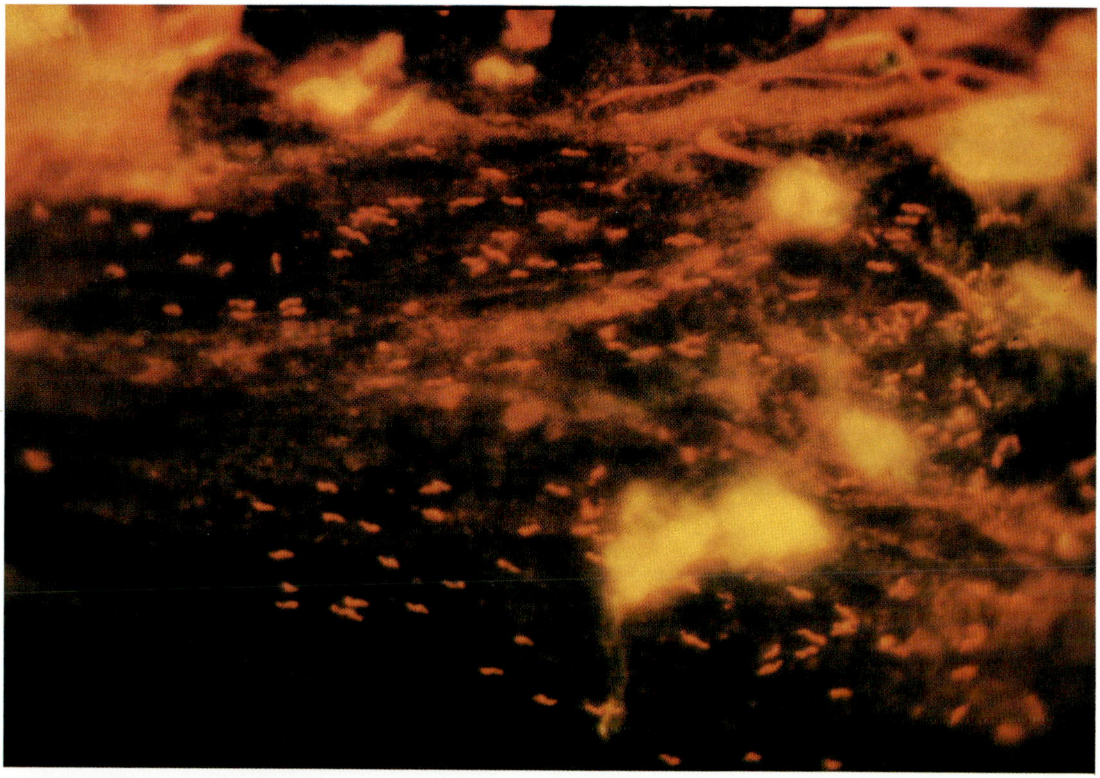

Plate 7.5 Acridine orange stain showing fluorescent spiral rods.

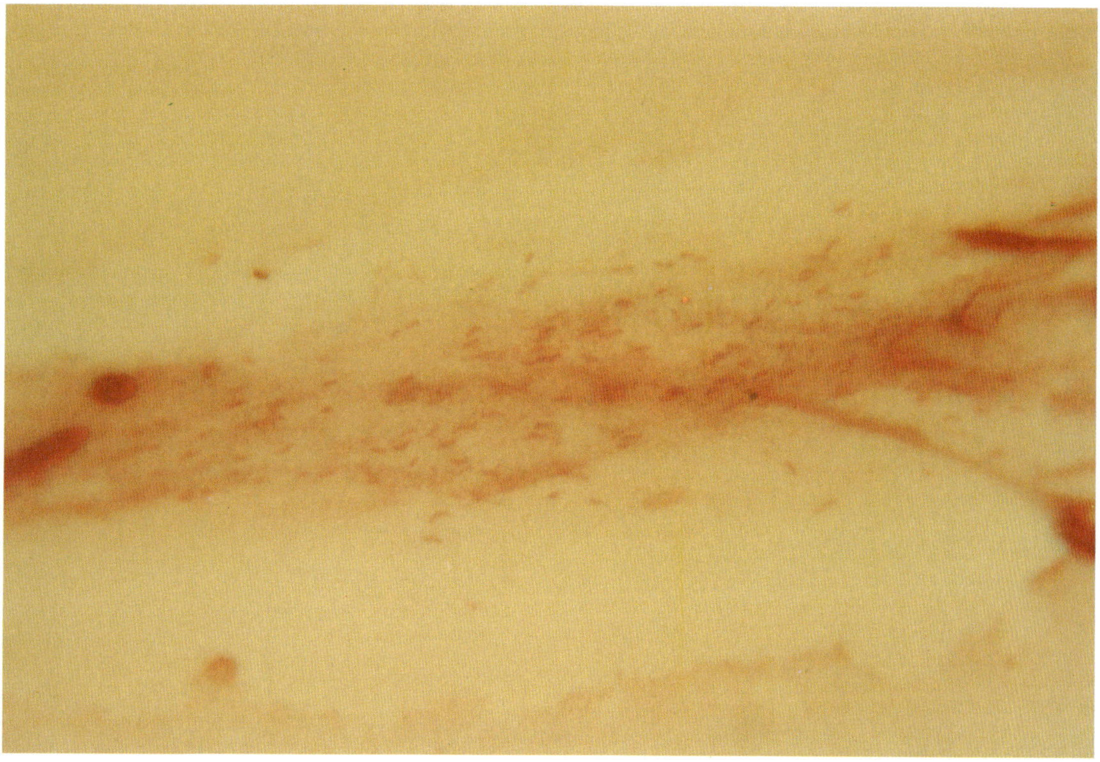

Plate 7.6 Modified Gram stain of smear from fresh gastric biopsy.

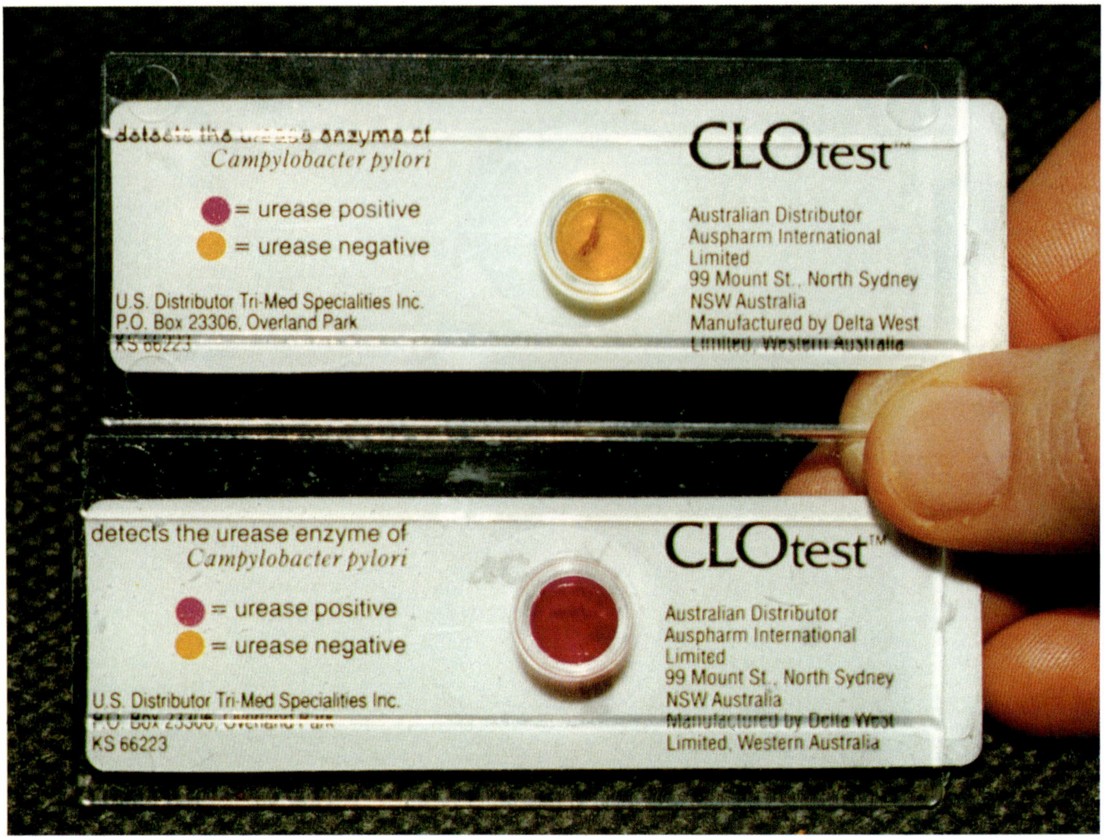

Plate 7.7 The CLOtest rapid urease test. CLOtest is approved by the FDA in the United States for the diagnosis of *H. pylori* in gastric biopsy specimens. Positive biopsies produce a red color, usually within 1 hour. If the gel remains yellow 24 hours after insertion of the biopsy, then *H. pylori* is not present (sensitivity 95%).

viable *H. pylori* for 10 days at both room temperature and 4 °C. However, its usefulness in transportation of fresh biopsies has not been evaluated.

Storage media

Most bacteria can be easily stored in −20 °C or −70 °C freezers for several years using a nutrient broth containing 20% glycerol. However, *H. pylori* seems to be more susceptible to freeze damage than other bacteria. Using traditional freeze media [35] or freeze-drying [32, 36] often results in low viability, and the isolates may be lost. An alternative medium, which has been proved effective, is whole defibrinated blood [35]. The blood may be of either horse, sheep, or bovine origin. *H. pylori* isolates frozen in whole blood have been successfully revived after more than 2 years of storage.

Nevertheless, whole blood is not a perfect medium. For seemingly erratic reasons, vials stored only a few months may sometimes fail to produce growth, while others stored much longer can result in profuse growth. This may be the result of differences between batches of blood, but it is not known which factors may be involved. A recovery rate of 70% can be expected within the first year using whole blood. For this reason it is recommended to save each isolate in more than one vial, preferably using different batches of blood. The blood should be as fresh as possible. Even though thawed and lysed blood may produce good growth on second or third thawing of the same vial, no controlled study has been done comparing it to fresh blood, and it is not recommended to use frozen blood if it can be avoided.

An alternative method for −70 °C storage was recently described by Drumm & Sherman [37]. They grew *H. pylori* in *Brucella* broth with 10% fetal bovine serum, then added 10% glycerol and an additional 10% serum before freezing the organisms in their original culture medium. This method has the advantage of a high bacterial concentration before freezing, and multiple freeze vials can be prepared from the same culture. Preliminary results from freezing 10 strains with this technique showed good growth in all of them after 6 months' storage [37].

Liquid nitrogen storage, if available, is usually more reliable than a regular freezer. Whole blood can be used as freezing medium for this purpose also. However, a medium consisting of *Brucella* broth, 10% serum, and 10% DMSO (dimethyl sulfoxide) has been shown to work just as well, when compared side by side (TU Westblom, unpublished data). Because *H. pylori* kept in −70 °C freezers have a limited lifespan, it is recommended to use liquid nitrogen if such a system is available. Whichever system is used, viability can be expected to increase if freezing is done as slowly as possible. Most freeze damage is caused by cellular membrane breakdown from formation of crystals. Agents such as DMSO reduce the formation of such crystals, but so does controlled slow freezing. Some sophisticated liquid nitrogen systems contain programmable units for slow freezing. If this is not available, one can use a three-step process by placing the vials in −20 °C and −70 °C freezers before final placement in liquid nitrogen.

Freeze-drying, which has been used successfully to store other bacteria for prolonged periods of time, does not work very well for *H. pylori*. If standard freeze-drying methods are used, there is a loss of viability of up to 7 log units [36]. The bacteria are exposed to damage from both the freezing and the drying, of which the latter seems to be the more important. This is not surprising, in view of the known growth requirements for *H. pylori*, which include a high humidity. Still, freeze-drying can be used for preservation if the procedure is modified to include a suspending fluid of 5% inositol-serum or 5% inositol-broth with 25% glucose. Using these suspending fluids, Owen *et al.* showed a short-term loss of viability of only 4 log units [36]. However, there is no information yet on the long-term viability of *H. pylori* preserved by freeze-drying.

Histologic diagnosis of *H. pylori*

Laboratory diagnosis of *H. pylori* should include some form of histologic staining of gastric biopsies, since cultures by themselves rarely achieve a sensitivity above 90%. In his original report, Warren recommended the Warthin–Starry stain [38]. This stain is very good at visualizing the organism, but has certain drawbacks. It is time-consuming and costly, and requires an experienced technician in order to reduce batch-to-batch variations. Furthermore, the silver impregnation sometimes gives the organism a granular appearance. This can lead to difficulty in differentiating it from silver precipitate in the mucus layer, thus leading to false-positive biopsy readings [39]. A modified Giemsa stain was reported by Gray *et al.* [40] and is a more consistent and less costly alternative. Other stains that have been proposed for *H. pylori* diagnosis include Brown–Hopps [41], cresyl fast violet [42], histologic half-Gram [43], Gimenez [44], carbol fuchsin [45], and acridine orange [46, 47].

The modified Giemsa stain, according to Madan *et al.* [39], uses a 2.5 ml solution of Giemsa concentrate (GamRad, San Juan Capistrano, California). Paraffin-embedded sections (5 μm) are placed in the solution for 15 minutes at room temperature and then rinsed in tap water for 2 minutes. The modified Giemsa stain provides a simple and economical method that is common to most histology laboratories. The organism is easy to identify, staining uniform purple–blue against a light blue background (Plate 7.1).

Brown–Hopps stain uses Gallego's differentiating solution, a 1.5% tartrazine solution and basic fuchsin as part of the counterstaining technique. The stain is best viewed using a microscope without a daylight blue filter. It shows the mucus yellow, and *H. pylori* can be observed as purple–red curved bacteria, often visualized within the mucus layer itself [41] (Plate 7.2).

Cresyl fast violet is a simple staining method that shows the organism and its characteristic morphology well (Plate 7.3). There is good definition of the inflammatory cells. It also stains intestinal mucins, which potentially can complicate the reading in patients with intestinal metaplasia [42]. However, the mucin is light pink in color, while *H. pylori* stains purple, and this rarely causes any problems.

The Gimenez technique uses carbol fuchsin with a counterstain of malachite green. The organism stains magenta against a blue–green background [44]. Compared to other stains it is fairly hard to perform, and can exhibit variations similar to those of Warthin–Starry; like the silver stain it is also prone to precipitations, which stain dark and can be confused with the organism.

The simplified carbol fuchsin staining method, on the other hand, uses no counterstain. After applying a carbol fuchsin solution for 5 minutes, the sections are decolorized with acetone and inspected under oil. The mucus is stained light pink to red and the organism purple. Inflammatory cells are well identified (Plate 7.4). When compared to culture, the sensitivity of this stain was 92% and the specificity 100% [45]. However, no comparison with other stains has been reported yet.

Acridine orange is a fluorochrome that binds to nucleic acids. A 0.01% solution is applied for 2 minutes, and the slides then examined with a fluorescent microscope. *H. pylori* is shown as bright orange fluorescent spiral rods [46] (Plate 7.5). The sensitivity of the stain is high. In a clinical study of 76 biopsies, it was more sensitive than culture and urease test [47]. However, no comparison with other stains has been reported.

Existing experience and resources in the laboratory will doubtlessly influence the choice of stain for *H. pylori*. However, when five stains were compared in a clinical material, the Giemsa and the Brown–Hopps were superior to Warthin–Starry, Brown–Brenn and hematoxylin and eosin [39]. The Brown–Hopps stain gave more information about the relative microbial density inside and outside the mucus, but the Giemsa was easier to perform. Based on simplicity and cost, the Giemsa was therefore recommended for routine use. In a similar comparison the Giemsa, the cresyl fast violet, and the simple carbol fuchsin stains all showed high correlation and were comparable in simplicity (E Madan & TU Westblom, unpublished data). Either is suitable for routine diagnostic use. If more information about the mucus and surrounding tissues is desired, the Brown–Hopps stain without daylight blue filtration is recommended.

Rapid tests for *H. pylori*

Culture and histology are both excellent ways of making the diagnosis, but they will not provide an answer while the patient is still in the endoscopy suite. There are rapid tests available, however, which can make a presumptive diagnosis within 30–60 minutes. Smears from biopsies can be inspected with direct microscopy after Gram staining, or immediately with phase contrast. Alternatively, a rapid urease test can be used.

Direct microscopy

Gram staining is simple to perform, but can require up to 20–30 minutes of technician time for each biopsy. One can either do an impression smear, or the biopsy can be rubbed over the surface of the slide. After heat fixation, a modified Gram staining is performed. *H. pylori* does not take up safranin well, and it is recommended to substitute carbol fuchsin for the counterstain. The slide is then inspected under oil for the presence of typical curved bacteria (Plate 7.6). The distribution of organisms can be patchy, and it will take 10–15 minutes before one can say with any certainty that a biopsy is negative. If many biopsies are performed each day, this test will take up a lot of technician time. However, if done routinely it can often provide a quick and accurate diagnosis. Montgomery *et al.* [48] reported a 92% sensitivity and 100% specificity with the Gram stain. Similar results have also been reported by Parsonnet *et al.* [49]. They found that, by Gram staining biopsies from both fundus and antrum, the sensitivity could be increased from 91% to near 100%.

Another form of direct examination that can be useful is phase contrast microscopy. The method reported by Pinkard *et al.* [13] calls for fine mincing of the biopsy in two drops of saline. One-quarter of this homogenate is pressed firmly between two glass slides. After application of a coverslip the slide is then examined under phase contrast using ×400 magnification. *H. pylori* is identified as characteristic black curved rods. When a clinical sample of 70 biopsies was examined with this technique, the investigators found it to be slightly superior to the Gram stain and equal to the Warthin–Starry stain in sensitivity [13].

Urease tests

H. pylori characteristically has a very strong urease reaction. Among *Campylobacter* spp., most species have no detectable urease activity [50]; only *C. nitrofigilis* [51], *C. laridis* [52] and a group of thermophilic *Campylobacter* spp. [53] are known to have any urease activity, but all are much weaker than *H. pylori*. Of these, only *C. laridis* has been shown rarely to infect humans. The urease of *H. pylori* has a much higher affinity for the urea substrate, and a significantly higher activity than ureases of other organisms including *Proteus* and *Providencia* [54]. This makes *H. pylori* easy to detect and has led to the development of rapid tests for identifying *H. pylori* in gastric biopsies.

With minor modifications, rapid urease tests are based on the ability of bacterial urease to convert urea to ammonia. Increasing levels of ammonia elevate the pH, which can be detected by an indicator such as phenol red. This conversion of urea to ammonia may have a physiologic function as a survival mechanism for *H. pylori*, enabling it to neutralize some of the hydrochloric acid in the stomach and promoting colonization [55].

The first clinical application of this test in detecting *H. pylori* infection was reported by McNulty & Wise [56]. They placed the biopsies in a 2% Christensen's urea broth which was kept at room temperature. The test was highly specific, but slow compared to later modifications. Only one-third of tests became positive within 3 hours, and half within 6 hours. With crushing of the biopsies, leading to a greater release of organisms into the medium, the same investigators were able to get more than half of their tests to turn positive within 1 hour [57]. Similar release of organisms can be achieved by 15 seconds of high speed vortexing of the vials.

The basic 2% Christensen's urea broth has been used by several other investigators [58–62], yielding similar results. When read at 1 hour it is 100% specific, but has only a sensitivity around 70% [61]. An increase in sensitivity and speed has been reported by Vaira *et al.* [63] by using a 6% urea concentration instead. Other modifications of the urea broth include the use of Stuart broth [64] and 2% urea–indole broth [65].

A different urease test has been developed by Marshall *et al.* [66]. The *Campylobacter*-like organisms test (CLOtest: Delta-West Ltd, Perth,

Western Australia) is commercially available and is made specifically for the diagnosis of *H. pylori* (Plate 7.7). It uses the same phenol red indicator as Christensen's urea broth, but is instead incorporated into a gel. There are several advantages to this approach: by keeping the biopsy in a fixed position in the gel, the indicator can turn red at the interface between the medium and the biopsy, and be visible faster than in a broth, where the pH change would be distributed throughout the medium and therefore dependent on the volume of the broth. The CLOtest has a higher sensitivity than the urea broth. Marshall *et al.* reported 75% of the infected biopsies to be positive within 20 minutes and 92% within 3 hours. Like most other urease tests it was 100% specific [66]. Sensitivities of 90% [67] and 91% [68] have been reported by other investigators using the CLOtest.

In a study performed at the University of Virginia by Dye *et al.* [69], the CLOtest was more sensitive than a single antral biopsy sent for histology and stained with Giemsa.

The choice of urease test for the individual laboratory will be dependent on factors such as economy and convenience. The CLOtest is reliable, standardized, and has a long shelf-life if refrigerated, but the Christensen's urea broth can be made cheaply by most laboratories. If the urea broth is used, the volume should be kept low, no greater than 0.5 ml [61], to achieve a high inoculum : reagent ratio. The test should be read at 1 hour to avoid false-positive reactions, which have been reported when reading times of up to 24 hours have been used [60, 61, 70, 71]. Incorporating selective antibiotics such as cefsulodin, trimethoprim, vancomycin, and amphotericin B (Table 7.1) in the urea broth may reduce the risk of false-positive reactions from other urease-producing organisms, but does not seem to be necessary if the reading time is kept at 1 hour [61]. Regardless of which test is used, it is recommended to keep it above room temperature, because of the enzyme's higher activity at increased temperatures. Both 37 °C [61, 64, 65] and 50 °C [63] have been used. The optimal temperature may however be 45 °C, which has been shown to be the temperature of maximum activity for the urease by spectrophotometric assay [54].

Other diagnostic tests for *H. pylori*

Other ways of diagnosing *H. pylori* include the use of serology and the urea breath test, which are described separately. Monoclonal antibodies have been raised against *H. pylori* and can be used for highly specific indirect immunofluorescence diagnosis [71]. Immunocytochemical techniques for diagnosis have been described [71–74]. Histologic sections are incubated with anti-*H. pylori* rabbit antibodies, which can then be visualized with peroxidase-labeled anti-rabbit antibodies. The specificity and sensitivity of such tests rely on the individual specificity of the anti-*H. pylori* antibodies. The use of monoclonal antibodies with this technique [71, 74] therefore promises to be a useful diagnostic tool.

References

1 Talley, NJ, Cameron, AJ, Shorter, RG, Zinsmeister, AR, & Phillips, SF. *Campylobacter pylori* and Barrett's esophagus. *Mayo Clin. Proc.* 1988;**63**:1176–80.
2 Paull, G, & Yardley, JH. Gastric and esophageal *Campylobacter pylori* in patients with Barrett's esophagus. *Gastroenterology* 1988;**95**:216–8.
3 Talley, R, Weinstein, WM, Marin-Sorensen, M, Schneidman, D, Reedy, TJ, & van Deventer, G. *Campylobacter pylori* colonization of Barrett's esophagus. *Gastroenterology* 1988;**94**:A454.
4 De Cothi, GA, Newbold, KM, & O'Connor, HJ. *Campylobacter*-like organisms and heterotopic gastric mucosa in Meckel's diverticula. *J. Clin. Pathol.* 1989;**42**(2):132–4.
5 Dye, KR, Marshall, BJ, Frierson, HF, Pambianco, DJ, & McCallum, RW. *Campylobacter pylori* colonizing heterotopic gastric tissue in the rectum. *Am. J. Clin. Pathol.* 1990;**93**:144–7.
6 Krajden, S, Fuksa, M, Anderson, J, *et al.* Examination of human stomach biopsies, saliva, and dental plaque for *Campylobacter pylori*. *J. Clin. Microbiol.* 1989;**27**:1397–8.
7 Rosenthal, LE, Smoot, D, Mobley, HLT, & Guisbert, W. *Campylobacter pylori* gastritis not related to periodontal disease. *Am. J. Gastroenterol.* 1988;**83**:202.
8 Westblom, TU, Madan, E, Midkiff, BR, Adkins, VA, & Subik, MA. Failure of *Campylobacter pylori* to grow in commercial blood culture systems. *J. Clin. Microbiol.* 1988;**26**:1029–30.
9 Goodwin, CS, Blincow, ED, Warren, JR, Waters, TE, Sanderson, CR, & Easton, L. Evaluation of cultural techniques for isolating *Campylobacter pyloridis* from endoscopic biopsies of gastric

mucosa. *J. Clin. Pathol.* 1985;**38**:1127–31.

10 Westblom, TU, Midkiff, BR, Madan, E, & Subik, MA. Transportation of gastric biopsies in a biphasic *Campylobacter pylori* medium. *J. Clin. Gastroenterol.* 1989;**11**:483–4.

11 Langenberg, ML, Tytgat, GNJ, Schipper, MEI, Rietra, PJGM, & Zanen, HC. *Campylobacter*-like organisms in the stomach of patients and healthy individuals. *Lancet* 1984;**i**:1348.

12 Buck, GE, Gourley, WK, Lee, WK, Subramanyam, K, Latimer, JM, & DiNuzzo, AR. Relation of *Campylobacter pyloridis* to gastritis and peptic ulcer. *J. Infect. Dis.* 1986;**153**:664–9.

13 Pinkard, KJ, Harrison, B, Capstick, JA, Medley, G, & Lambert, JR. Detection of *Campylobacter pyloridis* in gastric mucosa by phase contrast microscopy. *J. Clin. Pathol.* 1986;**39**:112–13.

14 Rollason, TP, Stone, J, & Rhodes, JM. Spiral organisms in endoscopic biopsies of the human stomach. *J. Clin. Pathol.* 1984;**37**:23–6.

15 Kasper, G, & Dickgiesser, N. Isolation of *Campylobacter*-like bacteria from gastric epithelium. *Infection* 1984;**12**:179–80.

16 Price, AB, Levi, J, Dolby, JM, *et al.* *Campylobacter pyloridis* in peptic ulcer disease: microbiology, pathology, and scanning electron microscopy. *Gut* 1985;**26**:1183–8.

17 McNulty, CAM, & Dent, JC. Rapid identification of *Campylobacter pylori* (*C. pyloridis*) by preformed enzymes. *J. Clin. Microbiol.* 1987;**25**:1683–6.

18 Megraud, F, Bonnet, F, Garnier, M, & Lamouliatte, H. Characterization of "*Campylobacter pyloridis*" by culture, enzymatic profile, and protein content. *J. Clin. Microbiol.* 1985;**22**:1007–10.

19 Jones, DM, Lessells, AM, & Eldridge, J. *Campylobacter*-like organisms on the gastric mucosa: culture, histological, and serological studies. *J. Clin. Pathol.* 1984;**37**:1002–6.

20 Krajden, S, Bohnen, J, Anderson, J, *et al.* Comparison of selective and non-selective media for recovery of *Campylobacter pylori* from antral biopsies. *J. Clin. Microbiol.* 1987;**25**:1117–8.

21 Marshall, BJ, & Warren, JR. Unidentified curved bacilli in the stomach of patients with gastritis and peptic ulceration. *Lancet* 1984;**i**:1311–15.

22 McNulty, CAM, & Watson, DM. Spiral bacteria of the gastric antrum. *Lancet* 1984;**i**:1068–9.

23 Buck, GE, & Smith, JS. Medium supplementation for growth of *Campylobacter pyloridis*. *J. Clin. Microbiol.* 1987;**25**:597–9.

24 Hirschl, AM. Frequency of occurrence of *Campylobacter pylori* and analysis of the systemic and local immune response. *Zbl. Bakt. Hyg. A* 1987;**266**:526–42.

25 Queiroz, DMM, Mendes, EN, & Rocha, GA. Indicator medium for isolation of *Campylobacter pylori*. *J. Clin. Microbiol.* 1987;**25**:2378–9.

26 Glupczynski, Y, Labbe, M, & Thibaumont, F. Comparative evaluation of a new selective culture medium for isolation of *Campylobacter pylori* from gastric biopsy specimens (abstract 126). *Vth International Workshop on Campylobacter Infections*, Puerto Vallarta, Mexico, February 25–March 1, 1989.

27 Dent, JC, & McNulty, CAM. New selective medium for *Campylobacter pylori* (abstract 127). *Vth International Workshop on Campylobacter Infections*, Puerto Vallarta, Mexico, February 25–March 1, 1989.

28 Westblom, TU, Madan, E, & Midkiff, BR. Egg yolk emulsion agar, a new medium for the cultivation of *Helicobacter pylori*. *J. Clin. Microbiol.* 1991;**29**:819–21.

29 Morgan, DR, Freedman, R, Depew, CE, & Kraft, WG. Growth of *Campylobacter pylori* in liquid media. *J. Clin. Microbiol.* 1987;**25**:2123–5.

30 Armstrong, JA, Wee, SH, Goodwin, CS, & Wilson, DH. Response of *Campylobacter pyloridis* to antibiotics, bismuth and an acid-reducing agent *in vitro* — an ultrastructural study. *J. Med. Microbiol.* 1987;**24**:343–50.

31 Hudson, MJ, & Newell, DG. Continuous culture of *C. pylori* (abstract 128). *Vth International Workshop on Campylobacter Infections*, Puerto Vallarta, Mexico, February 25–March 1, 1989.

32 Hartmann, D, & von Graevenitz, A. A note on name, viability and urease tests of *Campylobacter pylori*. *Eur. J. Clin. Microbiol.* 1987;**6**:82–3.

33 Thomas, JM, Poynter, D, Gooding, C, *et al.* Gastric spiral bacteria. *Lancet* 1984;**ii**:100.

34 Owen, RJ, On, SLW, & Costas, M. Potential transport medium for *Campylobacter pylori*. *J. Clin. Pathol.* 1988;**41**:1337–8.

35 Westblom, TU, Barthel, JS, Havey, AD, Gonzalez, FJ, Tarka, EF, & Everett, ED. Long-term freeze storage of *Campylobacter pyloridis*. *J. Clin. Pathol.* 1987;**40**:353.

36 Owen, RJ, On, SLW, & Costas, M. The effect of cooling rate, freeze-drying suspending fluid and culture age on the preservation of *Campylobacter pylori*. *J. Appl. Bacteriol.* 1989;**66**:331–7.

37 Drumm, B, & Sherman, P. Long-term storage of *Campylobacter pylori*. *J. Clin. Microbiol.*. 1989;**27**:1655–6.

38 Warren, JR. Unidentified curved bacilli on gastric epithelium in active chronic gastritis. *Lancet* 1983;**ii**:1273.

39 Madan, E, Kemp, J, Westblom, TU, Subik, M, Sexton, S, & Cook, J. Evaluation of staining methodologies for identifying *Campylobacter pylori*. *Am J. Clin. Pathol.* 1988;**90**:450–53.

40 Gray, SF, Wyatt, JI, & Rathbone, BJ. Simplified techniques for identifying *Campylobacter pyloridis*. *J. Clin. Pathol.* 1986;**39**:1279.

41 Westblom, TU, Madan, E, Kemp, J, Subik, MA, &

Tseng, J. Improved visualisation of mucus penetration by *Campylobacter pylori* using a Brown–Hopps stain. *J. Clin. Pathol.* 1988;**41**:232.
42 Burnett, RA, Brown, IL, & Findlay, J. Cresyl fast violet staining method for *Campylobacter*-like organisms. *J. Clin. Pathol.* 1987;**40**:353.
43 Trowell, JE, Yoong, AKH, Saul, KJ, Gant, PW, & Bell, GD. Simple half-Gram stain for showing presence of *Campylobacter pyloridis* in sections. *J. Clin. Pathol.* 1987;**40**:702.
44 McMullen, L, Walker, MM, Bain, LA, Karim, QN, & Baron, JH. Histological identification of *Campylobacter* using Gimenez technique in gastric antral mucosa. *J. Clin. Pathol.* 1987;**40**: 464–5.
45 Rocha, GA, Queiroz, DMM, Mendes, EN, Lage, AP, & Barbosa, AJA. Simplified staining for showing spiral microorganisms on gastric tissue section (abstract 136a). *Vth International Workshop on Campylobacter Infections*, Puerto Vallarta, Mexico, February 25–March 1, 1989.
46 Walters, LL, Budin, RE, & Paull, G. Acridine-orange to identify *Campylobacter pyloridis* in formalin-fixed, paraffin-embedded gastric biopsies. *Lancet* 1986;**i**:42.
47 Chodos, JE, Dworkin, BM, Smith, F, van Horn, K, Weiss, L, & Rosenthal, WS. *Campylobacter pylori* and gastroduodenal disease: a prospective endoscopic study and comparison of diagnostic tests. *Am. J. Gastroenterol.* 1988;**83**:1226–30.
48 Montgomery, EA, Martin, DF, & Peura, DA. Rapid diagnosis of *Campylobacter pylori* by Gram's stain. *Am. J. Clin. Pathol.* 1988;**90**:606–9.
49 Parsonnet, J, Welch, K, Compton, C, *et al.* Simple microbiologic detection of *Campylobacter pylori*. *J. Clin. Microbiol.* 1988;**26**:948–9.
50 Owen, RJ, Martin, SR, & Borman, P. Rapid urea hydrolysis by gastric campylobacters. *Lancet* 1985;**i**:111.
51 McClung, CR, Partriquin, DG, & Davis, RE. *Campylobacter nitrofigilis* sp. nov., a nitrogen fixing bacterium associated with roots of *Spartina alterniflora* Loisel. *Int. J. Syst. Bacteriol.* 1983;**33**: 605–12.
52 Megraud, F, Chevrier, D, Desplaces, N, Sedallian, A, & Guesdon, JL. Urease-positive thermophilic *Campylobacter* (*Campylobacter laridis* variant) isolated from an appendix and from human feces. *J. Clin. Microbiol.* 1988;**26**:1050–51.
53 Bolton, FJ, Holt, AV, & Hutchinson, DN. Urease-positive thermophilic campylobacters. *Lancet* 1985;**i**:1217–18.
54 Mobley, HLT, Cortesia, MJ, Rosenthal, LE, & Jones, BD. Characterization of urease from *Campylobacter pylori*. *J. Clin. Microbiol.* 1988; **26**:831–6.
55 Barrett, LJ, Marshall, BJ, Prakash, C, & Guerrant, RL. Protection of *Campylobacter pylori* but not *Campylobacter jejuni* against acid susceptibility by urea (abstract 1171). *27th Interscience Conference on Antimicrobial Agents and Chemotherapy*, New York, 4–7 October, 1987.
56 McNulty, CAM, & Wise, R. Rapid diagnosis of *Campylobacter*-associated gastritis. *Lancet* 1985; **i**:1443–4.
57 McNulty, CAM, & Wise, R. Rapid diagnosis of *Campylobacter pyloridis* gastritis. *Lancet* 1986;**i**: 387.
58 Hazell, SL, Borody, TJ, & Lee, A. *Campylobacter pyloridis* gastritis I: detection of urease as a marker of bacterial colonization and gastritis. *Am. J. Gastroenterol.* 1987;**82**:292–6.
59 Börsch, G, & Opferkuch, W. Schnelltest für *Campylobacter pylori*. *Dtsch. Med. Wochenschr.* 1987;**112**:780.
60 Das, SS, Bain, LA, Karim, QN, Coelho, LG, & Baron, JH. Rapid diagnosis of *Campylobacter pyloridis* infection. *J. Clin. Pathol.* 1987;**40**: 701–2.
61 Westblom, TU, Madan, E, Kemp, J, & Subik, MA. Evaluation of a rapid urease test to detect *Campylobacter pylori* infection. *J. Clin. Microbiol.* 1988;**26**:1393–4.
62 Warrelmann, DM, Hahn, H, Menge, H, & Schmidt, H. *Campylobacter pylori*: Nachweisverfahren. *Dtsch. Med. Wochenschr.* 1987;**112**: 821–2.
63 Vaira, D, Holton, J, Cairns, S, *et al.* Urease tests for *Campylobacter pylori*: care in interpretation. *J. Clin. Pathol.* 1988;**41**:812–13.
64 Czinn, SJ, & Carr, H. Rapid diagnosis of *Campylobacter pyloridis*-associated gastritis. *J. Pediatr.* 1987;**110**:569–70.
65 Riard, P, Hostein, J, Croize, J, *et al.* Le *Campylobacter pylori*: valeur diagnostique de l'urease test pratique en salle d'endoscopie. *Gastroenterol. Clin. Biol.* 1989;**13**:8–13.
66 Marshall, BJ, Warren, JR, Francis, GJ, Langton, SR, Goodwin, CS, & Blincow, ED. Rapid urease test in the management of *Campylobacter pyloridis*-associated gastritis. *Am. J. Gastroenterol.* 1987:**82**:200–10.
67 Borromeo, M, Lambert, JR, & Pinkard, KJ. Evaluation of "CLO-test" to detect *Campylobacter pyloridis* in gastric mucosa. *J. Clin. Pathol.* 1987; **40**:462–8.
68 Szeto, ML, Pounder, RE, Hamilton-Dutoit, SJ, & Dhillon, AP. Rapid urease test provides specific identification of *Campylobacter pylori* in antral mucosal biopsies. *Postgrad. Med. J.* 1988;**64**: 935–6.
69 Dye, KR, Marshall, BJ, Frierson, HF, Barrett, LJ, Guerrant, RL, & McCallum, RW. Is CLOtest alone adequate to diagnose *Campylobacter pylori*? *Am. J. Gastroenterol.* 1988;**83**:1032.
70 Bayerdörffer, E, Sommer, A, Ottenjann, R, & Kasper, G. CLO-tests zum Nachweis von *Campylobacter pylori*. *Dtsch. Med. Wochenschr.*

1987;**112**:902–3.

71 Engstrand, L, Påhlson, C, Schwan, A, & Gustavsson, S. Monoclonal antibodies for detection of *Campylobacter pylori* in biopsy smears and frozen sections. *Scand. J. Gastroenterol.* 1988;**23**(suppl 142):50–52.

72 Andersen, LP, Holck, S, & Povlsen, CO. *Campylobacter pylori* detected by indirect immunohistochemical technique. *APMIS* 1988; **96**:559–64.

73 Barbosa, AJA, Queiroz, DMM, Mendes, EN, Rocha, GA, Lima, GF, & Oliveira, CA. Immunocytochemical identification of *Campylobacter pylori* in gastritis and correlation with culture. *Arch. Pathol. Lab. Med.* 1988;**112**:523–5.

74 Negrini, R, Lisato, L, Cavazzini, L, *et al.* Monoclonal antibodies for specific immunoperoxidase detection of *Campylobacter pylori. Gastroenterology* 1989;**96**:414–20.

8: Immunology of Helicobacter pylori

M. KIST

Introduction

Colonization of mucosal surfaces by various microorganisms is a widespread phenomenon in biology, and predominantly functions as a biological barrier. Generally the immune response to this endogenous flora is low, and largely restricted to local phenomena. Colonizing microorganisms, which elicit a marked local and systemic immune response, are more readily assumed to be pathogenic in nature. The presence of *Helicobacter pylori* on human gastric mucosal surfaces, especially of the antral region, is usually accompanied by signs of local inflammation and a measurable systemic and local immune response. As Langenberg *et al.* [1] could demonstrate, *H. pylori* infections seem to be long-lasting and the level of systemic immune response remains constant during the presence of the causative agent.

This chapter describes the known facts about the *H. pylori*-specific immune response and furthermore deals with serologic methods, which allow the determination of peripheral antibodies, predominantly for diagnostic purposes.

Suitable serologic test systems could be helpful in replacing endoscopic procedures in special patient groups, allow monitoring of therapeutic intervention and, last but not least, could be a prerequisite for population-based epidemiologic studies or, as Marshall *et al.* have stated, [2]: "Serological testing may also help answer the question, 'How do you acquire pyloric campylobacters and from whom?'".

Systemic and local immune response

Systemic immune response

Colonization of the gastric mucosa by *H. pylori* is characterized by a significant mucosal accumulation of inflammatory cells, especially polymorphonuclear granulocytes (PMN), plasma cells and lymphocytes, the latter obviously predominantly T cells [3]. Furthermore, an increase of prominent lymphoid follicles was observed [4]. Such findings all indicate a more or less intensive immunologic host response to the infective agent, characterized by the occurrence of local and circulating antibodies.

Applying predominantly the enzyme-linked immunosorbent assay (ELISA) and the Western immunoblot techniques, most authors found immunoglobulin G (IgG) antibodies in more than 95% of patients with *H. pylori* detectable by histology or culture methods [5–9]. Using a urease preparation as ELISA antigen, Dent *et al.* [10] found IgG in all infected patients investigated. Further reported frequencies of an IgG response were 66–80% [11], 71.4% [12], 74–80% [13], or 90–93%, depending on the patient population investigated [14]. Other authors described significantly elevated IgG titers in infected patients when compared with controls [15, 16]. Steer *et al.* [17] investigated the IgG-specific immune response and found a marked elevation, predominantly of IgG1 and IgG4 and less frequently of IgG2, subclass antibodies. A finding of interest was, furthermore, a rather high IgG response in patients with peptic ulcers, possibly indicating a better penetration of antigens through mucosal lesions.

Very little is known about the occurrence of antibodies of various immunoglobulin classes in early stages of infection. Morris & Nicholson [18], who monitored the *H. pylori*-specific immune response after self-inoculation from day 22 to day 33, exclusively detected IgG-specific, but not IgA or IgM, antibodies.

Similar results were reported by Goodwin *et al.* [13] in 160 patients who underwent gastroscopy. Despite a marked IgG response, he was not able to detect IgA- or IgM-specific antibodies when applying an ELISA method. In contrast to such findings, many other authors underlined a particular role of circulating IgA antibodies in *H. pylori*-positive (HP+) patients. In most cases IgA antibodies were found to be significantly increased, but this was not a constant finding in patients with positive IgG responses [14, 15, 17, 19–23]. Von Wulffen & Grote [24] were not able to define a clear-cut conformity between the IgG and IgA response. On the other hand, workers such as Kosunen *et al.* [25] reported IgA antibodies as a constant finding, when the IgG response was high.

Furthermore, the presence of both IgG and IgA antibodies might indicate a more acute infection, compared with cases presenting with an isolated IgG or IgA immune response [14, 19, 23, 26, 27]. Hirschl [15] found IgA-specific antibody titers virtually non-absorbable by *C. jejuni*, possibly indicating a high degree of specificity of such an immune response.

In contrast to the obvious importance of an IgA immune response, IgM antibodies are found in less than 10% of *H. pylori*-infected patients [28], without any correlation with particular conditions. Most authors found the IgM response to be neither specific nor sensitive in serologic diagnosis of *H. pylori* infection [14, 15, 22, 24, 27].

Local immune response

Humoral immune response

Rathbone and coworkers investigated gastric juices of 22 fasting *H. pylori*-infected patients with an ELISA technique [4, 29, 30]. As a rule they found a significantly elevated IgA response and, to a lesser extent, IgG antibodies, probably due to their lack of protease resistance. IgM antibodies were seen as an exception. These results were confirmed by *in vitro* experiments, where biopsy specimens of patients with HP+ active chronic gastritis, or with normal mucosa, respectively, were monitored for antibody production over several days. Titers of *H. pylori*-specific IgA and IgG were significantly elevated in the HP+ group. IgM was only detected in one patient. The presence of both IgG and IgA antibodies correlated well with the initial density of plasma cells in the gastric mucosa [4].

In parallel to these findings, most microorganisms lining the mucosa surface of infected patients showed an immunoglobulin coating when stained with immunoperoxidase antiglobulin. IgA-coated bacteria were detectable in 100% of patients with active chronic gastritis, and in 60% of cases with inactive gastritis; IgG were found in 62% and 16% respectively. Interestingly enough, bacteria located at the base of gastric pits were only rarely antibody-coated [4]. The reason for this finding is still unclear.

Cellular immune response

The presence of a local humoral immune response correlates well with cellular findings, such as accumulation of submucosal lymphoid follicles consisting of plasma cells and lymphocytes [4]. The lymphocytes can be characterized predominantly as T cells, which are positive for CD3 and CD4 receptors [3], or as helper cells bearing predominantly CD7 receptors [31, 32]. An increase of transplantation antigens on the surface of epithelial cells, predominantly of the HLA-DR class, was also confirmed [3], possibly indicating a certain autoimmune activity. Interestingly enough, in cases of lymphoid gastritis possibly representing a stage of autoimmunity, *H. pylori* are only rarely detected [33].

Protein pattern of *H. pylori*

Methods

Sodium dodecylsulfate–polyacrylamide gel electrophoresis (SDS–PAGE), after the method

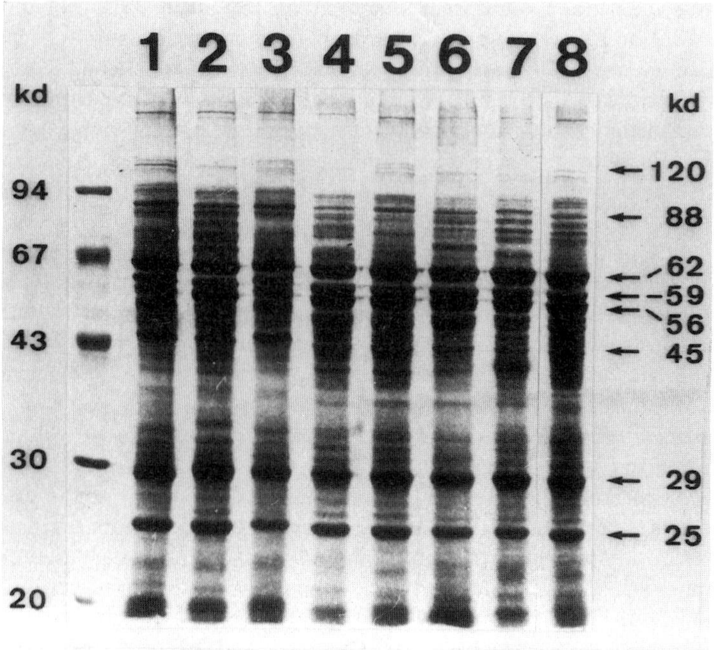

Fig. 8.1 Protein profiles of eight *H. pylori* strains, isolated from different patients and analyzed by SDS–PAGE. ← indicates major protein bands.

of Laemmli [34], is currently the most widely established method to identify the protein patterns of microorganisms. Briefly, *H. pylori* is grown on solid blood-containing media without antibiotics, and harvested in saline after 2–4 days. Alternatively, culture in liquid media for 1–2 days is possible.

The microorganisms are pelleted by centrifugation and the pellet washed in phosphate-buffered saline (PBS). Finally, the sample (2–10 mg ml^{-1} protein) is boiled at 100 °C for 5 minutes with a tris-hydrochloride buffer containing 2-β-mercaptoethanol, sodium dodecylsulfate (SDS), glycerol and bromophenol blue. Then the proteins are separated on a SDS–PAGE system consisting of 3–4.5% stacking gel, and a running gel in concentrations between 7% and 14%. Several authors prefer gradient gels, i.e. with concentrations increasing from 6% to 18% [13]. High concentration gels allow better discrimination of low molecular weight bands, whereas low concentration gels are more suitable for separation of high molecular weight proteins.

The unidimensional SDS–PAGE method can be preceded by an isoelectric focusing step to get a two-dimensional separation of proteins, which allows additional differentiation of proteins of identical molecular weights [35].

Proteins

Pearson *et al.* [36] were the first to investigate the protein profiles of 15 *H. pylori* strains. They found similar patterns in all strains, predominately proteins of 62, 53, 50, 39, 25, 21 and 14 kDa. For technical reasons, proteins of larger molecular weights were not detected.

Later investigations applying SDS–PAGE systems with various gel concentrations or gradients showed three main groups of proteins (Fig. 8.1) in whole cell lysates:

1 High molecular weight proteins between about 200 and 80 kDa.

2 Medium weight proteins between about 66 and 44 kDa.

3 Proteins of lower molecular weights between 39 and 14 kDa [15, 22, 37–42].

With the exception of the high molecular weight range, which was probably missed due to technical reasons, Dunn *et al.* [35] could also confirm such findings in a two-dimensional gel electrophoresis technique.

Recently, Evans *et al.* [43] detected very high

molecular weight proteins (700–400 kDa) when whole cell lysates were extracted with 1.0% *N*-octylglucoside.

In general, with increasing molecular weight, the degree of antigenic specificity seems to increase, and the occurrence of interspecies cross-reactions to decrease [37].

In the high molecular weight group, protein banding around 120 kDa (range 110–128 kDa) is well established [7, 15, 22, 24, 37, 38, 44]. Apel *et al.* [22] were the first to analyze a 120 kDa protein, and found it to be species-specific and surface located (see below). This protein is probably identical with the 110 kDa protein described by von Wulffen *et al.* [44] and Kist *et al.* [45].

A protein triplet between 88 and 82 kDa also seems to be a constant finding [26].

The medium weight group of proteins is characterized by bands around 66, 63, 61 and 60 kDa, correlated with "flagella sheet" structures [35, 39, 46], and by proteins in the 59–50 kDa region, of which 56 kDa [39], 54 kDa [35, 37, 39, 46] and a 51 kDa protein [47] have been described as *H. pylori* flagellin proteins (see below).

Antigens of *H. pylori*

Methods of detection

To detect constituents of *H. pylori* which are antigenic in humans or animals, two main procedures are in use: (1) the Western immunoblot method (see below); and (2) isolation of bacterial constituents followed by serologic tests such as the ELISA or comparable techniques [37, 38]. Both sera of infected humans [7, 22, 26, 28, 35, 48] and sera of immunized animals [35, 46, 49, 50] can be used for antigen detection.

Most investigations were done with the Western immunoblot method [7, 22, 26, 28, 46, 48, 49, 50]. In brief, after an initial SDS–PAGE step, the separated proteins are transferred from the slab gel to nitrocellulose membranes by electrotransfer. Free protein binding sites have to be blocked, e.g. with skimmed milk or gelatine, to avoid subsequent non-specific binding of antibodies. After incubation of the nitrocellulose with diluted serum which contains antibody, excess immunoglobulin is washed out and individual protein bands, to which antibodies have bound, are visualized by means of immunoenzymatic methods, applying alkaline phosphatase or horse radish peroxidase as labels. To ascertain the molecular weights of the separated protein antigens, the bands are compared with reference proteins of known molecular weight. Cross-reacting antigens are detected by immunoblotting with antisera against other, related bacterial species.

Proteins

Specific protein antigens

High molecular weight proteins

High molecular weight (>80 kDa) *H. pylori* proteins with antigenic activity have not been consistently reported in the literature. This may be mainly due to technical reasons connected with the preparation of the SDS–PAGE gels, where larger molecules are difficult to separate in gels of more than 10% concentration. In a few publications, high molecular weight proteins are faintly visible in the protein patterns demonstrated, but are not mentioned by the authors [13, 15]. On the other hand, as shown by Hirschl *et al.* [37], antigens of higher molecular weights are generally of more use for serologic tests. These special features may be due to good immunogenicity [22] and/or the presence of a relatively large number of epitopes, which are able to bind antibodies.

Recently, Evans *et al.* [43] described a 400–700 kDa protein, without urease activity, which seems to be a good candidate antigen for a sensitive and specific ELISA. The high molecular weight proteins were extracted from a washed cell pellet using 1% *N*-octylglucoside over 20 minutes at room temperature. After a centrifugation step, the supernatant was dialyzed and cleared by a second centrifugation step. When analyzing isolated antigens in an ELISA with a set of positive and negative sera, Hirschl *et al.* [37] observed a 128.8 kDa protein and five protein bands ranging from 79–106 kDa, both exhibiting a rather good discrimination between positive and negative sera.

Apel and coworkers [22, 45] were the first to investigate an *H. pylori* protein of 120 kDa molecular weight, which might be identical to a 110 kDa protein reported earlier by von Wulffen *et al.* [44] and Kist *et al.* [45]. To visualize the 120 kDa protein, samples of 20 μg of the heated cell suspension were separated by SDS–PAGE using a 5% stacking gel and a 12% running gel. The separated proteins were blotted on nitrocellulose membranes and incubated with human sera (1:100), after blocking of free non-specific binding sites with skimmed milk–PBS. Fixed antibodies were detected with rabbit anti-human-IgG, -IgA, or -IgM respectively, and visualized with a rabbit horse radish peroxidase–antiperoxidase complex [22]. Besides the 120 kDa protein, protein bands of 75, 62, 59, and 56 kDa were most frequently seen. The 120 kDa protein was not a constant finding, either in the strains tested or from the antibody response of the patients. On the other hand, it exhibits good antigenicity and specificity, as could be demonstrated by incubation with sera of patients infected with a range of other related bacteria.

Absorption experiments of anti-120 kDa-positive sera with living 120 kDa-positive *H. pylori* strains, and furthermore mild trypsinization of such *H. pylori* cells, revealed the 120 kDa protein to be surface-exposed [22].

Under slightly modified conditions, Reiff *et al.* [26] were also able to demonstrate a protein triplet of 88, 86, and 82 kDa, which were nearly always positive in patients with prominent anti-*H. pylori* immune responses. Von Wulffen *et al.* [7] described an 89 kDa protein which was highly reactive, especially with patient IgA antibodies. A 110 kDa protein was also reported [7, 23, 44], most probably identical with the 120 kDa antigen, and besides that a 94 kDa protein with antigenic activity [23, 44]. Hirschl *et al.* [37] eluted a total of five bands between 106 and 79 kDa exhibiting good discrimination capacity between HP+ and HP− patients' sera.

Low molecular weight proteins (≤66 kDa)

The proteins of the molecular weight range between 66 and 14 kDa should be differentiated with respect to their species-specificity. Proteins predominantly exhibiting cross-reactions with antisera to more or less related microorganisms are described below.

Dunn *et al.* [35] analyzed the protein pattern of three *H. pylori* strains with a two-dimensional gel electrophoresis technique (TDGE), and detected proteins with antigenic activity by immunoblotting experiments, applying rabbit and human antisera respectively. They demonstrated two prominent proteins of molecular weight 66 kDa (protein 2) and 63 kDa (protein 3), both also present in partially purified preparations of urease and flagella respectively. Both proteins additionally were labeled by ^{125}I surface labeling. While the 66 kDa protein exhibited excellent species-specificity, the 63 kDa protein was detected by rabbit antisera to *C. jejuni*, *C. coli* and *C. fetus fetus*. The latter was also seen by von Wulffen *et al.* [23] reacting with sera of infected patients. Dunn *et al.* [35] speculated that their 63 kDa protein probably was identical to a 61 kDa protein described by Newell [46, 48], who found it reacting strongly, but not consistently, with patients' sera. This latter protein was present in partially purified flagella [48], and recently was also described in urease preparations. The same protein was immunoprecipitable from ^{125}I surface-labeled bacteria in six out of 10 cases.

Further proteins were of 56 kDa and 45 kDa, probably identical with an *H. pylori* flagellin, the latter exhibiting strong cross-reactions with sera of *C. jejuni*-infected patients (see below); also a 48 kDa protein, not consistently labeled by *H. pylori*-seropositive sera; and finally a 31 kDa protein which was not cross-reactive with rabbit antisera to *C. jejuni* [46, 48]. The latter protein may be identical with a 30 kDa protein described by Hirschl [15], and by von Wulffen *et al.* [44], and probably also with a 29 kDa protein [37] and 28 kDa protein [23], both exhibiting remarkable antigenic activity in humans.

In the low molecular weight region a 22 kDa protein seems to be of further interest. It was strongly labeled by seven of eight sera of patients with gastritis [44]. This observation is in line with the finding of Dunn *et al.* [35], of a group of proteins below 29 kDa, which were strongly labeled by rabbit antisera.

Proteins with urease activity

Urease activity is a characteristic feature of *H. pylori*, different in nature from other microbial ureases. *H. pylori* urease was characterized by Mobley *et al.* [51] as a protein of 625±15 kDa molecular weight, with an isoelectric point of 5.9 and a pH optimum of 8.2. Evans *et al.* [52], applying *N*-octylglycoside extraction, were able to isolate in total a protein of about 600 kDa which exhibited strong urease activity.

Dunn *et al.* [35] analyzed a partially purified urease preparation of three strains of *H. pylori* in a TDGE technique. The urease-enriched proteins were prepared after disruption of a cell suspension in a French press, by chromatography of the concentrated supernatant on a 4000 SW spherogel LTSK of the centrifuged sample (10 000 *g* for 25 minutes). Dunn *et al.* identified two proteins of 66 and 63 kDa molecular weight respectively, both exhibiting marked urease activity. Both proteins were also associated with outer membrane material and with a flagella preparation. This 63 kDa protein may be identical to a 61 kDa protein of similar characteristics described by Newell [46, 48].

Clayton *et al.* [53], who were able to clone two *H. pylori* polypeptides with urease activity in an *Escherichia coli* vector, determined their molecular weights at 66 and 31 kDa respectively. Dunn *et al.* [35] missed a corresponding 31 kDa protein in their TDGE, but observed it in their SDS–PAGE preparations.

Proteins with adhesin activity

Evans *et al.* [54] first observed a surface-associated fibrillar hemagglutinin which binds to a specific isomer of neuramine lactose, i.e. *N*-acetylneuraminyl-(2-3)-β-D-galactopyranosyl-(1-4)-glucopyranose. Its molecular weight was roughly determined to lie between 150 and 66 kDa by elution from an agarose A 1.5 m column. In a follow-up investigation, Evans *et al.* [52] could demonstrate antibodies against this adhesin in about 75% of infected patients.

Flagellar proteins

Proteins associated with *H. pylori* flagella preparations are generally localized between 73 and 51 kDa molecular weight. Newell [46] isolated flagella of *H. pylori* by differential centrifugation and observed an SDS–PAGE pattern of three main proteins banding at 73, 61, and 54 kDa, and an additional "distorted" band of proteins between 50 and 40 kDa. These 73 and 61 kDa proteins may possibly be identical with the two proteins described above, which were observed by Dunn *et al.* [35], migrating as 66 and 63 kDa in a TDGE of a partially purified flagella preparation. Furthermore, a 29 kDa protein was seen in those preparations. Interestingly, all three showed no cross-reaction with rabbit antisera against *C. jejuni* flagella preparations.

On the other hand, Lee *et al.* [40] observed a strong cross-reactivity of rabbit sera against *C. jejuni* flagellin with two *H. pylori* polypeptide bands at 58 and 59 kDa. They speculated that those antibodies should cross react with *H. pylori* flagellin, identical with strongly conserved regions common in several spiral bacteria species. In contrast to that finding, antibodies against a 63 kDa molecular weight flagellin of *C. jejuni* did not exhibit any cross-reactivity. Such differing observations concerning cross-reactivity between flagellins of different *Campylobacter* spp. can possibly be explained by partial homologies between such proteins. So Newell [42] found only one monoclonal antibody in a panel of nine, generated against *C. jejuni* flagellin, which reacted with flagellar proteins of all *Campylobacter* spp. tested, including two *H. pylori* strains.

In contrast to other authors, Geis *et al.* [47], who isolated *H. pylori* flagellin by sucrose density gradient centrifugation followed by sepharose CL-4B gel chromatography, determined its molecular weight as 51 kDa. The observed differences in the molecular weights of flagellins described by different groups are not yet clarified, but may be partly due to different preparation procedures.

Outer membrane proteins

In contrast to *C. jejuni*, *C. coli*, and *C. fetus fetus* [55], characteristic major outer proteins are obviously lacking in *H. pylori* [35, 46]. Nevertheless, some proteins seem to occur more or less regularly in *N*-laurolyl sarconisate cell extracts, such as a 61, 54, and 31 kDa triplet [46], a protein doublet of 57 and 52 kDa, sometimes accompanied by a 44 kDa protein [49], and two common major antigens of 66 and 63 kDa, together with "surface-exposed" proteins, detected by ^{125}I surface labeling, of 44, 24, and 16 kDa [35], and a low molecular weight surface protein of 20 kDa, detected regularly by Engstrand with a monoclonal antibody [3].

Apel *et al.* [22] characterized their 120 kDa protein as surface-exposed, but not as a quantitatively-dominant protein.

Non-specific and cross-reacting proteins

The diagnostic quality of serologic tests is characterized by their sensitivity and specificity. Microbial antigens used in such tests, which cross-react with other species, markedly reduce the specificity of serologic test procedures. Therefore, it is obviously an advantage to purify such antigen preparations to a certain degree by elimination of cross-reacting protein fractions. In the case of *H. pylori*, such proteins are predominantly localized in the 65–55 kDa region. Newell [46, 48] described two *H. pylori* proteins of 56 and 54 kDa, which were detected by antisera to *C. jejuni* flagellin and by sera of patients with *C. jejuni* infections. On the other hand, antisera against *H. pylori* exhibited marked cross-reaction with an 18 and 62 kDa protein of *C. jejuni*, the latter probably representing *C. jejuni* flagellar protein.

Both proteins are possibly identical with two *H. pylori* antigens of 59 and 57 kDa, observed by Lee *et al.* [40], which strongly cross-reacted with the flagellin of different *Campylobacter* spp., and with the 59 kDa protein described by Dunn *et al.* [35], also cross-reacting with anti-*C. jejuni* flagellin antibodies.

Furthermore Dunn *et al.* [35] and Perez-Perez & Blaser [49] reported proteins of 63 or 62 kDa respectively, which both cross-reacted strongly with antisera to *C. jejuni*, *C. coli* and *C. fetus fetus*. Kist *et al.* [45] also tested, by immunoblotting, sera of patients with *C. jejuni*, *C. coli*, and *C. fetus fetus* infection, and found marked seroreactivity with *H. pylori* protein bands of 75, 62, 59, and 56 kDa. A synopsis of *H. pylori* proteins identified by different authors as species-specific or cross-reacting, respectively is given in Fig. 8.2.

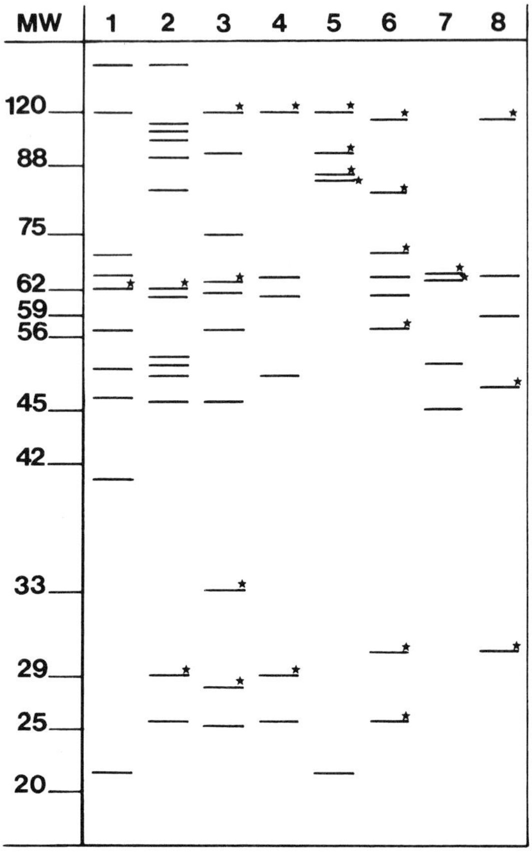

Fig. 8.2 Immunoblot pattern of *H. pylori* protein antigens detected with human and animal antisera. Comparison of different studies. *Bands which were reported probably species-specific. References: [15], [22], [26], [35], [37], [38], [39], [44].

Lipopolysaccharides

Information about the outer membrane polysaccharides of *H. pylori* is limited. Perez-Perez & Blaser [49] extracted lipopolysaccharides (LPS) of *H. pylori* by proteinase K treatment to eliminate contaminating proteins, followed by a heating step. They found remarkable variability among the lipopolysaccharide profile of the *H. pylori* strains tested, ranging from rough to smooth and with multiple repeating side chains. By immunoblot analysis they observed cross-reactivity between LPS core regions but not between side chains. The authors suggested a minor degree of conservation of LPS structures, but the influence of different growth conditions should also be taken into account.

Detection of the human immune response to *H. pylori*

Antigen preparations

Whole cell preparations

In order to establish serologic tests for the detection of the human immune response to *H. pylori*, the correct choice of microbial antigens is essential. A broad range of antigen preparations has been used, from whole cell suspensions to defined antigens like urease or special adhesins. Whole cell suspensions were, in most cases, harvested after growth on solid media, and used for direct coating of ELISA microtiter plates, either without further treatment [28, 56], or after formalin fixation [1, 19]. Jones *et al.* [57] and Bolton *et al.* [27] applied whole cell preparations for microagglutination procedures. Because of the disadvantage of a high degree of serologic cross-reactions, whole cell antigens have not enjoyed common use [5]. Most investigators, therefore, tried to improve the sensitivity and specificity of their serologic tests by the use of cell sonicates.

Marshall *et al.* were the first to use a whole cell sonicate of *H. pylori* for a passive hemagglutination test [2]. Sonicates without further treatment, mostly of a strain pool, were also used to establish complement fixation tests [28, 57, 58], and more recently to coat ELISA microtiter plates as solid phase antigens [8, 12, 14, 15, 59]. Kaldor *et al.* [16], in order to coat ELISA plates, preheated their "dense milky" cell mixture, prepared from 12 *H. pylori* strains, before sonication. Schaub *et al.* [60] used only the pellet of a centrifuged sonicate as ELISA antigen, while other groups preferred the use of sonicate supernatants after various centrifugation steps to coat ELISA titer plates [9, 11, 27, 37], or to establish a complement fixation test [27].

Acid cell extracts

The preparation of an acid antigen extract of *C. jejuni*, for use in an ELISA for detection of human serum antibodies, was originally described by Blaser & Duncan [61]. When applying such an acid extract, they were able to improve markedly the sensitivity and specificity of the test characteristics. Based on such experience, acid extracts of *H. pylori* strains were used by several other authors with the aim of improving the specificity of serologic tests. An acid extract of 11 *H. pylori* strains was first introduced in the ELISA by Goodwin *et al.* [13]. Following the method of Newell *et al.* [39], the acid extraction method can be briefly described as follows. Intact bacteria (4 g wet weight 100 ml^{-1}) were incubated in 0.2 mol glycine HCl buffer, pH 2.2 (15 minutes, 20 °C). After a centrifugation step, the supernatant was neutralized with 1 mol sodium hydroxide, dialyzed against water and finally stored at −20 °C. The protein profiles of such acid extractable preparations differ to a variable extent from the whole cell protein patterns [48].

While Newell *et al.* [39] described a 110 kDa band in the SDS–PAGE pattern of acid extracts, and a 116 kDa band is visible in the illustrations of Goodwin *et al.*'s communication [13], von Wulffen *et al.* [24] (Fig. 8.3), and Hirschl *et al.* [37], reported instead a reduction of high molecular weight proteins in the acid extracted preparations. Bands of 84 kDa and 83 kDa were described by Goodwin *et al.* [13] and von Wulffen *et al.* [24], respectively; the latter was obviously predominantly detected by IgA class antibodies (Fig. 8.3). Further bands between 69 and 53 kDa — 69, 64, 63, 62, 61, 58, 57, 56, 54, and 53 kDa — were inconsistently observed by different groups [13, 24, 37, 39, 46, 48, 49]. The 63, 62, and 61 kDa proteins reported seem to be identical, as do the the 58, 57, and 56 kDa proteins, the latter exhibiting marked cross-reaction when immunoblotted with control sera [48]. A protein determined as 31, 30, or 29 kDa seems to be consistently found in acid extracts [24, 37, 39, 46, 48, 49].

Newell in particular reported improvement in antigen specificity by using acid extracts in the immunoblot technique [48], whereas other authors, such as Hirschl *et al.* [37] and von Wulffen *et al.* [24], could not confirm that observation. They observed predominantly a loss of the more species-specific high molecular weight antigens between 130 and 80 kDa, and furthermore a loss of sensitivity.

Czinn *et al.* [11] finally compared three antigen preparations for their suitability in an IgG ELISA with childrens' sera: namely a whole cell sonicate, an outer membrane preparation (OMP) and a lipopolysaccharide (LPS) extract. The outer membranes were isolated by treatment of cell suspensions with DNase and RNase, followed by sonication and centrifugation of the sonicate (150 000 *g* for 1 hour). Finally the pellet was extracted with sodium-*N*-laurolyl sarcosine and the outer membranes were recovered by ultracentrifugation. The main proteins found in the OMP preparation were localized at the 61, 54, 31, and 14 kDa regions. These findings were comparable to the previously reported protein triplet of OMP migrating at 61, 54, and 31 kDa, which was described by Newell [46].

Czinn *et al.* [11] found results with the whole cell sonicate and the OMP preparation to be comparable; nevertheless the sensitivity of the OMP preparation was slightly reduced. By contrast, the LPS preparation revealed itself to be a rather poor antigen and was not capable of differentiating between HP+ and HP− patient sera.

Defined antigens

Three kinds of more or less defined antigens have been reported, namely a urease preparation [10], a protein of adhesin character [52], and a high molecular weight cell-associated protein (HM-CAP) exhibiting urease activity [43, 52].

Dent *et al.* [10] reported 100% sensitivity and 79% specificity for his partially purified urease preparation, which appeared as "one major band" in the SDS–PAGE. Evans *et al.* [52] isolated two to three fractions of about 600 kDa molecular weight exhibiting urease activity, using 1% octoglucoside extraction of *H. pylori* cells. These urease-rich preparations were used in an HM-CAP ELISA test. They compared this method with another ELISA (anti-NLBH ELISA), where an *N*-acetylneuraminyllactose-binding hemagglutinin (NLBH) was used as a solid phase antigen. While only 75% of sera of patients with *H. pylori* infection were reactive in the anti-NLBH ELISA, the anti-urease ELISA, using HM-CAP as antigen, showed markedly better sensitivity (98.7%) and specificity (100%).

Serologic methods

Various serologic tests were employed to monitor human immune response to *H. pylori.* The huge diversity of methods applied, of antigen preparations used, of evaluation of the results, of definition of HP+ and HP− patients, and of control groups investigated, and last but not least the different procedures to define and control test specificity and sensitivity, make reviewing of this subject difficult.

The first attempt to measure human antibodies to *H. pylori* was undertaken by Marshall *et al.* [2], by use of a positive hemagglutination test with erythrocytes sensitized with a cell sonicate. This first attempt was hampered by a remarkable degree of background reactivity, concerning which Goodwin *et al.* [13] commented that "unsensitized erythrocytes hemagglutinated as well as sensitized erythrocytes."

Further studies were done, using microagglutination, by Jones *et al.* [57], and recently by Bolton *et al.* [27], who reported a sensitivity of 96% and a specificity of 78% when titers of ≥320 were taken as cut-off points (COP). The same group found 93% sensitivity and 68% specificity, using a complement fixation test (CFT) with an *H. pylori* "surface antigen." Other communications regarding CFT indicate a lower degree of specificity [28, 57, 58], and a higher degree of cross-reactions, especially with *C. jejuni* antibodies [57].

Two methods appear to be of greater interest regarding their use in *H. pylori* routine serology, namely the ELISA and the Western immunoblot. The advantages of the ELISA method are the possibility of generating quantitative results, their evaluation by relatively inexperienced personnel, automatization of the method, and use as a screening test employing a limited number of serum dilutions. Furthermore the ELISA allows an Ig class-specific evalu-

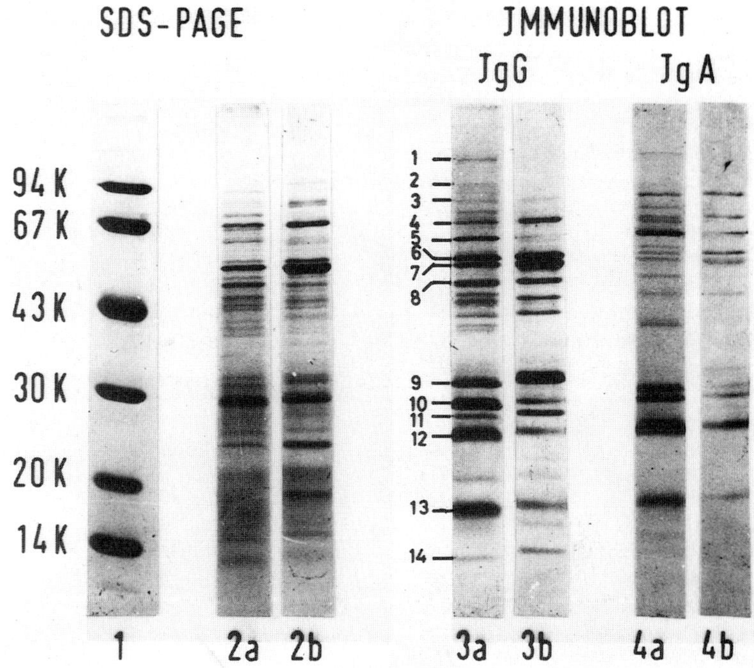

Fig. 8.3 SDS–PAGE and immunoblots of whole cell lysate (lanes a) and acid–glycine preparation (lanes b) of *H. pylori*, strain CLO 185. Lane 1, marker proteins; lane 2, Coomassie stains; lane 3, IgG immunoblot; lane 4, IgA immunoblot. Numbered *H. pylori* proteins (hp) have the following calculated molecular weights: hp1, 120 kDa; hp2, 94 kDa; hp3, 83 kDa; hp4, 69 kDa; hp5, 63 kDa; hp6, 58 kDa; hp7, 54 kDa; hp8, 49 kDa; hp9, 31 kDa; hp10, 29 kDa; hp11, 27 kDa; hp12, 25 kDa; hp13, 17 kDa; hp14, 13 kDa. (From von Wulffen & Grote [24].)

ation of the immune response. Problems to be solved include: how to define the cut-off point; how to select the most suitable antigen; how to verify the day-to-day test reliability; and how to reduce the relatively high cost of the equipment necessary.

In comparison to the ELISA, the Western immunoblot technique allows analysis of the immune response to a number of defined antigens, and also the differentiation between species-specific and cross-reacting proteins. Further, it allows monitoring of the development of antibody patterns with ongoing disease. Disadvantages of the method are the lack of quantitative results, the relative difficulty of interpretation of the blot pattern, which needs experienced personnel, and technical problems with regard to test automatization.

Enzyme-linked immunosorbent assay (ELISA)

The most commonly used systems to detect anti-*H. pylori* antibodies in patients' sera are based on enzyme-linked immunosorbent assay techniques (ELISA). The sensitivity and specificity of such test systems, and therefore their positive (PPV), or negative (NPV) predictive values, are strongly dependent upon the specific features of the antigen(s) bound to the solid phase. A large variety of antigen preparations are used in practice. Newell & Stacey [62] have defined the prerequisites to be fulfilled by suitable preparations, which should: (1) have a high proportion of microbial components of good antigenicity; (2) be common to all strains; (3) exhibit a low or better negative background of cross-reacting material; (4) be easy to isolate and to purify; and (5) bind effectively to the solid phase support.

The question as to whether one representative strain or a sample of strains should be used for antigen preparation was investigated by Bauernfeind *et al.* [63] with acid–glycine extracts of 13 strains, and also by Hirschl [15]. These authors did not find significant differences between the two approaches. Probably, various immune response patterns between different patients are more related to host factors than to marked strain-to-strain variability. Furthermore, the sensitivity and specificity of different ELISA test approaches seem to be largely dependent on the patient population investigated. So, von Wulffen & Grote [24] found decreasing sensitivity values, but increas-

Table 8.1 Mean values (%) of sensitivity and specificity of ELISAs with various antigen preparations

Antigen preparation	No. of studies	Sensitivity (range)	Specificity (range)	References
Whole cells	3	97 (96–97)	85 (74–91)	[1, 28, 56]
Whole cell sonicates	6	86 (66–100)	95 (88–100)	[8, 11, 12, 14, 19, 59]
Supernatants				
of whole cells	2	100 (100)	66 (44–79)	[9, 64]
of sonicated cells	1	76	98	[15]
of ultrasonicated cells	1	84	95	[37]
Acid–glycine extract	9	88 (70–100)	88 (63–100)	[13, 21, 25, 37, 39, 62, 64, 67, 70]
Urease	3	89 (66–100)	86 (73–100)	[10, 62, 64]
HM-CAP	1	99	100	[43]
NLBH	1	75	98	[52]
Protein 120 kDa + ultracentrifuged sonicates	1	97	100	[69]
Protein 120 kDa + acid–glycine extract	1	97	100	[69]

HM-CAP, high molecular weight cell-associated proteins.
NLBH, *N*-acetylneuraminyllactose-binding hemagglutinin.

ing specificity, in patients with a normal antrum, in comparison with cases with severe gastritis. A similar trend was seen by other authors [9, 13, 14].

In the beginning of serologic studies, mainly whole bacteria, without further modification as well as after formalin fixation or freeze-drying, were applied as ELISA antigens [1, 19, 28, 56]. The sensitivity of such tests was remarkably good (96–97%), but they suffered mainly from a lack of specificity (74–91%) (Table 8.1). Further problems were antigenic cross-reactivity with other *Campylobacter* spp., resulting in a relatively high background activity [19], or broad overlapping between HP– and HP+ test groups [56].

Instead of whole cell preparations, cell sonicates without further modification [8, 11, 12, 14, 30, 60], or after heating to 60 °C [16], were used by several authors. Overall, such preparations exhibited increased specificity but reduced sensitivity, when compared to whole cells (Table 8.1).

On the other hand, Mitchell *et al.* [8] reported a marked influence on test results due to the prevalence of anti-*C. jejuni* antibodies in the study population. After absorption of patients' sera with *C. jejuni* the proportion of *H. pylori*-seropositive samples was markedly reduced, especially in a population with high *C. jejuni* prevalence. This was particularly true for borderline titers, and was not seen to such an extent in high titer samples. This could be the reason that other authors did not observe such an effect after absorption of anti-*H. pylori*-positive sera with different bacteria species [14, 16, 60]. Steer *et al.* [17], who investigated serologic cross-reactions between sera seropositive for *C. jejuni* or *H. pylori*, described a marked cross-reactive activity of sera from *C. jejuni*-positive patients with *H. pylori* acid–glycine extracted antigens, but not vice versa.

Supernatants of centrifuged whole cell preparations [9, 27, 64], or of whole cell preparations boiled for 2 hours [65], exhibited good sensitivity (94%) but reduced specificity (73%), whereas supernatants of centrifuged or ultracentrifuged sonicates [15, 37] were characterized by a good specificity (97%), accompanied, however, by reduced sensitivity (80%).

The preparation of acid–glycine extract as solid phase antigen, using 0.2 M acetic acid, as described by Goodwin *et al.* [13], was reported to reduce marked serological cross-reactivity with *C. jejuni*-positive sera [17], and therefore seemed to be a promising approach to increase ELISA sensitivity and specificity. It was used by many workers [13, 17, 21, 24, 25, 38, 39, 64, 66, 67] with different modifications. Von Wulffen & Grote [24], and Hirschl *et al.* [37], who compared whole cell sonicates with acid–glycine extracts, could demonstrate a qualitatively similar protein pattern in both preparations, but quantitative differences, especially a relative loss of high molecular weight bands. This might be one reason for the overall reduction in sensitivity (88%) and specificity (88%) seen with such preparations (Table 8.1). Nevertheless, in the hands of some investigators the use of acid–glycine extracts yielded a remarkably good specificity of about 97% [13, 37, 62]. Alternative preparations such as OMP, which were proposed by Czinn *et al.* [11], have not enjoyed extended use.

Based on experiences with poorly-defined antigen preparations, the use of antigens with defined properties seemed to be promising. Examples of such an approach were the use of HM-CAP by Evans *et al.* [43], or of an *N*-acetylneuraminyllactose-binding hemagglutinin (NLBH) by the same group [54]. While for the latter antigen only 75% sensitivity but 98% specificity were found, the HM-CAP ELISA was described as exhibiting 100% specificity and 99% sensitivity. These results need confirmation by other groups.

Various attempts were made to use *H. pylori* urease preparations of varying purity as solid phase antigens [10, 52, 62, 64, 68]. Most authors reported antigens of 61, 56, and 31 kDa in their urease-positive fractions. The broad range of sensitivity (66–100%) and specificity (73–100%) values seen by the different authors can probably be attributed to the varying degrees of urease purity. As Newell & Stacey [62] could demonstrate, rather crude urease preparations were characterized by high sensitivity but poor specificity, while highly-purified urease exhibited good specificity but suffered from a markedly reduced sensitivity (66%).

The 120 kDa protein, as first described by Apel *et al.* [22], was tested by Hirschl *et al.* [69], and compared with other antigen preparations. Hirschl *et al.* reported a test sensitivity of 84% and a specificity of 98%. The reduced sensitivity was probably due to a small proportion of strains lacking the 120 kDa protein [22], therefore Hirschl *et al.* [69] proposed the use of the 120 kDa protein together with antigen mixtures such as acid–glycine extract or ultracentrifuged sonicate. For both mixed preparations the sensitivity (97%) and the specificity (100%) were remarkably good (Table 8.1).

In respect of test-to-test standardization, a broad variety of reference methods are still in use (Table 8.2). Most frequently one positive or negative control serum [1, 60, 67], or a panel of positive, negative or weakly positive control sera [8, 13, 24, 43, 56], serve as standards. Other authors prefer the end-point titration up to a lower optical density (OD) limit [9, 10, 11, 25, 27], or compare their test results with the mean OD "of control sera" [12, 14, 16, 30]. A reasonable approach to measuring the immune response, as demonstrated by Newell *et al.* [39, 62] and other authors [17, 66], seems to be to determine the total Ig mass bound specifically to the antigen, by comparing the test OD with

Table 8.2 Test-to-test standardization of ELISA results

Reference methods	References
One positive and/or negative control serum	[1, 60, 67]
Panel of positive and negative (and weakly positive) control sera	[8, 13, 24, 43, 56]
End-point titration up to a lower OD limit	[9, 10, 11, 27]
Mean OD of control sera	[12, 14, 16, 19]
Total immunoglobulin mass standardized with ^{125}I-labeled protein	[17, 39, 62,66]

OD, optical density.

a standard curve of serially diluted ^{125}I-labeled reference immunoglobulins. When the total Ig mass is determined, the cut-off point (COP) which discriminates between positive and negative sera can be clearly set. Newell *et al.* [39] and Steer *et al.* [17] propose a COP of 2.0 $\mu g\,ml^{-1}$ for their test systems, whereas Przyklenk *et al.* [66] used a much lower COP of 0.5 $\mu g\,ml^{-1}$.

Compared with the various methods of test-to-test standardization, there are rather more discrepancies to be found in the literature concerning the definition of further COPs in the different ELISA test systems (Table 8.3). Most authors arbitrarily define one OD value as the COP, mostly between 0.200 and 1.000 [8, 10, 15, 28, 43, 52, 59], or the OD of a reference serum at a constant dilution [25, 38], whereas others define different OD limits as COPs for the different Ig classes [14, 27].

Goodwin *et al.* [13] and von Wulffen & Grote [24], respectively proposed COPs defined as ELISA units (EU), which were defined according to the OD of reference sera at distinct dilutions. Other groups define the COP of their test systems as borderline titers, which must be reached or exceeded by positive sera [9, 11, 27, 60].

Other authors simply compared OD values [16, 19, 30, 65] or titer values [1, 9, 11, 15, 25, 27, 28, 37, 60] of different patient groups, applying various statistical tests to evaluate statistical differences. A good method seems to be that of Dwyer *et al.* [12], who used the 99% lower confidence interval of the mean OD of sera of culture-positive patients.

Overall, such a large variety of test parameters makes it difficult to draw definitive conclusions, when different test systems are compared in respect of their accuracy and practical value. Until highly specific and sensitive antigens are in common use, the question of whether absorption with cross-reacting strains is necessary or not will remain [8, 13, 15, 16, 17, 19, 27, 59].

Table 8.3 Methods of definition of the cut-off points (COPs) in ELISAs

Definition of the COP	References
One arbitrarily defined OD value	[8, 10, 15, 28, 43]
OD of a reference serum at a constant dilution	[25, 38]
Different OD limits as COPs for different Ig classes	[14, 64]
COP defined as EU	[7, 13]
Borderline titers which have to be reached or exceeded	[9, 11, 27, 60]
Only comparison of OD values and/or titer of different sera	[1, 9, 11, 15, 16, 19, 21, 27, 28, 37, 60, 65]

OD, optical density.
EU, ELISA units.

Western immunoblot

For the principal method of performing the Western immunoblot see p. 95.

ELISA or Western immunoblots applied to detect an anti-*H. pylori* immune response in patients with or without *H. pylori* infection reveal comparable results [70]. Overall, the immunoblot has not enjoyed such broad use for routine serology as ELISA. This is most probably due to technical problems in respect of standardization and automatization. Therefore in the majority of studies the immunoblot serves predominantly as a reference method, or as an approach to analyzing the antigen pattern of the ELISA antigen preparation used.

Most authors used a 10–12% running gel for the PAGE as the first step of the immunoblot procedure [7, 23, 26, 28, 71]. The screening dilutions of patients' sera vary from 1 : 20 [71] to 1 : 50 [26] for IgA detection, and 1 : 100 for IgG detection [7, 23, 26, 28]. Von Wulffen *et al.* [7] described the following bands as being relevant for IgG detection — 110, 94, 63, and 28 kDa — and the following as being characteristic for IgA — 100, 94, 89, and 63 kDa. The 110 kDa protein antigen mentioned by von Wulffen is most probably identical with the 120 kDa protein used as index marker by Reiff *et al.* [26], who furthermore identified an 88 kDa protein as being a specific antigen marker. Von Wulffen *et al.* [7] found antibodies to the 110 kDa protein in 81% of patients with severe gastritis, in contrast to only 11% of patients with normal antrum mucosa.

On the other hand, in earlier studies by Kaldor *et al.* [71], or Jones *et al.* [28], predominantly protein bands of lower molecular weight (28–70 kDa) were described as marker proteins. This was probably mostly due to technical reasons in preparing the gels, which did not demonstrate bands of higher molecular weight. As well as a simple visual evaluation of bands as being present or not, von Wulffen *et al.* [7] established a score, which was related to the presence of certain IgG or IgA banding, and provided good discrimination between patients with or without gastritis, and, further, between cases of different severity.

Seroepidemiology

Putative routes of transmission of *H. pylori* are the person-to-person route, either oral–oral or fecal–oral, transmission from animals to humans, and food- or water-borne spread of infection. One important approach for investigating such questions is the use of population-based prevalence studies, as well as case-control studies in putative risk groups and controls. In the case of *H. pylori* infection, invasive methods of detection such as gastroscopy and biopsies are not well suited for investigating large study groups, but non-invasive methods, such as serologic tests or the ^{14}C or ^{13}C breath test, are of important practical usefulness for such purposes. Therefore, both these test procedures are most commonly used for population-based epidemiologic investigations.

Until now, serologic studies have generally shown that the frequency of seropositive samples increases markedly with the age of the population samples tested [2, 14, 15, 21, 26, 28, 60, 71, 72]. Schaub *et al.* [60], in Switzerland, described a 17% prevalence of seropositive sera in a 21–30-year age group, increasing to about 50% in persons older than 60 years. Kosunen *et al.* [25] detected 20% positive with IgG in 16–25-year-old controls. Eldridge & Jones [72] found a very low prevalence of only 3.3% in school children aged up to 17–18 years. These findings are in line with data reported by Brassens-Rabbe *et al.* [73], who found a 3.5% seropositivity of French children aged 0–10 years, and in contrast to the results of Bolton *et al.* [27], who detected 15% positive sera in children younger than 5 years. Reiff *et al.* [26] reported 8.3% IgG-positive controls in a 0–16-year age group, the frequency increasing to 50% in older age groups. Reiff *et al.* [26], as well as Hirschl [15], both observed a much stronger age dependency for the IgG response compared with the IgA response.

All the studies reviewed above were carried out in developed countries. However, the overall prevalence of *H. pylori*, correlated with the time of the first infection, seems to differ in different geographical regions, e.g. Brassens-Rabbe *et al.* [73] found markedly higher prevalences in developing countries such as Vietnam, Algeria, and the Ivory Coast, when compared to France. While French children of the first decade were 3.5% seropositive, comparable age groups in Vietnam, Algeria and Ivory Coast showed seroprevalences of 13.1%, 45% and 55% respectively.

A similar increase of age-corrected prevalences was reported by Graham *et al.* [74] from United States blacks, Chinese, Indians, Mexicans, and Columbians (see Graham *et al.* [74] for further literature). Despite such impressive data, the increased prevalence of enteropathogenic *Campylobacter* spp. in those developing countries should be kept in mind, and the possibility of serologic cross-reactions between *H. pylori* antigen and anti-*Campylobacter* antibodies should be carefully controlled.

Besides such geographical, racial, and probably socioeconomic features influencing the overall prevalence of *H. pylori* infection in the population, other groups with increased risk of oral–oral or fecal–oral spread exist also in developed communities. This was shown by a number of interesting seroepidemiologic studies carried out in putative risk groups, such as endoscopists [26, 59], dental staff [26], general practitioners [59], family contacts of infected adults [26] and infected children [26, 32, 75, 76, 77], mentally retarded patients [78], chronic psychiatric inpatients [26], orphanage children [26], and patients with chronic polyarthritis [79] or chronic renal failure [23].

The most important risk factor for acquiring infection seems to be contact with infected patients, followed by performing of gastroscopies, and by residence for a long time in relatively closed communities, such as orphanages, or psychiatric clinics. On the other hand dentists, dealing with the normal population, or patients with renal failure or chronic polyarthritis, seem not to be at increased risk [26, 79].

To investigate the possibility of animal-borne infection of humans, Vaira *et al.* [80] serologically studied abattoir workers with and without contact with freshly cut meat. They observed a significant increase of seropositive reactions in abattoir workers with direct animal contacts, but the seroreaction pattern paralleled largely the antibody responses to *C. jejuni* and *C. coli*, so that serologic cross-reactivity between microorganisms should be kept in mind when considering such data.

Conclusions

H. pylori colonization of the gastric mucosa is accompanied by an inflammatory response, characterized by accumulation of plasma cells, polymorphonuclear granulocytes and T lymphocytes, predominantly of the helper cell type. Signs of a local immune response, with detection of immunoglobulins, predominantly IgA, in gastric secretions, and the occurrence of immunoglobulin-coated bacteria, are observed. The systemic humoral immune response is characterized by the occurrence of IgG as a rule, not always accompanied by an IgA response, and with a nearly total lack of specific IgM antibodies.

The protein patterns of *H. pylori*, when analyzed with the SDS–PAGE technique, do not differ markedly between strains of different origin. Proteins of higher (about 130–80 kDa), medium (about 70–50 kDa), and lower (<40 kDa) molecular weights are typically found. Besides these proteins, extraction procedures with *N*-octylglucoside yield high molecular weight cell-associated proteins of between 700 and 400 kDa. Urease activity is detectable predominantly in 63–61 kDa and 31 kDa fractions; flagellin proteins are found between 56 and 51 kDa.

The species-specific antigens of *H. pylori* are predominantly located in the protein spectrum of about 130–80 kDa, possibly due to the relatively large amount of epitopes present in these proteins, which could improve their overall antigenicity. Such antigens are found predominantly in the regions of 120, 88, 86 and 83 kDa molecular weight proteins, as well as around 63 and 31 kDa, where urease activity is concentrated, while flagellar proteins occur around 76–54 kDa. Most antigens which cross-react with other more or less related organisms are found between 65 and 55 kDa.

The analysis of the human immune responses to *H. pylori*, for predominantly diagnostic purposes, has been carried out with antigen preparations consisting of whole cells without further treatment, with various supernatant preparations, and with acid–glycine extracts which, in respect of their protein pattern, did not differ markedly from other preparations.

More or less defined antigens, such as urease preparations, proteins of adhesin character, and so-called HM-CAP, were also investigated and showed in this order increasing test specificity. ELISAs or the Western immunoblot are the serologic test systems generally in use. The sensitivity and specificity of most of the tests investigated vary between 70 and 100%. Increasing specificity in most cases is accompanied by a decrease of sensitivity, and vice versa. Mixtures of defined antigens of good specificity (e.g. 120 kDa, urease or others), with more general antigens such as acid–glycine extracts, seem to be the most promising approach. The seroepidemiology of the *H. pylori* infection is characterized by an increasing seroprevalence with increasing age of the population tested. Population groups with higher probability of person-to-person contacts are obviously at high risk of acquiring the *H. pylori* infection.

References

1 Langenberg, W, Rauws, EAJ, Houthoff, HJ, *et al.* Follow-up study of individuals with untreated *Campylobacter pylori*-associated gastritis and of non-infected persons with nonulcer dyspepsia. *J. Infect. Dis.* 1988;**157**(6):1245–8.

2 Marshall, BJ, McGechie, DB, Francis, GJ, & Utley, PJ. Pyloric campylobacter serology. *Lancet* 1984;**ii**:281.

3 Engstrand, L, Scheynius, A, Pahlson, C, Grimelius, L, Schwan, A, & Gustavsson, S. Association of *Campylobacter pylori* with induced expression of class II transplantation antigens on gastric epithelial cells. *Infect. Immun.* 1989; **57**:827–32.

4 Wyatt, JI, & Rathbone, BJ. Immune response of the gastric mucosa to *Campylobacter pylori*. *Scand. J. Gastroenterol.* 1988;**23**(suppl 142):44–9.

5 Newell, DG, & Rathbone, BJ. The serodiagnosis of *Campylobacter pylori* infection. *Infect. Dis.* 1989;**3**:172–5.

6 Vaira, D, Cairns Holton, J Sr, Falzon, M, Polydorou, A, Dowsett, JF, & Salmon, PR. Antibody titres to *Campylobacter pylori* after treatment for gastritis. *Br. Med. J.* 1988;**297**:397.

7 von Wulffen, H, Grote, HJ, Gatermann, S, Löning, T, Berger, B, & Buhl, C. Immunoblot analysis of immune response to *Campylobacter pylori* and its clinical associations. *J. Clin. Pathol.* 1988;**41**: 653–9.

8 Mitchell, HM, Lee, A, Berkowicz, J, & Borody, T. The use of serology to diagnose active *Campylobacter pylori* infection. *Med. J. Austr.* 1988;**149**:604–9.

9 Musgrove, C, Bolton, FJ, Krypczyk, AM, *et al.* *Campylobacter pylori*: clinical, histological and serological studies. *J. Clin Pathol.* 1988;**41**: 1316–21.

10 Dent, JC, McNulty, CAM, Uff, JS, Gear, MWL, & Wilkinson, SP. *Campylobacter pylori* urease: a new serological test. *Lancet* 1988;**i**:1002.

11 Czinn, S, Carr, H, Sheffler, L, & Aronoff, S. Serum IgG antibody to the outer membrane proteins of *Campylobacter pylori* in children with gastroduodenal disease. *J. Infect. Dis.* 1989; **159**:586–9.

12 Dwyer, B, Nanxiong, S, Kaldor, J, *et al.* Antibody response to *Campylobacter pylori* in an ethnic group lacking peptic ulceration. *Scand. J. Infect. Dis.* 1988;**20**:63–8.

13 Goodwin, CS, Blincow, E, Peterson, G, *et al.* Enzyme-linked immunosorbent assay for *Campylobacter pyloridis*: correlation with presence of *C. pyloridis* in the gastric mucosa. *J. Infect. Dis.* 1987;**155**:488–99.

14 Perez-Perez, GI, Dworkin, BM, Chodos, JE, & Blaser, MJ. *Campylobacter pylori* antibodies in humans. *Ann. Intern. Med.* 1988;**109**(1):11–17.

15 Hirschl, AM. Frequency of occurrence of *Campylobacter pylori* and analysis of the systemic and local immune response. *Zbl. Bakt. A* 1987;**266**:526–42.

16 Kaldor, J, Tee, W, McCarthy, P, Watson, J. & Dwyer, B. Immune response to *Campylobacter pyloridis* in patients with peptic ulceration. *Lancet* 1985;**i**:921.

17 Steer, HW, Hawtin, PR, & Newell, DG. An ELISA technique for the serodiagnosis of *Campylobacter pyloridis* infection in patients with gastritis and benign duodenal ulceration. *Serodiagn. Immunother.* 1987;**1**:253–9.

18 Morris, A, & Nicholson, G. Ingestion of *Campylobacter pyloridis* causes gastritis and raised fasting pH. *Am. J. Gastroenterol.* 1987; **82**:192–9.

19 Rathbone, BJ, Wyatt, JI, Worsley, BW, *et al.* Systemic and local antibody response to gastric *Campylobacter pyloridis* in non-ulcer dyspepsia. *Gut* 1986;**27**:642–7.

20 Booth, L, Holdstock, G, McBride, H, *et al.* Clinical importance of *Campylobacter pyloridis* and associated IgG and IgA antibody responses in patients undergoing upper gastrointestinal endoscopy. *J. Clin. Pathol.* 1986;**39**:1215–19.

21 Kosunen, TU, Höök, J, Rautelin, HI, Vainio, U, & Seppälä, K. Correlation of circulating antibodies with the presence of culturable *Campylobacter pylori* in biopsy specimens. In: Mégraud F, & Lamouliatte, H (eds), *Gastroduodenal Pathology and Campylobacter pylori*. Amsterdam: Elsevier, 1989, pp. 223–6.

22 Apel, I, Jacobs, E, Kist, M, & Bredt, W. Antibody response of patients against a 120 kDa surface protein of *Campylobacter pylori*. *Zbl. Bakt. A* 1988;**268**:271–6.

23 von Wulffen, H, Grote, HJ, & Krämer-Hansen, H. Serological screening for *Campylobacter pylori* in candidates for renal transplantation. *Lancet* 1987; **i**:1140–1.

24 von Wulffen, H, & Grote, HJ. Enzyme-linked immunosorbent assay for detection of immunoglobulin A and G to *Campylobacter pylori*. *Eur. J. Clin. Microbiol. Infect. Dis.* 1988;**7**:559–65.

25 Kosunen, TU, Höök, J, Rautelin, JI, & Myllylä, G. Age-dependent increase of *Campylobacter pylori* antibodies in blood donors. *Scand. J. Gastroenterol.* 1989;**24**:110–14.

26 Reiff, A, Jacobs, E, & Kist, M. Seroepidemiological study of the immune response to *Campylobacter pylori* in potential risk groups. *Eur. J. Clin. Microbiol. Infect. Dis.* 1989;**8**:592–6.

27 Bolton, FJ, Hutchinson, DN, Hinchliffe, PM, & Holt, AV. Distribution in various clinical groups of antibody to *C. pylori* detected by enzyme-linked immunosorbent assay, complement fixation and microagglutination tests. *Serodiagn. Immunother. Infect. Dis.* 1989;**3**:41–50.

28 Jones, DM, Eldridge, J, Fox, AJ, Sethi, P, & Whorwell, PJ. Antibody to the gastric campylobacter-like organism ("*Campylobacter pyloridis*") — clinical correlations and distribution in the normal population. *J. Med.*

Microbiol. 1986;**22**:57–62.
29 Wyatt, JI, Rathbone, BJ, & Heatly, RV. Local immune response to gastric campylobacter in non-ulcer dyspepsia. *J. Clin. Pathol.* 1986;**39**: 863–70.
30 Rathbone, BJ, Wyatt, J, Tompkins, D, Heatly, RV, & Losowsky, MS. Diagnostic IgG ELISA for gastric *Campylobacter pyloridis* infection using serum samples. *Gut* 1986;**27**:A607.
31 Rathbone, BJ, Wyatt, JI, & Heatly, RV. Local response of the host to *Campylobacter pylori. Gastroenterol. Clin. Biol.* 1989;**13**:75B–77B.
32 Jones, DM, Eldridge, J, & Whorwell, PJ. Antibodies to *Campylobacter pyloridis* in household contacts of infected patients. *Br. Med. J.* 1987; **294**:615.
33 Dixon, MF, Wyatt, JI, Burke, AD, & Rathbone, BJ. Lymphocytic gastritis — relationship to *Campylobacter pylori* infection. *J. Pathol.* 1988; **154**:125–32.
34 Laemmli, UK. Cleavage of structural proteins during the assembly of the head of bacteriophage T4. *Nature* 1970;**227**:680–86.
35 Dunn, BE, Perez-Perez, GI, & Blaser, MJ. Two-dimensional gel electrophoresis and immunoblotting of *Campylobacter pylori* proteins. *Infect. Immun.* 1989;**57**:1825–33.
36 Pearson, AD, Bamforth, J, Booth, L, *et al.* Polyacrylamide gel electrophoresis of spiral bacteria from the gastric antrum. *Lancet* 1984;**i**:1349–50.
37 Hirschl, AM, Pletschette, M, Hirschl, MH, Berger, J, Stanek, G, & Rotter, ML. Comparison of different antigen preparations in an evaluation of the immune response to *Campylobacter pylori. Eur. J. Clin. Microbiol. Infect. Dis.* 1988;**7**: 570–75.
38 Höök, J, Blomberg, B, Danielsson, D, & Kosunen, TU. Detection of antibody responses in rabbits hyperimmunized with *Campylobacter pylori. Acta Pathol. Microbiol. Scand.* 1989;**97**:56–60.
39 Newell, DG, Johnston, BJ, Ali, MH, & Reed, PI. An enzyme-linked immunosorbent assay for the serodiagnosis of *Campylobacter pylori*-associated gastritis. *Scand. J. Gastroenterol.* 1988; **142**(suppl):53–7.
40 Lee, A, Logan, SM, & Trust, TJ. Demonstration of a flagellar antigen shared by a diverse group of spiral-shaped bacteria that colonize intestinal mucus. *Infect. Immun.* 1987;**55**:828–31.
41 Danielsson, D, Blomberg, B, Järnerot, G, & Kosunen, TU. Heterogeneity of *Campylobacter pylori* as demonstrated by co-agglutination testing with rabbit antibodies. *Scand. J. Gastroenterol.* 1988;**23**(suppl 142):58–63.
42 Newell, DG. Monoclonal antibodies directed against the flagella of *Campylobacter jejuni*: cross-reacting and serotypic specificity and potential use in diagnosis. *J. Hyg. Camb.* 1986; **96**:377–84.
43 Evans, DJ Jr, Evans, DG, Graham, DY, & Klein, PD. A sensitive and specific serologic test for detection of *Campylobacter pylori* infection. *Gastroenterology* 1989;**96**:1004–8.
44 von Wulffen, H, Heesemann, J, Bützow, GH, Löning, T, & Laufs, R. Detection of *Campylobacter pyloridis* in patients with antrum gastritis and peptic ulcers by culture, complement fixation test, and immunoblot. *J. Clin. Microbiol.* 1986;**24**:716–20.
45 Kist, M, Apel, I, & Jacobs, E. Protein antigens of *Campylobacter pylori*: the problem of species-specificity. In: Menge, H, Gregor, M, Tytgat, GNJ, & Marshall BJ (eds), *Campylobacter pylori. Proceedings of the First International Symposium on Campylobacter pylori*, Kronberg, June 12–13, 1987. Berlin: Springer Verlag, 1987, pp. 19–26.
46 Newell, DG. Identification of the outer membrane proteins of *Campylobacter pyloridis* and antigenic cross-reactivity between *C. pyloridis* and *C. jejuni. J. Gen. Microbiol.* 1987;**133**: 163–70.
47 Geis, G, Leying, H, Suerbaum, S, Mai, U, & Opferkuch, W. Ultrastructure and chemical analysis of *Campylobacter pylori* flagella. *J. Clin. Microbiol.* 1989;**27**:436–41.
48 Newell, DG. Human serum antibody responses to the surface protein antigens of *Campylobacter pyloridis. Serodiagn. Immunother.* 1987;**1**: 209–17.
49 Perez-Perez, GI, & Blaser, MJ. Conservation and diversity of *Campylobacter pyloridis* major antigens. *Infect. Immun.* 1987;**55**:1256–63.
50 Burnie, JP, Lee, W, Dent, JC, & McNulty, CAM. Immunoblot fingerprinting of *Campylobacter pylori. J. Med. Microbiol.* 1988;**27**:153–9.
51 Mobley, HLT, Cortesia, MJ, Rosenthal, LE, & Jones, BD. Characterization of urease from *Campylobacter pylori. J. Clin. Microbiol.* 1988; **26**:831–6.
52 Evans, DJ Jr, Evans, DG, Smith, KE, & Graham, DY. Serum antibody responses to the *N*-acetylneuraminyllactose-binding hemagglutinin of *Campylobacter pylori. Infect. Immun.* 1989; **57**:664–7.
53 Clayton, CL, Wren, BW, Mullany, P, Topping, A, & Tabaqchali, S. Molecular cloning and expression of *Campylobacter pylori* species-specific antigens in *Escherichia coli* K-12. *Infect. Immun.* 1989;**57**:623–9.
54 Evans, DG, Evans, DJ Jr, Moulds, JJ, & Graham, DY. *N*-Acetylneuraminyllactose-binding fibrillar hemagglutinin of *Campylobacter pylori*: a putative colonization factor antigen. *Infect. Immun.* 1988;**56**:2896–906.
55 Dunn, BE, Martin, MJ, & Snyder, EL. Two-dimensional gel electrophoresis and immuno-

blotting of *Campylobacter* outer membrane proteins. *Infect. Immun.* 1987;**55**:1564–72.

56 Schaber, E, Umlauft, G, Stöffler, G, Aigner, F, Paulweber, B, & Sandhofer, F. Indirect immunofluorescence test and enzyme-linked immunosorbent assay for detection of *Campylobacter pylori*. *J. Clin. Microbiol.* 1989;**27**:327–30.

57 Jones, DM, Lessells, AM, & Eldridge, J. *Campylobacter*-like organisms on the gastric mucosa: culture, histological, and serological studies. *J. Clin. Pathol.* 1984;**37**:1002–6.

58 Eldridge, J, Lessells, AM, & Jones, DM. Antibody to spiral organisms on gastric mucosa. *Lancet* 1984;**i**:1237.

59 Mitchell, HM, Lee, A, & Carrick, J. Increased incidence of *Campylobacter pylori* infection in gastroenterologists: further evidence to support person-to-person transmission of *C. pylori*. *Scand. J. Gastroenterol.* 1989;**24**:396–400.

60 Schaub, N, Stalder, H, Stalder, GA, *et al. Campylobacter pylori*, Gastritis und Ulcuskrankheit. *Schweiz. Med. Wschr.* 1988;**118**:293–301.

61 Blaser, MJ, & Duncan, DJ. Human serum antibody response to *C. jejuni* infections as measured in an enzyme-linked immunosorbent assay. *Infect. Immun.* 1984;**44**:292–8.

62 Newell, DG, & Stacey, A. Antigens for the serodiagnosis of *Campylobacter pylori* infections. *Gastroenterol. Clin. Biol.* 1989;**13**:37B–41B.

63 Bauernfeind, A, Przyklenk, B, Hörl, G, & Otto, U. Representative *Campylobacter pylori* antigen for IgG-ELISA and diagnostic significance of antibody titres. In: Mégraud, F, & Lamouliatte, H (eds), *Gastroduodenal Pathology and Campylobacter pylori*. Amsterdam: Elsevier, 1989, pp. 185–8.

64 Bolton, FJ, & Hutchinson, DN. Evaluation of three *Campylobacter pylori* antigen preparations for screening sera from patients undergoing endoscopy. *J. Clin. Pathol.* 1989;**42**:723–6.

65 Andersen, LP. *Campylobacter pylori* antibodies measured by indirect ELISA using O-antigen. In: Mégraud, F, & Lamouliatte, H (eds), *Gastroduodenal Pathology and Campylobacter pylori*. Amsterdam: Elsevier, 1989, pp. 201–3.

66 Przyklenk, B, Bauernfeind, A, Bornschein, W, Emminger, G, Heilmann, K, & Schweighart, S. The role of *Campylobacter (Helicobacter) pylori* in disorder of the gastrointestinal tract. *Infection* 1990;**18**:9–13.

67 Gobert, B, Bene, MC, Faure, G, et al. IgG, IgA and IgM antibodies to *Campylobacter pylori* detected by dot-ELISA and ELISA. In: Mégraud, F, & Lamouliatte, H (eds), *Gastroduodenal Pathology and Campylobacter pylori*. Amsterdam: Elsevier, 1989, pp. 219–22.

68 Hawtin, PR, Stacey, A, & Newell, DG. The antigenicity of *Campylobacter pylori* urease. In: Mégraud, F, & Lamouliatte, H (eds), *Gastroduodenal Pathology and Campylobacter pylori*. Amsterdam: Elsevier, 1989, pp. 189–91.

69 Hirschl, AM, Rathbone, BJ, Wyatt, JI, Berger, J, & Rotter, ML. Four different antigen preparations for serodiagnosis of *Campylobacter pylori* infection. *Klin. Wochenschr.* 1989;**67**(suppl XVIII):30.

70 von Wulffen, H, & Grote, HJ. Serodiagnosis of *Campylobacter pylori* infection using an enzyme-linked immunosorbent assay. In: Mégraud, F, & Lamouliatte, H (eds), *Gastroduodenal Pathology and Campylobacter pylori*. Amsterdam: Elsevier, 1989, pp. 231–5.

71 Kaldor, J, Tee, W, Nicolacópolous, C, Demirtzoglou, K, Noonan, D, & Dwyer, B. Immunoblot confirmation of immune response to *Campylobacter pyloridis* in patients with duodenal ulcers. *Med. J. Austr.* 1986;**145**:133–5.

72 Eldridge, J, & Jones, DM. Longitudinal study of the incidence of antibody to *Campylobacter pylori* in school children. In: Mégraud, F, & Lamouliatte, H (eds), *Gastroduodenal Pathology and Campylobacter pylori*. Amsterdam: Elsevier, 1989, pp. 419–21.

73 Brassens-Rabbe, MP, Mégraud, F, Denis, F, *et al.* Seroepidemiology of *Campylobacter pylori* infection in four populations which differed in their ethnic and geographical characteristics. In: Mégraud, F, & Lamouliatte, H (eds), *Gastroduodenal Pathology and Campylobacter pylori*. Amsterdam: Elsevier, 1989, pp. 427–9.

74 Graham, DY, Adam, E, Klein, PD, *et al.* Epidemiology of *Campylobacter pylori* infection. *Gastroenterol. Clin. Biol.* 1989;**13**:84B–89B.

75 Cadranel, S, Conti-Nibali, S, van Tricht, L, Verhas, M, Glupczynski, Y, & de Prez, C. *Campylobacter pylori* in parents of children with *C. pylori*-positive gastritis and primary ulcers. In: Mégraud, F, & Lamouliatte, H (eds), *Gastroduodenal Pathology and Campylobacter pylori*. Amsterdam: Elsevier, 1989, pp. 447–50.

76 Oderda, G, Boero, M, Ponzetto, A, Bellis, D, & Ansaldi, N. *Campylobacter pylori* in families of children with relapsing gastroduodenal disease due to *C. pylori* infection. In: Mégraud, F, & Lamouliatte, H (eds), *Gastroduodenal Pathology and Campylobacter pylori*. Amsterdam: Elsevier, 1989, pp. 443–5.

77 Mitchell, HM, Bohane, TD, Berkowicz, J, Hazell, SL, & Lee, A. Antibody to *Campylobacter pylori* in families of index children with gastrointestinal illness due to *C. pylori*. *Lancet* 1987;**ii**:681–2.

78 Berkowicz, J, & Lee, A. Person-to-person transmission of *Campylobacter pylori*. *Lancet* 1987;**ii**:680–1.

79 Kist, M, Reiff, A, Jacobs, E, Lang, B, & Peter, HH. *Campylobacter pylori* antibodies in patients with rheumatoid arthritis. *Klin. Wochenschr.* 1989;**67**

(suppl XVIII):34.
80 Vaira, D, D'Anastasio, C, Holton, J, Dowsett, JF, Londei, M, Salmon, PR, & Gandolfi, L. A possible source of *Campylobacter pylori*? ELISA testing of abattoir workers. In: Mégraud, F, & Lamouliatte, H (eds), *Gastroduodenal Pathology and Campylobacter pylori*. Amsterdam: Elsevier, 1989, pp. 431–4.

9: Molecular biology and its application to Helicobacter pylori

L.S. TOMPKINS

Introduction

This chapter outlines the applications of molecular biology and molecular techniques to *Helicobacter pylori*, focusing on the genetic and molecular basis of pathogenicity and the utility of molecular diagnostic reagents. Since little is currently known about the genes encoding pathogenic properties of *H. pylori*, our experience in developing genetic systems to study *Campylobacter* spp. will serve as a foundation and model for the approach to *H. pylori*. Coupled with a rather philosophical discussion of pathogenicity, the author hopes to address potentially fertile areas for future research into molecular genetics and to discuss the significance of some data that have already been collected.

Molecular Koch's postulates and *H. pylori*

Since the advent of recombinant DNA methods, and their application to the study of prokaryotic pathogens, it is now possible to take a rather different look at the basis of virulence and to redefine a "pathogen". Bacterial pathogens generally possess specific genetic properties that provide them with the ability to establish infection and, infrequently, to cause disease. The first goal of the molecular geneticist is to isolate and characterize the genes responsible for infection and disease, as the first step in the proof of pathogenicity. Falkow [1] has recently reformulated Koch's original postulates into molecular terms, as shown in Table 9.1.

Some alternative molecular tricks that also demonstrate the role of each genetic determinant include:

1 The gene associated with the trait must be isolated by molecular methods. Specific inactivation or deletion should lead to loss of function.

2 Replacement of the modified gene for its allelic counterpart in the strain of origin should lead to loss of function and concomitant virulence.

The steps involved in these genetic experiments are outlined as follows. First, the DNA containing the genes encoding each polypeptide must be extracted, cut into fragments using restriction endonucleases, and cloned into a vector, such as a plasmid or bacteriophage, creating a library of genes now contained within recombinant vectors. Next, these recombinant molecules must be introduced (cloned) into a suitable recipient cell, such as *Escherichia coli*, which will be able to maintain and replicate the foreign DNA.

Depending upon the desired result, plasmid vectors can be constructed so that they replicate in the cytoplasm of the *E. coli* recipient and remain as extrachromosomal elements. Alternatively, the vectors may be of the "suicide" type, so that upon entry into the recipient, the inserted DNA is "rescued" by genetic recombination into the chromosome of the recipient cell. The recipient cells must next be screened for the presence of the recombinant vector. Usually, the plasmid contains an antibiotic resistance gene, which serves as a marker that can be selected following plating of recipient bacteria onto antibiotic-containing media. This step ensures that the recipients contain the plasmid, but does not select for the

Table 9.1 Molecular Koch's postulates

1 The phenotype or property thought to play a role in pathogenesis should be associated with pathogenic members of a genus or pathogenic strains
2 Specific inactivation of the gene should lead to a measurable loss in pathogenicity or virulence
3 Reversion of the mutated gene, or allelic replacement, should restore pathogenicity

desired gene *per se.* In the final selection step, the cells containing recombinant vectors are screened for expression of the foreign protein (enzyme, polypeptide, etc.). Although it is often possible to obtain expression (i.e. transcription and translation) of foreign genes in *E. coli*, this often depends on the degree of relatedness between the donor DNA and the recipient cell DNA. Since the guanine and cytosine (G + C) content of *Campylobacter* (32–38%) is so different from *E. coli* (50%), it has been difficult to detect expression of some cloned genes. Other barriers to expression can also be encountered, including restriction of incoming foreign DNA.

Having obtained recombinant clones containing and expressing the foreign DNA insert, a series of molecular methods is then used to characterize the gene. Methods include mapping by restriction endonucleases, subcloning, characterization of polypeptides by gel electrophoresis, and finally by DNA sequence analysis. These analyses are all essential to the proof that the correct gene has been cloned and is producing the appropriate product.

The next step is to develop stable isogenic mutants of the pathogen, each deficient in a single gene. As outlined above, this step is essential in fulfilling molecular Koch's postulates, since by examining the behavior of isogenic mutants in comparison with the wild-type strain in relevant models of infection, it should be possible to dissect out the contribution of each toward the process. Mutants can be constructed either by inactivating genes in the pathogenic cells directly, usually by insertion of transposons, or by exchanging the wild-type gene with a modified gene that has been constructed and inactivated *in vitro.* Exchange of genes requires a system to introduce the modified sequence back into the donor strain. The usual methods are by transformation of wild-type strains with "suicide" plasmids containing a transposon, or by conjugation with *E. coli* cell donors containing recombinant "suicide" plasmids.

Molecular studies in *Campylobacter jejuni*: a model for the molecular and genetic approach to *H. pylori*

Development of genetic exchange systems

Our laboratory has approached the genetic determinants of virulence in *Campylobacter jejuni* in an analogous manner. When we began genetic studies of *C. jejuni*, we found that there were no methods to accomplish genetic exchange. Although some strains of *C. jejuni* contained plasmids, some of which contained antibiotic resistance genes, and others which were cryptic, encoding for no known functions other than to ensure autonomous replication, it had not been possible to mobilize these from *Campylobacter* into *E. coli* or other bacterial recipients, nor had it been possible to introduce foreign plasmids, even those that had a broad host range, into *Campylobacter* by bacterial conjugation.

Our first goal in the research was to develop a series of plasmids that could be used to shuttle DNA back and forth between *E. coli* and *Campylobacter*. These recombinant plasmids would contain *Campylobacter* DNA inserts encoding the putative virulence determinants or transposons, and thus they were designed to overcome the barriers to entry (restriction) and replication. In order to introduce them by conjugation, these recombinant shuttle vectors had to be able to replicate in *E. coli*, and *E. coli* donors had to have the necessary genetic functions to permit mobilization of the plasmids into *Campylobacter* by conjugation. The essential elements of such shuttle plasmids were:

1 Replication in *E. coli* provided by pBR322, a Gram-negative bacterial plasmid that replicates to high copy number in *E. coli*.

2 Replication in *C. jejuni*, provided by the cryptic plasmid isolated from a *C. coli* strain.

3 A suitable marker that would be expressed in both *E. coli* and *Campylobacter*; we used the kanamycin-resistance determinant from a *C. coli* strain for this purpose.
4 A DNA sequence (*ori*T) permitting mobilization.
The recombinant shuttle plasmids were constructed to contain all of these elements, using the usual molecular and genetic techniques of "cutting and pasting". These plasmids were then transformed into *E. coli* donor cells that also contained a broad host range plasmid carrying essential mobilization functions. In matings between the *E. coli* donors (kanamycin-resistant) and *C. jejuni* recipients (kanamycin-susceptible), carried out under reduced oxygen conditions, we were able to select *Campylobacter* transconjugants that had become kanamycin-resistant. Analysis of the recombinant plasmids contained in the cytoplasm of the recipients showed that they had not been modified in the process of mobilization, and were stably maintained as extra-chromosomal elements [2].

The next goal was to construct "suicide" plasmid vectors that could be employed to introduce either transposons or modified genes into *Campylobacter* recipients. We removed the portion of the shuttle plasmid obtained from the *Campylobacter* cryptic plasmid by restriction digestion deletion, creating a recombinant that could replicate in *E. coli*, but which would "suicide" upon entry into *Campylobacter*. Prior to loss of the plasmid during cell division, a transposon could "jump" into the chromosome, thus creating disruption of the gene into which it inserted, and a modified gene could be rescued in exchange for the complementary, wild-type gene. Since we were not able to find any known transposons that were able to transpose and express an antibiotic-resistance marker in *Campylobacter*, we tested the suicide plasmid system using a modified *Campylobacter* gene. For this purpose, we selected the gene encoding the 16S ribosomal RNA (the gene is referred to as the 16S rDNA).

In *C. jejuni*, as in all other bacteria, the ribosomal genes are present in multiple copies on the bacterial chromosome, and therefore the exchange of a single modified, non-functional gene, for a wild-type gene would not be a lethal modification. As shown in Fig. 9.1, the gene was modified *in vitro* by inserting a kanamycin-resistance gene into the 16S rDNA gene. The entire cassette was then inserted into the suicide plasmid and introduced into *Campylo-*

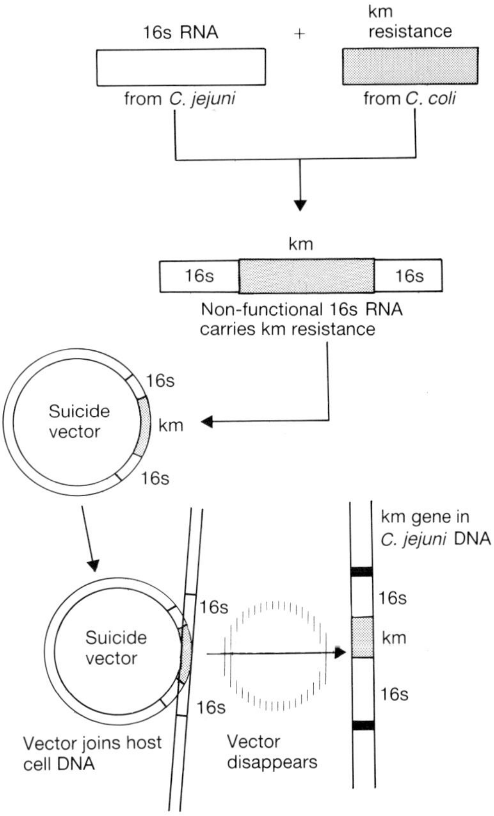

Fig. 9.1 Diagrammatic representation of scheme used to construct an isogenic mutant of *Campylobacter jejuni*. A kanamycin (km) resistance determinant has been ligated *in vitro* into the fragment of DNA encoding 16S RNA in the first step. Next, this sequence was cloned into a suicide vector. Transfer of the recombinant suicide vector into *Campylobacter* via conjugation with *E. coli* donors then provides for the opportunity for recombination to occur with the homologous copy of a 16S RNA gene in the chromosome of *Campylobacter*. The vector cannot replicate in the *Campylobacter* host, and thus disappears. In this final step the mutant contains a modified copy of the km-resistant gene, stably integrated into its chromosome. The mutants can then be detected by plating of *Campylobacter* recipients onto medium containing kanamycin.

bacter recipients by conjugation with *E. coli* donors. Analysis of the kanamycin-resistant mutants showed that the "cassette" had been recombined into the chromosome in exchange for one of the intact, functional 16S rDNA genes [3].

We have also devised a second method to introduce recombinant plasmids into *C. jejuni*, by transformation using high voltage electroporation [4]. The application of high voltage electrical energy creates pores in the bacterial cell membrane, through which intact plasmids can pass. This method has been especially useful for *Campylobacter*, since transformation cannot be accomplished using other methods and no transducing phages have been discovered for this species.

H. pylori molecular genetic studies

These methods of accomplishing genetic exchange in *C. jejuni* and *C. coli* have served as a foundation for a genetic approach to *H. pylori*. Labigne-Roussel & Courcoux have recently reported the successful isolation of the genetic sequence encoding the *H. pylori* urease, using a modified shuttle plasmid (cosmid) that they originally constructed for *C. jejuni* [5, 6]. They constructed a genetic library of *H. pylori* chromosomal DNA in a cosmid shuttle plasmid, pILL590, by ligating large chromosomal restriction fragments from *H. pylori* into the shuttle plasmid containing a selectable antibiotic resistance marker (km). The recombinant cosmid was then transfected into *E. coli* donors, where it replicated autonomously. Although the kanamycin-resistance marker was expressed in *E. coli*, indicating the presence of the plasmid, none of the *E. coli* clones produced an active urease. However, when these plasmids were mobilized into *C. jejuni* by conjugation with *E. coli* donors, a small number of kanamycin-resistant transconjugants were formed. One out of 160 transconjugants was detected which produced urease. Analysis of the recombinant cosmid isolated from this clone revealed that it contained *H. pylori* DNA, from which two specific polypeptides having urease activity were synthesized and elaborated. Thus, the cosmid shuttle vector system was useful in identifying and cloning the DNA sequence containing the urease operon.

Having identified the urease operon in *C. jejuni*, Labigne & Courcoux then reintroduced the plasmid into a strain of *E. coli* that produces "mini-cells" during cell division. Each mini-cell contains a copy of the plasmid but has no chromosome. When mini-cells are grown in the presence of ^{35}S-labeled amino acids, polypeptides that are made in the mini-cells can be specifically labeled, and subsequently detected by autoradiography of polyacrylamide gels containing the proteins segregated by electrophoresis. Even though they were unable to detect urease activity in *E. coli*, the mini-cell strain was capable of transcribing and translating two polypeptides derived from the *H. pylori* DNA, and thus they concluded that *E. coli* cells could indeed express *H. pylori* genes, but that there was a block at the level of activity, perhaps related to problems in protein processing or a deficiency of an essential cofactor [6]. Work is continuing to further characterize this operon (A. Labigne-Roussel, personal communication).

These experiments reveal several important features about *H. pylori*. First, the recombinant plasmid initially constructed for the purpose of shuttling genes into *C. jejuni* can also serve this function for *H. pylori*, even though the two species are not closely related. Therefore, it should be possible to construct a suicide plasmid from this cosmid that could be used to introduce a modified urease gene into *H. pylori*, thereby creating an isogenic mutant. It should also be possible to construct *H. pylori* shuttle and suicide plasmids using an *H. pylori* cryptic plasmid and a *C. jejuni* kanamycin-resistance gene, in combination with *E. coli* plasmid functions, in the same way the *C. jejuni* shuttle plasmids were constructed.

Construction of *H. pylori* mutants

The analysis of isogenic mutants in relevant models of infection will be critically important in the assessment of the role that specific genes play in establishing colonization or in disease. It seems likely that the *H. pylori* urease is an essential determinant in the natural lifecycle, even though it may have nothing to do with colonization of the stomach *per se*. Possibly, the primary function of this enzyme system is to derive nutrients from the natural environment, wherever that may be, or from the milieu of the stomach. It may even have an effect upon chemotaxis of the cell. Thus, the behavior of isogenic mutants in the mucus-colonization model developed by Lee *et al.* [7] may be substantially different in comparison with wild-type strains.

Similarly, the functional knock-out of the urease gene might affect that ability of isogenic mutants to induce gastritis in animal models. The urease gene could also serve as a probe to identify the distribution of closely related genes among *H. pylori* strains and other related urease-producing bacteria. These studies would also add to our understanding of the role of urease in the natural history of infection. Comparison of the urease genes from other species, by DNA sequence analysis, would also provide another measurement that would be useful in assigning the taxonomic position of the species.

Other genes that would be relevant targets for cloning and genetic analysis would include those that encode for *H. pylori* flagella, neuraminic acid receptors and putative toxins. The role of each of these in the pathogenesis of infection or disease could then be assessed.

Application of molecular methods to *H. pylori*

Nucleic acid hybridization

The isolation of specific *H. pylori* genes also opens up a new avenue to the diagnosis of *H. pylori* infection by DNA hybridization. DNA probes have been developed to detect a large number of pathogenic bacteria using a variety of formats to accomplish hybridization between the probe nucleic acid and the complementary target nucleic acids in clinical specimens. Fig. 9.2 represents the process of hybridization between a labeled probe and a target DNA molecule.

The sensitivity of DNA probes depends, in large part, upon the number of target nucleic acid sequences that are present in the specimen. The prototype toxin gene probes, developed by Moseley *et al.* to detect enterotoxigenic *E. coli* in fecal samples, were highly sensitive because the target toxin genes were carried on multiple copy plasmids in *E. coli* cells, and thus the actual concentration of the target molecules was sufficiently great to be detected after an overnight amplification of the *E. coli* cells [8]. The sensitivity of the nucleic acid probes falls dramatically when the number of target molecules is less than 10^7 per specimen. A recently developed method to accomplish amplification of the number of target molecules enzymatically, called polymerase chain reaction (PCR) amplification, is dramatically expanding the application of nucleic acid probes.

The PCR method (Fig. 9.3) utilizes specific oligonucleotide primers that flank the target DNA sequence. These oligonucleotides serve to prime the enzymatic polymerization of complementary strands in the presence of polymerase enzyme and nucleotide base substrates, thereby creating a copy of each strand at the end of one round of amplification. Following this, the double-stranded target molecules are denatured to expose each single strand to the addition of new primers and polymerase, creating another round of amplification, and so forth. Theoretically, 60 rounds of amplification would produce a million-fold amplification of the target DNA. In practice, the number of rounds of amplification is usually set between 20 and 30, a level that can detect approximately 10–100 target molecules. If the target nucleic acid sequence is encoded as a single copy in each bacterial cell, this means that approximately 50 bacteria could be detected after 30 rounds of amplification. Following amplification, a single nucleic acid fragment (the target) of known molecular size is thereby produced at detectable concentrations. At the conclusion of the amplification process, target DNA may be detected by hybridization with a labeled probe.

How could DNA hybridization and PCR technology be employed to address the issues of *H. pylori* diagnosis, pathogenesis, and virulence, or prove Koch's postulates? Although *H. pylori* can be isolated from the majority of gastric biopsy specimens showing histologic gastritis, culture is only a moder-

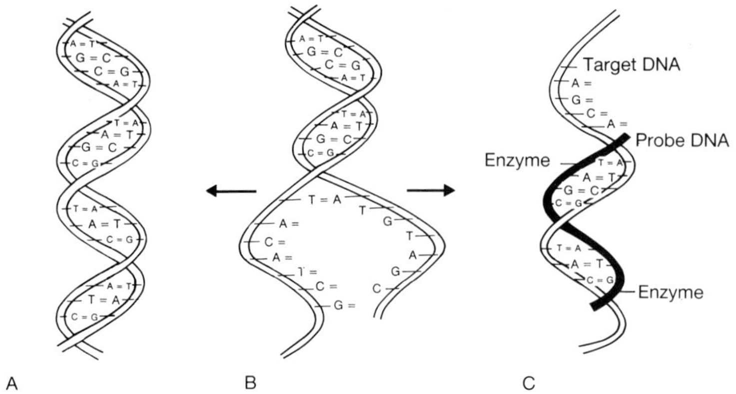

Fig. 9.2 DNA hybridization technique. A, structure of DNA; B, denaturation of DNA; C, binding of a probe to DNA. (From Tenover, FC. Clin. Microbial. Rev. 1988;**1**:82–101.)

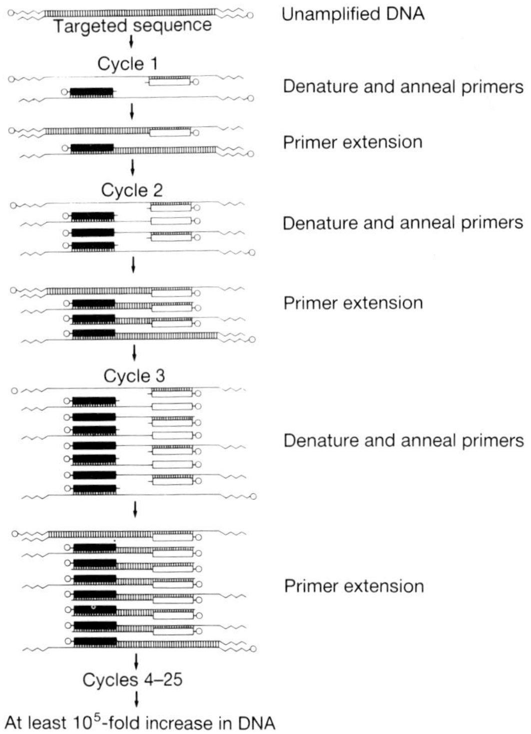

Fig. 9.3 Polymerase chain reaction (PCR) amplification of specific target nucleic acid, using specific primers in conjunction with polymerase to denature and anneal primers; extend primers by synthesizing complementary strands; and denature double-stranded molecules to prepare for another round of replication. (From Oste, C. *Biotechniques* 1988; **6**:162–7.)

ately sensitive test of infection. Identification of *Campylobacter*-like microorganisms by tissue stain is useful, but not necessarily specific. Infected tissue can be tested for urease activity, and a breath test that detects the production of $^{14}CO_2$ from the action of urease is a specific method of detection, but the sensitivity is not necessarily high.

Labigne-Roussel *et al.* recently reported the application of two DNA probes to identify *H. pylori* [9, 10]. The probes were derived from a portion of the sequence encoding the *H. pylori* urease; probe A encompassed an 8.1 kilobase (kb) fragment, while probe B consisted of a 294 base pair (bp) fragment. When tested on DNA extracted from colonies of 32 *H. pylori* strains and strains of *C. jejuni*, *C. coli*, and *C. fetus*, these investigators found that both probes gave 100% sensitivity and specificity. Neither probe reacted with strains of 13 species of other urease-producing bacteria.

In order to apply these probes to gastric biopsies, some sort of amplification of target sequences will be necessary, since the urease gene is found in a single copy in each bacterial chromosome. Experiments are underway to amplify target sequences in biopsies by PCR amplification, followed by hybridization with the urease gene probes (A. Labigne-Roussel, personal communication).

In addition to testing gastric biopsy specimens, it will also be interesting to apply DNA probes and PCR amplification to fecal samples, dental plaque, and saliva, again looking for the natural reservoir of *H. pylori*. Most of the evidence, primarily based upon culture results, suggests that humans without gastritis are not infected. However, the sensitivity of culture for any bacterial pathogen is poor when the concentration of microorganisms is low, as in asymptomatic gonococcal infection in females, for instance. Therefore, it is possible that humans could in fact be the natural reservoir for *H. pylori*.

Currently, it is thought that *H. pylori* is causally related to gastritis in humans. Part of the evidence which supports this conclusion is based on the absence of *H. pylori* in normal gastric mucosa, whereas *H. pylori* is almost always present in gastritis. Another explanation for these findings, however, could be that *H. pylori* is a normal inhabitant of the stomach, but is present in very low concentrations not detectable by culture. Probing gastric biopsies from normal controls and from individuals with gastritis with an *H. pylori*-specific probe should provide interesting results which could settle this issue.

Molecular fingerprinting

Genotyping systems, such as restriction endonuclease analysis (REA) and plasmid analysis, have contributed substantially to epidemiologic investigations of other bacterial species. Langenberg *et al.* analyzed the REA patterns derived from *H. pylori* strains isolated from several patients with recurrent infections [11], as shown in Fig. 9.4. These data were quite revealing in several respects. First, this study definitively showed that recurrence of infection in a single individual is primarily due to relapse with the original infecting strain; strains recovered over several months or years from the same patient exhibited molecularly similar fingerprints. Second, strains from different patients were all molecularly distinct, including isolates obtained from two members of the same household.

These data are particularly intriguing because they strongly suggest that *H. pylori* infections are produced by a large number of different clones. In fact, no two isolates yet studied appear to be alike. The discovery of the *absence* of clonality in *H. pylori* casts doubt on the intrinsic virulence of this species. It has been shown that most true bacterial pathogens are clonal, meaning that only a limited number of clones (strains) are associated with disease, as opposed to infection. For example, among all the serogroups of *E. coli* that naturally inhabit the gastrointestinal tract, only a small number of serogroups are capable of causing extra-intestinal tract infections, such as meningitis or bacteremia. Among enteric pathogens, this is also true for *Salmonella* and *Shigella*, although not for *C. jejuni*.

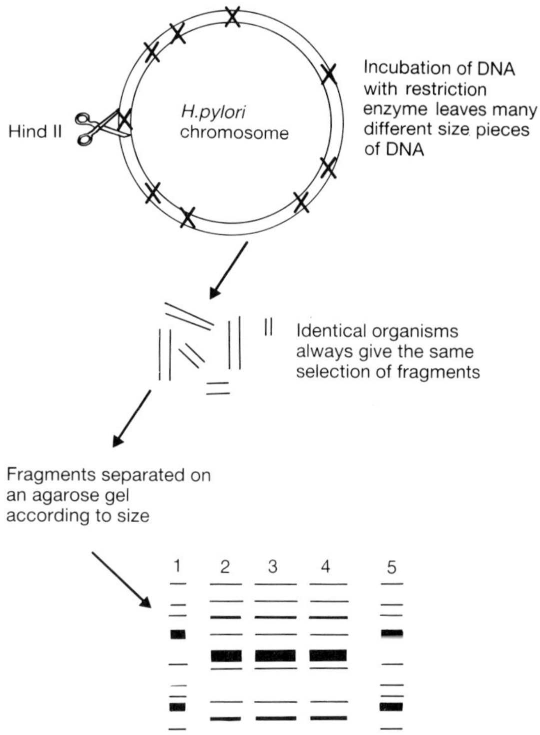

Fig. 9.4 Restriction digestion fingerprinting of a *Helicobacter pylori* isolate. The genomic DNA from the isolate is extracted and incubated with a restriction endonuclease (Hind II). The fragments are next electrophoretically separated on the basis of size in an agarose gel. Staining with ethidium bromide permits one to identify each unique strain by a distinctive pattern or "fingerprint." Strains 1 and 5 are identical as are strains 2, 3, and 4.

The genotypic data suggest that all *H. pylori* strains are equally competent at establishing infection, and that none are particularly pathogenic. Therefore, it would behove investigators to learn more about those properties of the species that permit it to become established in its natural reservoir, since these would be the traits that would most likely be highly conserved among all strains. Presumably the urease gene will be found in virtually all strains of *H. pylori*, indicating that it is an essential "housekeeping" gene.

While restriction endonuclease analysis of chromosomal DNA is an excellent tool to distinguish among strains, the number of fragments produced is far too large to examine adequately on a single gel. DNA probing of restriction digestion fragments, by the method of Southern hybridization, produces a discrete number of bands that are easier to analyze, and thus this method has been especially useful in highlighting restriction site polymorphism. One of the urease gene probes developed by Labigne-Roussel *et al.* appears to identify a restriction fragment length polymorphism (RFLP) of the urease region of *H. pylori* strains [10]. Coupled with REA, this technique should be quite useful in epidemiologic studies, and could also serve as a basis for a strain typing scheme.

Summary

Although little is currently known about the genetic and molecular basis of *H. pylori* infection or disease, molecular studies in *C. jejuni* have laid a foundation for the current and future genetic approach. Isolation and characterization of genes encoding *H. pylori* pathogenic properties, and construction of isogenic mutants by genetic exchange, should provide insights into the role of this species in the pathogenesis of gastric disease and into its natural history. The application of molecular methods such as molecular fingerprinting, DNA probe detection and DNA target amplification will help to elucidate the epidemiology of *H. pylori*, and hopefully will provide definitive answers to questions about the relationship between this microbe and human disease.

Glossary of terms for recombinant DNA methods

allelic replacement. A gene coding for a certain enzyme (e.g. urease) may have slight variations (alleles) in different strains. The original gene may be replaced by a modified gene (allele). When digested with restriction enzymes, the resulting pieces are different lengths (allelic polymorphism).

bacteriophage ("phage"). A virus, usually with a specific bacterial host. Recombinant DNA can be injected into a bacterial host by attaching it to the bacteriophage DNA.

cloned. This term is used when a gene is isolated and amplified by splicing it into a vector (a plasmid or a bacteriophage) and introducing the recombinant DNA molecule into a new host.

cosmid. A type of shuttle vector that can package large fragments of foreign DNA.

cryptic. These plasmids are present in bacteria (e.g. *C. jejuni*), but their function is unknown. They replicate in *C. jejuni*, whereas plasmids introduced from *E. coli* may not.

DNA probe. A manufactured, usually radiolabeled, piece of DNA or RNA which will attach to matching DNA in a test sample if such is present.

electroporation. The art of applying high voltage electrical energy to a bacterial culture to cause non-lethal damage to bacterial cell walls, which allows passage of plasmids into the cell via pores in the cell membranes.

G+C. In all DNA, bases are adenine (A), thymine (T), guanine (G), and cytosine (C), and A=T and G=C (because of complementary base pairs). G+C content is independent of A+T content. However, within the same genus, G+C content of DNA is similar (e.g. ≈35% for *C. jejuni* and *C. coli*). The melting point of DNA reflects its G+C content.

gene. The biologic unit of heredity. It occupies a defined position on the chromosome and is capable of reproduction. At its simplest level, one gene codes for one protein product.

genetic library. A random collection of DNA fragments contained within a vector, representing each gene. For example, a (bacterial) chromosome is cut into many small pieces with endonuclease so that the ends are "sticky." These pieces are inserted into plasmid or bacteriophage DNA, which also has been digested to give matching "sticky" ends. The joints are welded with ligase. After reinsertion into bacterial cells, each bacterial cell line will have a plasmid containing one small segment of the original DNA. All these cell lines form the "library."

isogenic mutant. A mutant bacterium created by replacing a normal gene with a similar "engineered" gene which is not transcribed (expressed), thus functionally deleting the gene.

ligate. Refers to action of DNA ligase. After pieces of DNA are cut with restriction enzymes, they usually have "sticky ends" (like Velcro), which means pieces of DNA from different sources can attach to each other via hydrogen bonding between matching base pairs at the ends. DNA ligase catalyzes the formation of covalent diester bonds and makes the join permanent. Ligases are used to weld fragments of DNA into plasmids after both have been cut with the same restriction enzyme (Fig. 9.5).

nucleic acid hybridization. The formation of double-stranded molecules of nucleic acid (DNA or RNA) that are complementary. Thus, a single-stranded probe molecule can react with a single-stranded, complementary target molecule, to form hybrids (duplexes).

operon. A collection of adjacent genes which are transcribed together, and result in different segments of the same metabolic pathway. An example is the lac-operon of *E. coli*, which codes the three enzymes necessary for the optimal utilization of lactose.

phenotype. The outward visible expression of the genetic constitution of an organism.

plasmid. Autonomously replicating circular DNA "mini-chromosomes" in bacteria. Multiple copies may be present, allowing the bacterium to produce large amounts of a protein product (e.g. penicillinase).

polymerase chain reaction. This is a method of amplifying tiny amounts of specific "target" DNA (1–50 pieces) so that they can be detected on gels or by DNA hybridization. DNA polymerase will produce the complementary DNA strand if a piece of single-stranded DNA is present and the necessary nucleotides are available. By attaching an engineered fragment of DNA to the polymerase enzyme, the polymerase is made specific and will only attach to an exact matching complementary strand of DNA. After this action, if the solution is heated, the strands separate, and new (excess) polymerase attaches to the original specific DNA sequence, and also to its complement. When cooled, two double-stranded DNA molecules are constructed. Each heating and cooling sequence doubles the amount of specific target DNA. Twenty cycles result in amplification by 10^6.

prime. Refers to the single-stranded DNA sequence which is attached to DNA polymerase prior to the polymerase chain reaction (PCR). This DNA is designed to be the complement of the DNA being probed for.

prokaryotic. Organisms without a nuclear membrane (e.g. bacteria). Their DNA corresponds directly to linear mRNA and linear amino acid sequences in proteins. In eukaryotes (e.g. man), DNA cannot be translated directly, as it contains "introns", sequences which must be excised before translatable RNA is obtained.

recombinant. Pieces of DNA which have been genetically engineered.

restriction endonucleases. These are enzymes which bacteria possess which chop up extraneous DNA. Restriction endonucleases (RE) probably protect the bacterial cell from incoming bacteriophage DNA. REs do not destroy the "good" host DNA, because only specific base sequences can be attacked by most REs. Susceptible sequences of host bacterial DNA may be protected by being methylated (the 5-methylcytosine is formed after the DNA is made). REs cut at specific base sequences and leave sticky (cohesive) ends (Eco R1 from *E. coli*) or blunt ends (Hind II from *Haemophilus influenzae*) (see Fig. 9.5).

restriction of foreign DNA. Refers to the ability of bacteria to destroy foreign DNA with bacterial restriction endonucleases.

16S ribosomal RNA. This is the RNA which makes up a part of the RNA of ribosomes. Its DNA is called 16S rDNA. It is duplicated 3–5 times in the chromosomal DNA of most bacteria, whereas there are thousands of copies of 16S ribosomal RNA in each cell. Bacteria contain 16S, 23S, and 5S molecular rRNA species; eukaryotic ribosomes have slightly different molecular weights.

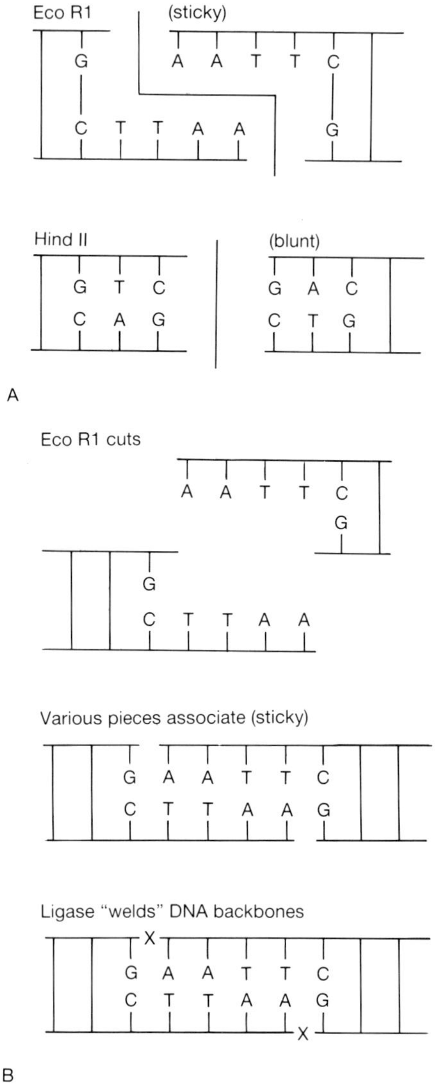

Fig. 9.5 A, Mechanism of action of two restriction endonucleases, Eco R1 and Hind II. B, The association of two strands of DNA, each restricted with Eco R1, creating "sticky ends." The enzyme DNA ligase then seals the single-strand breaks, joining the sticky ends to create a recombinant molecule.

shuttle (vector). A plasmid (e.g. pBR322) or a bacteriophage, which has the ability to carry DNA between species. Used to insert and retrieve segments of DNA into or from the bacterial chromosome.

suicide plasmid vector. A plasmid which does not survive in the host cell. It is used to exchange a modified gene with the wild-type gene, inactivating or reactivating it. It may also contain a transposon.

transposon. A segment of DNA containing a gene flanked by insertion elements. Has the ability to duplicate itself and insert somewhere else in an adjacent DNA molecule ("jumping gene"). In fact, the process occurs by a complicated crossover with staggered (sticky) DNA cuts and ligation rather than simply "jumping" (discovered by Barbara McClintock).

vector. Bacteriophages or plasmids into which engineered DNA is inserted so that it can be carried into host cells.

virulence. The degree of pathogenicity of an organism, as determined by its ability to produce pathogenic effects.

wild-type gene. The naturally occurring, original form of the gene, before it was tampered with.

References

1 Falkow, S. Molecular Koch's postulates applied to microbial pathogenicity. *Rev. Infect. Dis.* 1988;**10** (suppl):S274–6.

2 Labigne-Roussel, A, Harel, J, & Tompkins, LS. Gene transfer from *E. coli* to *Campylobacter* species: development of shuttle vectors for the genetic analysis of *Campylobacter jejuni*. *J. Bacteriol.* 1987;**169**:5320–23.

3 Labigne-Roussel, A, Courcoux, P, & Tompkins, LS. Gene disruption and gene replacement as a feasible approach for the mutagenesis of *Campylobacter jejuni*. *J. Bacteriol.* 1988;**170**: 1704–8.

4 Miller, JF, Dower, W, & Tompkins, LS. High-voltage electroporation of bacteria: genetic transformation of *Campylobacter jejuni* with plasmid DNA. *Proc. Natl. Acad. Sci. USA* 1988; **85**:856–60.

5 Labigne-Roussel, A, Cussac, V, & Courcoux, P. Shuttle cloning of genes responsible for urease activity from *Helicobacter pylori* and nucleotide sequence determination. *J. Bacteriol.* 1991;**173**: 1920–31.

6 Labigne-Roussel, A, & Courcoux, P. Cloning and expression of the urease genes from *Campylobacter pylori*. In: Mégraud, F, & Lamouliatte, H (eds), *Gastroduodenal Pathology and Campylobacter pylori*. Amsterdam: Elsevier, 1989.

7 Lee, A, O'Rourke, JL, Barringon, PJ, & Trust TJ. Mucus colonization as a determinant of pathogenicity in intestinal infection by *Campylobacter jejuni*: a mouse cecal model. *Infect. Immun.* 1986;**51**:536–46.
8 Moseley, SL, Huq, I, Alim, ARMA, So, M, Samapour-Motalebi, M, & Falkow, S. Detection of enterotoxigenic *Escherichia coli* by DNA colony hybridization. *J. Infect. Dis.* 1980;**142**: 892–8.
9 Courcoux, P, & Labigne, A. Identification of a specific nucleotide sequence for the detection of *Campylobacter pylori* by hybridization (abstract). *The Vth International Workshop on Campylobacter Infections*, Puerta Vallarta, Mexico, 1989.
10 Labigne-Roussel, A, Courcoux, P, & Moyen, E. Development of gene probes for the detection and characterization of *Campylobacter pylori*. In: Mégraud, F, & Lamouliatte, H (eds), *Gastroduodenal Pathology and Campylobacter pylori*. Amsterdam: Elsevier, 1989.
11 Langenberg, W, Rauws, EAJ, Widjojokusumo, A, Tytgat, GNJ, & Zanen, HC. Identification of *Campylobacter pyloridis* isolates by restriction endonuclease DNA analysis. *J. Clin. Microbiol.* 1986;**24**:414–17.

10: Randomized controlled trials of peptic ulcer therapy in the Helicobacter pylori era

W.L. PETERSON

Introduction

Randomized controlled trials (RCTs) of therapeutic agents for peptic ulcer have undergone a number of refinements during the past 10–20 years, but since the acceptance of endoscopy as the "gold standard" for diagnosis and follow-up, there have been few major changes. Whether the agent being studied reduced acid secretion, neutralized gastric acid, or had a mechanism of action other than an effect on gastric acidity, the design of RCTs has been virtually the same.

Recently, however, it has been suggested that *Helicobacter pylori* gastritis may play a role in the natural history of peptic ulcer disease [1]. Thus, the design of trials may need to be changed to incorporate an assessment of *H. pylori*. While some changes in the design of RCTs of peptic ulcer therapy are in order, the thrust of this discussion is that the crucial aspects of such trials have not changed. The goals of any randomized controlled trial should still be to answer a specific question or questions, to mimic "real life" situations regarding the patients studied and the conduct of the trial, and to arrive at a *confident* answer. The most important factors regarding the confidence with which someone can view a randomized controlled trial are the number of patients studied, the blinding process, and statistical considerations.

Studies designed to measure acute ulcer healing

Patient selection and exclusions

Carrying out randomized controlled trials is a difficult task at best, but overly restrictive exclusions make the trials even more difficult to complete in a timely fashion. In addition, trials should include the spectrum of patients who will ultimately be candidates for therapy with the new agent. Thus, as few patients as possible should be excluded.

The exclusion group should include patients with prior gastric surgery (other than simple oversew) and ulcers persisting or occurring under medical therapy (since such patients represent a special subgroup of ulcer patients to be studied separately); patients with a malignant ulcer; those who could not realistically complete the study; those with a contraindication to mucosal biopsy (e.g. anticoagulant therapy); and those in whom a medical illness presents a contraindication to the blinded administration of one drug or another. For example, patients with renal insufficiency might need altered dosing of drugs, which could not be accomplished in the blinded situation. Traditionally, patients with important bleeding from ulceration are also excluded.

In point of fact, no pharmacologic agent has been proved to prevent short-term recurrent bleeding, so this should be less of a problem. On the other hand, one would be reluctant to place a person whose ulcer has recently bled on a placebo for a 4–8 week period. Even though short-term bleeding is not an issue, it would seem desirable at least to initiate ulcer healing. Thus, if bleeders are used, they should be enrolled only in studies where no placebo arm is included.

Definition of ulcer being studied

Although the histology of an ulcer is basically the same regardless of its location in the stomach or duodenum, and although the pathogenic mechanisms are similar, the healing rates of ulcers differ depending upon their location. For example, ulcers in the prepyloric region tend to heal more slowly than duodenal ulcers of the same size [2]. Therefore, ulcer location should be strictly defined, with gastric ulcers defined as ulcers which are more than 2–3 cm proximal to the pylorus, prepyloric ulcers those which lie within the 2–3 cm proximal to the pylorus, channel ulcers those in the pyloric canal, and duodenal ulcers those ulcers confined to the duodenal bulb. Ulcers should be at least 4–5 mm in diameter, and are differentiated from erosions by the presence of depth.

Medications

Many future studies of ulcer healing will be directed toward the evaluation of a regimen or regimens designed to eradicate *H. pylori*. The control group for these studies will, in most instances, be a currently-available H2 (histamine) receptor antagonist. The use of a placebo should depend upon the question being asked. If the study is designed primarily to assess the acute healing of an ulcer, there are three reasons why at least some patients should be treated with a placebo. First, the proportion of patients healing on a placebo provides a "reference standard" of the study population compared to patients studied in other controlled trials. Second, since early studies suggest that H2 receptor antagonists and regimens designed to eradicate *H. pylori* will heal ulcers equally well [3], the natural inclination for an endoscopist at the follow-up endoscopy would be to assume that almost all ulcers will have healed. Thus, there may be a less-than-wholehearted attempt to examine the area of previous ulceration if no ulcer appears at first glance. The knowledge that a placebo group is included in the RCT will tend to make the endoscopist more thorough. Third, it is easier statistically to prove a regimen superior to placebo than it is to prove the regimen equal to another active agent.

On the other hand, if the hypothesis is that a regimen which eradicates *H. pylori* will produce *better* results than the H2 receptor antagonist (for example, in long-term remission) the need for a placebo is less important. Concern that treating a patient with placebo places a patient at undue risk is not supported by data [4].

Duration of therapy

Two factors should be considered in determining the duration of therapy. One factor is the length of time necessary to heal ulcers independent of the effect of medication on *H. pylori*. For gastric ulcers this is 8 weeks [5], and for duodenal ulcers 4–6 weeks [6]. The majority of patients will experience complete symptom relief *and* ulcer healing by these times. An interval endoscopy before these times is not recommended, since the standard of practice in "real life" is not to do so.

The second factor is the time required for eradication of *H. pylori*. Studies are now being conducted which will shed light on this issue.

Balance among treatment groups

There are several factors apart from therapeutic agents which have been suggested as important determinants of ulcer healing and/or ulcer recurrence. For example, a large ulcer will heal more slowly than a small ulcer [7]; ulcers in smokers tend to heal less rapidly than in non-smokers [8]; and ulcers in patients who have taken non-steroidal antiinflammatory drugs (NSAIDs) *may* be more likely to heal quickly (if the NSAID is discontinued) than ulcers in patients who have not taken NSAIDs previously. Therefore, a randomization scheme must be established to ensure that the treatment groups are balanced for these factors. Any imbalance between groups will possibly bias the results in favor of one treatment group or the other. For example, if all the smokers in a study were randomly assigned to group A, that study would be biased in favor of group B.

Gastric acid hypersecretion is another factor which may influence healing with an anti-secretory medication [9]. However, secretory testing is too time-consuming to be performed prior to randomization.

H. pylori status may also have an impact on short-term healing. Although determination of

H. pylori status will be important in future studies, it is not necessary to have this information prior to randomization in patients with duodenal ulcer. The reasoning for this is that virtually all patients with duodenal ulcer disease are already colonized with *H. pylori* [1], hence the chance of unbalanced treatment groups will be small in any study with adequate sample sizes. With gastric ulcers, there may be a substantial subgroup not colonized with *H. pylori* (e.g. NSAID-induced). Thus, knowledge of *H. pylori* status is necessary for proper randomization.

Determination of *H. pylori* status

All studies which have as one treatment arm a regimen designed to eradicate *H. pylori* should include an assessment of the presence or absence of the organism. At least in initial studies, it is important that information be gathered using all available diagnostic techniques. Thus, the presence of *H. pylori* should be demonstrated by reliable methods such as histology [10] and culture [11], supplemented by serology [12]. Where a breath test is available [13, 14], it should also be utilized to compare the results of therapy with the other diagnostic modalities. It is especially important at this stage of investigation that serum samples and, if resources are available, cultured organisms be saved for future analysis. For example, pathogenic factors may some day be found which differentiate strains of *H. pylori* which induce ulceration from those which do not.

End points

The primary end point in acute ulcer healing studies is, of course, healing of the ulcer. This is best defined as complete reepithelialization of the prior ulcer crater. Ulcer symptoms should also be assessed, although even patients taking placebo usually achieve rapid relief of ulcer symptoms. Even if symptoms persist, a healed ulcer satisfies the primary end point. At the time of follow-up endoscopy, mucosal biopsies of the antrum and fundus may be collected to assess the effect of therapy on mucosal histology. If the study is to be concluded after the acute phase, biopsy may also be taken of the duodenal bulb. However, if the patient is to be followed for ulcer recurrence, off therapy, the mucosal defect created by the biopsy may cloud the picture. Finally, it is important to determine the status of *H. pylori* after therapy. As mentioned above, this is best done by using all available modalities.

It should be pointed out that the absence of *H. pylori* immediately after therapy may reflect, in some patients, suppression of the organism rather than eradication. If that is the case, reexamination during long-term follow-up will again disclose the organism.

Blinding

It is incumbent upon those who design randomized controlled trials of ulcer therapy to do their absolute best to ensure that all study personnel associated with the study determine the various end points with as little potential bias as possible. Patients should also be blinded to the regimen they are receiving, not only to prevent an effect on ulcer healing, but also to prevent unintentional bias of study personnel. For example, patients may have less faith in one regimen or another and, either through poor compliance or psychologic factors, experience slower healing than they might otherwise experience if they did not know which medication they were receiving. In addition, if the patient is aware of which treatment he or she is receiving, it is eminently possible for that individual to unintentionally alert one of the study personnel. Thus, all medications should ideally be administered in a fashion that precludes the individual from knowing which he or she is receiving. This is commonly done by the concomitant administration of a dummy placebo for the medication to which the patient has not been assigned. For example, in a study comparing ranitidine against a bismuth compound, one group of patients would receive active ranitidine plus a bismuth dummy (placebo bismuth which is identical in appearance to active bismuth), while the other group receives active bismuth plus a ranitidine dummy.

A special problem with studies of bismuth compounds is the tendency of bismuth to stain the tongue and darken the stools. Until innovative methods are devised to produce such effects in patients not taking bismuth, these studies can never be considered completely blinded.

Separate personnel should be used for different aspects of the study. For example, the individual assessing ulcer symptoms must not be aware of the endoscopic status of the patient's ulcer (healed or unhealed). Likewise, the endoscopist assessing the presence or absence of the ulcer crater must have no knowledge of the patient's symptomatic response or, if adequate blinding for bismuth cannot be carried out, the color of the patient's stools. To blind the endoscopist it has been suggested that a charcoal mouth rinse be administered to patients before endoscopy and, in addition, it would seem prudent that a second physician sedate and intubate the patient. Then, the endoscopist of record can enter the room at a time when the patient will be less likely to inadvertently disclose any information.

Studies designed to measure long-term remission

Patient selection and exclusions

As with acute studies, the fewer exclusions the better. Indeed, any patient with an endoscopically documented history of ulcer disease, who is ulcer-free and symptom-free at the time of entry, is eligible. Exceptions include inability to take blinded medication, very short life expectancy, the need to take NSAIDs (unless that is the focus of the study), or the need to take any medication known or suspected to influence peptic ulcer.

Duration of study

Traditionally, patients are followed for 6–12 months. However, the longer the blinded follow-up, the better. The goal of therapy against *H. pylori* is cure of the disease, and in this situation, anything less than long-term remission is unsatisfactory.

Balance among treatment groups

Once one chooses the variable to be studied (e.g. prior acute therapy, *H. pylori* status at the time of enrollment, or maintenance therapy), one must then make sure that the two groups are balanced for other factors. For example, if one is assessing the effect of maintenance prostaglandin therapy, the groups should be balanced regarding prior acute therapy and *H. pylori* status. Other factors which must be considered include a history of excess alcohol intake or smoking, a history of early onset and/or severe ulcer disease, and the presence of duodenal scarring [15].

Medications

There are two types of long-term studies. In one, patients who have recently completed therapy are followed off all medications (or on placebo) to determine the relapse rate as a function of acute therapy and/or *H. pylori* status. In the other, patients without current ulcer are randomly assigned to a maintenance drug or to placebo. In either instance, the presence or absence of *H. pylori* must be determined.

Determination of *H. pylori* status

The crucial issues in future long-term studies of peptic ulcer are: (1) does prior eradication (or absence) of *H. pylori* predict prolonged remission?; and (2) does recrudescence of *H. pylori* infection herald relapse of ulcer? It is, therefore, mandatory to assess the presence or absence of *H. pylori* at the start and throughout the long-term study. Indeed, to ensure that any beneficial long-term effect of previous acute healing therapy on recurrence is not due to the drug *per se* (e.g. bismuth's presumed beneficial long-term effect might be related to bismuth itself, rather than to eradication of *H. pylori*), determination of *H. pylori* status is critical.

Definition of relapse

Three end points are of importance. One, for those who are initially *H. pylori*-negative, is continued freedom from infection or recrudescence. *H. pylori* status should be assessed independently of ulcer or symptom recurrence periodically throughout the study, with one time period about 4 weeks after completion of acute therapy, to define success or failure of antimicrobial therapy. A second end point is symptom recurrence, which is also determined independently from endoscopic ulcer recurrence. Such recurrence must be more than an occasional twinge of dyspepsia. If symptoms recur, endoscopy is done to confirm the presence of an ulcer (third end point). Presence of an ulcer indicates a symptomatic ulcer recurrence, while absence of ulceration indicates an ulcer-negative symptomatic recurrence. If such patients will require therapy with an interdicted medication, they must be removed from the study, otherwise they should continue.

Finally, while the importance of asymptomatic recurrences is problematic, it seems reasonable, at least early on, to acquire information on such recurrences. Thus, endoscopy should be performed routinely every 3–6 months to determine point prevalence of asymptomatic ulceration. Patients with asymptomatic ulceration should be continued on protocol, without therapy, as if an endoscopy had not been done. Such ulcers are of little concern and would never have been detected unless the patient was part of a study.

Blinding

Patients and study personnel alike must be unaware of prior therapy and unaware of *H. pylori* status throughout the study. Of course, any maintenance therapy given during the follow-up period must be blinded.

Statistical considerations and sample sizes

There are two factors to be considered when planning the sample sizes for RCTs: (1) enough patients must be enrolled to ensure statistical reliability; (2) there must be enough patients studied to provide clinical believability. For example, it may be possible to show a statistically significant difference between drug A and drug B with only 20 patients per group. However, a study with 40 patients per group would be more believable. Investigators must balance these two goals, since every patient beyond the minimum necessary for statistical purposes adds to the expense and duration of the study.

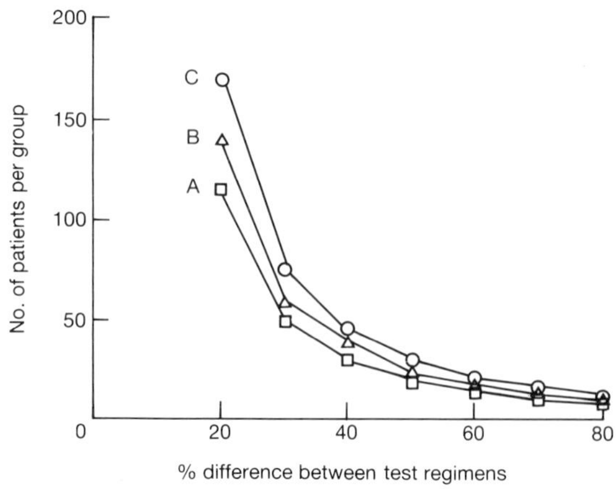

Fig. 10.1 Approximate number of patients needed per group for a study of two regimens. A, $\alpha = 0.05$, $\beta = 0.20$; B, $\alpha = 0.05$, $\beta = 0.10$; C, $\alpha = 0.02$, $\beta = 0.10$. As an example, if one predicts that ulcers will heal in 40% of one group and in 80% of the other group (difference = 40%), 40 patients must be enrolled in each group to ensure an α error of no more than 5% and a β error of no more than 10%.

In planning the minimum sample size of a study necessary for statistical purposes, one must take into account type I (α) and type II (β) (see Fig. 10.1). A type I error is the likelihood

Table 10.1 Healing study: comparison of a new ulcer therapy against placebo. The new therapy has an actual 8-week healing rate equal to that of ranitidine (≈80%). Placebo has a healing rate of 40% or less

Level of significance	Probability (power)	Sample size* required for each treatment: One-sided	Two-sided
0.05	0.70	19	23
0.05	0.80	23	28
0.05	0.90	29	35
0.05	0.95	35	41
0.01	0.70	29	33
0.01	0.80	34	39
0.01	0.90	42	47
0.01	0.95	49	55

* The number of patients required on each treatment to secure the indicated probability of obtaining a significant effect at indicated level.

that results of a study which are statistically significantly different occurred by chance, the recognized maximum for which is 5% (the *P* value). A type II error is the likelihood that a study which finds no significant difference (i.e. *P* value > 0.05) missed a true difference of a given amount. In general, one would like the type II error to be no more than 10–20%.

In planning ulcer healing studies, one first makes an assumption regarding results with the control regimen, and then what results one would consider clinically important for the test regimen. With these figures in hand, one consults standard tables to determine sample sizes necessary to limit type I and II errors to appropriate levels [16]. The smaller the difference between the two regimens, the larger the sample sizes needed (Fig. 10.1).

A more exact estimation of sample sizes can be derived from statistical packages. Tables 10.1–6 are derived from a printout of sample size calculations from the Clinstat package [17]. These samples may be of use in planning clinical studies of *H. pylori* therapy.

Table 10.2 Healing study: comparison of a new ulcer therapy with an H2 receptor antagonist (80% healing in 8 weeks). Sample sizes required to show if the new drug is at least 20% less effective than H2 receptor antagonists (less than 60% healing)

Level of significance	Probability (power)	Sample size required for each treatment	
		One-sided	Two-sided
0.05	0.70	59	74
0.05	0.80	74	91
0.05	0.90	98	119
0.05	0.95	121	144
0.01	0.70	95	110
0.01	0.80	114	131
0.01	0.90	145	164
0.01	0.95	173	194

Table 10.3 Same study as Table 10.2, sample sizes required to show if the drug is 10% less effective than H2 receptor antagonists (less than 70% healing)

Level of significance	Probability (power)	Sample size required for each treatment	
		One-sided	Two-sided
0.05	0.70	196	251
0.05	0.80	251	313
0.05	0.90	339	412
0.05	0.95	423	505
0.01	0.70	324	380
0.01	0.80	395	457
0.01	0.90	506	576
0.01	0.95	608	685

Table 10.4 Healing study: comparison of healing rate for a new drug against standard H2 receptor antagonist therapy. Study designed to detect a healing rate 10% better than that of H2 receptor antagonists (90% healing vs 80% in 8 weeks)

Level of significance	Probability (power)	Sample size required for each treatment	
		One-sided	Two-sided
0.05	0.70	139	177
0.05	0.80	177	219
0.05	0.90	237	286
0.05	0.95	293	349
0.01	0.70	227	264
0.01	0.80	275	317
0.01	0.90	350	397
0.01	0.95	419	471

Table 10.5 Relapse study: comparison of an H2 receptor antagonist against therapy which eradicates *H. pylori*. Study design assumes an actual 12-month relapse rate in the H2 receptor antagonist group of 80%, vs 20% or less in the *H. pylori* evadicated group. Note that the sample sizes are very small and, regardless of the significance of the result, would be unlikely to convince the average physician

Level of significance	Probability (power)	Sample size required for each treatment	
		One-sided	Two-sided
0.05	0.70	9	11
0.05	0.80	11	13
0.05	0.90	14	16
0.05	0.95	16	19
0.01	0.70	14	16
0.01	0.80	16	18
0.01	0.90	19	22
0.01	0.95	22	25

Table 10.6 Relapse study: comparison of an H2 receptor antagonist against *Helicobacter pylori* therapy in a population susceptible to reinfection. Relapse rate in the *H. pylori*-treated group is worsened by a 30% per annum reinfection rate.

Level of significance	Probability (power)	Sample size required for each treatment: One-sided	Two-sided
0.05	0.70	17	21
0.05	0.80	21	25
0.05	0.90	27	32
0.05	0.95	32	38
0.01	0.70	27	31
0.01	0.80	31	36
0.01	0.90	38	43
0.01	0.95	45	50

Regardless of the statistical significance of the result, sample sizes must be sufficient to convince clinicians that a new therapy has been adequately evaluated. In the United States, trials with less than 150 patients are unlikely to draw much attention. An example of this principle is the recent study reported by Rauws & Tytgat [18]. Fifty patients were treated for duodenal ulcer using bismuth subcitrate alone (26 patients) or bismuth plus antibiotic (24 patients). *H. pylori* was eradicated in 17 patients, none of whom relapsed in 12 months. In patients with continuing *H. pylori*, relapse occurred in 89%. The difference was highly significant ($P < 0.001$), but the number of patients in the successfully treated group was very small. In future studies it is hoped that larger numbers will be included.

References

1 Graham, D. *Campylobacter pylori* and peptic ulcer disease. *Gastroenterology* 1989;**96**:615–25.
2 Lauritsen, K, Bytzer, P, Hansen, J, Bekker, C, & Rask-Madsen, J. Comparison of ranitidine and high-dose antacid in the treatment of prepyloric or duodenal ulcer. A double-blind controlled trial. *Scand. J. Gastroenterol.* 1985;**20**:123–8.
3 Marshall, BJ, Goodwin, CS, Warren, JR, *et al.* Prospective double-blind trial of duodenal ulcer relapse after eradication of *Campylobacter pylori*. *Lancet* 1988;**ii**:1437–42.
4 Schiller, LR, & Fordtran, JS. Ulcer complications during short-term therapy of duodenal ulcer with active agents and placebo. *Gastroenterology* 1986; **90**:478–81.
5 Isenberg, JI, Peterson, WL, Elashoff, JD, *et al.* Healing of benign gastric ulcer with low dose antacid or cimetidine: a double-blind, randomized, placebo-controlled trial. *N. Engl. J. Med.* 1983;**308**:1319–24.
6 Jones, DB, Howden, CW, Burget, DW, Kerr, GD, & Hunt, RH. Acid suppression in duodenal ulcer: a meta-analysis to define optimal dosing with antisecretory drugs. *Gut* 1987;**28**:1120–27.
7 Scheurer, V, Witzel, L, Halter, F, Keller, H, Huber, R, & Galeazzi, R. Gastric and duodenal ulcer healing after placebo treatment. *Gastroenterology* 1977;**72**:838–41.
8 Sonnenberg, A, Muller-Lissner, S, Vogel, E, *et al.* Predictors of duodenal ulcer healing and relapse. *Gastroenterology* 1981;**81**;1061–7.
9 Collen, MJ, Stanczak, VJ, & Ciarleglio, CA. Refractory duodenal ulcers (nonhealing duodenal ulcers with standard doses of anti-secretory medication). *Dig. Dis. Sci.* 1989;**34**:233–7.
10 Peterson, WL, Lee, E, & Feldman, M. Relationship between *Campylobacter pylori* and gastritis in healthy humans after placebo or indomethacin. *Gastroenterology* 1988;**95**:1185–97.
11 Goodwin, CS, Blincow, ED, Warren, JR, Waters, TE, Sanderson, CR, & Easton L. Evaluation of cultural techniques for isolating *Campylobacter pyloridis* from endoscopic biopsies of gastric mucosa. *J. Clin. Pathol.* 1985;**38**:1127–31.
12 Evans, DJ, Evans, DG, Graham, DY, & Klein PD. A sensitive and specific serologic test for detection of *Campylobacter pylori* infection. *Gastroenterology* 1989;**96**:1004–8.
13 Graham, DY, Klein, PD, Evans, DJ, *et al.* *Campylobacter pylori* detected noninvasively by the ^{13}C-urea breath test. *Lancet* 1987;**i**:1174–7.
14 Marshall, BJ, & Surveyor, I. Carbon-14 urea breath test for the diagnosis of *Campylobacter pylori* associated gastritis. *J. Nucl. Med.* 1988;**29**:11–16.
15 van Deventer, GM, Elashoff, JD, Reedy, TJ, Schneidman, D, & Walsh, JH. A randomized study of maintenance therapy for ranitidine to prevent the recurrence of duodenal ulcer. *N. Engl. J. Med.* 1989;**320**:1113–9.
16 Fleiss, JL. *Statistical Methods for Rates and Proportions*, New York: Wiley, 1973, pp. 176–94.
17 Chassan, JB, & Clinstat, JB Chassan Consultations, 763 Bloomfield Avenue, Montclair, New Jersey 07042, USA (201) 746-9555.
18 Rauws, EAJ, & Tytgat, GN. Cure of duodenal ulcer associated with eradication of *Helicobacter pylori*. *Lancet* 1990;**335**:1233–5.

11: Helicobacter pylori and duodenal ulcer

C.P. DOOLEY

Introduction

Duodenal ulcer is viewed as the common end point of a group of heterogeneous disorders [1, 2]; the multiple pathophysiologic abnormalities described in patients with duodenal ulcer have supported this hypothesis [1, 3]. Some authors have maintained, however, that peptic ulcer disease (including gastric ulcers) is a homogeneous disorder [4]. This hypothesis is based on a number of factors, including the uniform response to medical therapy and the similar natural history noted with almost all ulcers.

The discovery and isolation of *Helicobacter pylori* [5] has added significant support to the hypothesis that duodenal ulcer disease is a homogeneous disorder: *H. pylori* has been isolated from the gastric antrum in up to 100% of cases of duodenal ulcer [6–13] suggesting that *H. pylori* infection is an essential component of duodenal ulcer disease.

Much of the research examining the role of *H. pylori* in duodenal ulcer disease has focused on the effect treating the infection has on the course of the syndrome in the short term [14, 15]. However, much information has been generated about duodenal ulcer in the pre-*H. pylori* era [1]. It is important that these data be integrated with, and reassessed in the light of, data emerging since the recognition of *H. pylori*. This chapter highlights important areas of disagreement between what is known about *H. pylori* and what is known about duodenal ulcer disease, in the hope of stimulating research that will reconcile these differences.

Epidemiology

Epidemiologically, duodenal ulcer disease is extremely dynamic [1]. There is some evidence to suggest that the incidence of duodenal ulcer disease is declining in developed countries, and that the male : female ratio also has been declining [1]. In developed countries, duodenal ulcers are more common than gastric, the incidence of ulcer disease increases with age, ulcers are more common in urban compared to rural areas, and also more common in lower occupational classes. There is a significant familial aggregation in duodenal ulcer disease, with up to 50% of patients having a positive family history. Subjects with blood group O, and subjects who are non-secretors of blood group substances, also have an increased risk of developing duodenal ulcer disease.

The development of non-invasive tests for the diagnosis of *H. pylori* infection has provided information on the epidemiology of the infection (see Chapter 4). These data show that *H. pylori* infection is more common and occurs at an earlier age in populations of developing countries [16, 17]. Although peptic ulcer is common in these populations, accurate data on the incidence of duodenal ulcer are difficult to obtain. Even between developed nations there appear to be differences in the prevalence of the infection [18, 19], which have not been correlated with differences in the prevalence of duodenal ulcer.

The incidence of duodenal ulcer increases with increasing age, paralleling an age-related increased prevalence of *H. pylori* infection in developed nations [16, 18]. In all studies of the epidemiology of *H. pylori* infection, no differences in the rates of infection of males and females have been noted. If the incidence of duodenal ulcer disease is indeed declining in the West, it should reflect a decline in the incidence of the infection. While some familial aggregation has been reported in cases of *H. pylori* infection [20, 21], there have been no reports of an association between the infection and blood group and secretor status. Of some interest too, is the reversal of the duodenal : gastric ulcer ratio in Japan [22], a country for which few data are available on *H. pylori* infection rates.

It is important to note that there are significant discrepancies between what is known about the epidemiology of duodenal ulcer disease and the preliminary data available concerning the epidemiology of *H. pylori* infection. Future studies on the epidemiology of duodenal ulcer disease should incorporate the population prevalence of *H. pylori* infection as a stratifying variable, so that comparisons may be made with other countries.

Another important point that emerges from the study of the epidemiology of *H. pylori* infection is that, at any point in time, the majority of infected subjects do not have clinical disease [16–19]. In postulating a significant role for *H. pylori* in the pathogenesis of duodenal ulcer disease, it must therefore be explained why such is the case. Much of the research to date has ignored the important question — what factors, if any, distinguish *H. pylori* infection in duodenal ulcer from the infection in subjects who fail to develop ulcer disease?

H. pylori infection in patients with duodenal ulcer

H. pylori is a genetically diverse organism [23] and thus one could hypothesize that certain strains might be "ulcerogenic." Alternatively, the host response to the infection might differ between patients who develop ulcers and those who remain asymptomatic. The following sections examine the evidence that *H. pylori* infection is a different disease in patients who develop ulcer disease.

The infection

Numerous virulence factors have been postulated for *H. pylori* infection. These include motility [24], abundant urease production [25], production of proteases [26] and lipases [27], cell penetration [28], *N*-acetylneuraminyllactose-binding hemagglutinin [29] and a number of cytotoxins [30–32]. To date, there is little information concerning possible differences in these virulence factors between isolates from ulcer patients and infected subjects without ulcers. Bode *et al.* have described penetration of the bacteria into cells of the duodenal bulb in patients with duodenal ulcer only [28]. This interesting finding has not been reported by others but suggests that ultrastructural studies of the duodenal bulb should be performed. *In vitro* studies with cultured cell lines might provide a model for studying this property of *H. pylori* isolates.

Cytotoxic activity has been noted in supernatants of isolates of *H. pylori* [30–33]. Of significant interest is the report by Figura *et al.* [33] that cytotoxic activity is more common in isolates from duodenal ulcer patients than in isolates from patients with non-ulcer dyspepsia. Similarly, Cover *et al.* have reported [32] that antibodies directed against *H. pylori* cytotoxin are found more commonly in serum from patients with duodenal ulcer disease than in the serum of infected asymptomatic subjects. Preliminary data suggest [34, 35] that *H. pylori* may also elaborate proteins which suppress acid secretion from the parietal cell. It is not known if isolates from symptomatic and asymptomatic groups differ in their ability to synthesize these proteins. Given the central role of acid secretion in duodenal ulcer, the interactions between the bacterium and parietal cell function deserve further scrutiny.

Currently, there are few studies that have attempted to define differences between *H. pylori* isolates from different groups of infected subjects. At the least, authors should report on the source of *H. pylori* isolates used for studies of virulence factors, and ideally, all studies should be stratified according to differing sources of isolates. Demonstrating significant differences in virulence among isolates from patients with duodenal ulcer would add support to the contention that *H. pylori* plays a causative role in this disease.

The host response

It is accepted that *H. pylori* elicits an inflammatory response in the laminal propria of the underlying gastric mucosa [36, 37], and such is seen in both symptomatic [6–13] and asymptomatic [13, 18, 38, 39] subjects. Are there quantifiable differences in the host response between those who develop ulcers and those who do not? In discussing this question, gastric histology, duodenal histology, and the immune response are examined.

Gastric histology

Prior to the discovery of *H. pylori*, antral gastritis had been noted in almost all duodenal ulcer patients [40–45], and this has now been correlated with the presence of *H. pylori* [6–13]. There is some evidence that the antral gastritis in patients with duodenal ulcer is more severe than antral gastritis observed in asymptomatic controls [43, 44]. It has also been noted that antral gastritis may be more severe in patients who develop prepyloric ulcers when compared to those with duodenal ulcers [40].

Of note too are the reports of fundic histology in patients with duodenal ulcer [40, 42–45]. Compared to asymptomatic controls with gastritis, the corpus is much less inflamed in patients with duodenal ulcer [40, 42–45]. *H. pylori* may be present on the uninflamed corpus [46] (Fig. 11.1). Furthermore, it is noteworthy that gastritis progresses rapidly in the corpus after duodenal ulcer surgery [42, 45].

It is not known if these differences in histology can be correlated with the differences in gastric function that have been noted between patients with ulcers and asymptomatic controls, specifically the high acid output observed in a significant minority of patients with duodenal ulcer [1]. The study by Meikle *et al.* failed to demonstrate a relationship between gastric histology and gastric acid output in patients with duodenal ulcer [45]. Studies of acid secretion in patients with duodenal ulcer should now be stratified by histology and acid-modulating factors produced by the patient's isolate. The *H. pylori* status and gastric histology of controls utilized in studies of gastric function should also be defined. It is our experience that subjects who undergo repeated gastrointestinal intubation have a high rate of infection with *H. pylori* (Dooley, CP, & Cohen, H, unpublished data), and this may be the experience in other laboratories [47].

Duodenal histology

In attempting to explain why a gastric pathogen might cause disease in the duodenum, researchers have focused their attention on the histology of the duodenal bulb. Findings of

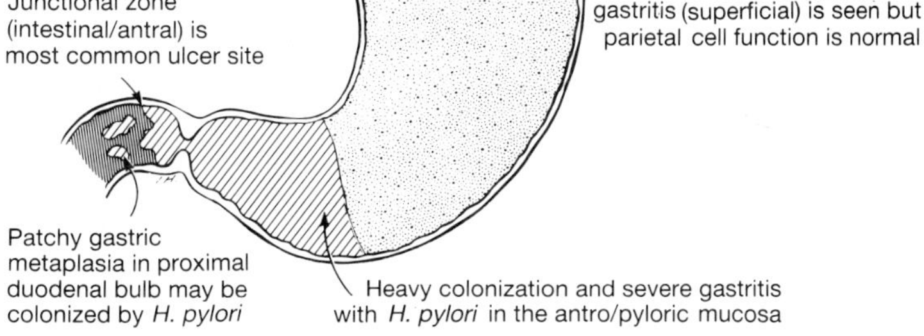

Fig. 11.1 Model of duodenal ulcer disease.

note are gastric metaplasia (GM), *H. pylori*, and duodenitis (Fig. 11.1).

Gastric metaplasia. Gastric metaplasia (GM) is defined as the replacement of the absorptive columnar cells, which normally cover the duodenal villi, by columnar cells rich in neutral mucin similar to those normally seen lining the stomach. The importance of GM is that it acts as a focus for *H. pylori* infection of the bulb. Gastric metaplasia has been noted in the bulb of almost every patient with a duodenal ulcer [15, 48, 49]. The etiology of this finding is unknown.

Gastric metaplasia is common in the asymptomatic population, suggesting that it may be a normal (primary) finding [50, 51]. However, there is good evidence that GM may be a response to increased acid loads in the duodenum [48, 49, 52–54]. Conversely, the author has been unable to demonstrate a correlation between serum levels of pepsinogen I and GM in asymptomatic subjects (CP Dooley & H Cohen, unpublished data). Alternatively, GM may be the consequence of chronic inflammation [55–57], although this, again, has not been noted in asymptomatic subjects [51]. I suspect that GM is found in many subjects, symptomatic and asymptomatic, but that its extent is greater in patients with duodenal ulcer. The cause-and-effect relationships between increased acid load, duodenitis, and GM need to be defined. There are some data to suggest that treatment of duodenal ulcer with a bismuth preparation may induce a regression of GM [58, 59], implying that inflammation may be the significant factor in these patients.

Is the presence or extent of GM a risk factor for the development of duodenal ulcer disease in infected subjects? We have found GM in the bulb of asymptomatic Hispanics less frequently than in asymptomatic Caucasians [39]. Does this finding explain the discrepancy between prevalence rates of *H. pylori* infection and duodenal ulcer in these populations? More studies of GM and its relationship to the natural history of duodenal ulcer are required.

It is important to note at this point that there is some confusion in the literature as to the distinction between GM and gastric heterotopia (GH) of the duodenum. Gastric heterotopia is defined as the presence of full-thickness body-type gastric mucosa with chief and parietal cells in the duodenum. Some authors describe the finding of GH in the same setting as GM [53, 60], and I believe that some heterotopia will be found in all cases of GM if a careful examination is made. In this setting, I believe that the heterotopia is a minor finding. Alternatively, it has been suggested that GM, as described above, might be associated with pyloric gland metaplasia, which would not be distinguishable from Brunner's gland hyperplasia [61]. Therefore, all GM would be associated with a degree of glandular metaplasia. True GH is, I believe, a congenital lesion with specific macroscopic and microscopic findings and is not of clinical significance [61–63].

H. pylori. The bacterium is found associated with GM in the bulb of the majority of patients with duodenal ulcer [15, 48] (Fig. 11.2). We have never found the bacterium associated with GM in asymptomatic subjects [39, 51]. There are no data available concerning the factors that favor duodenal colonization with *H. pylori*.

Duodenitis. Typically, the findings of GM and *H. pylori* are associated with duodenitis in patients with duodenal ulcer [15, 48]. However, duodenitis is not a finding that is specific for duodenal ulcer: we have noted duodenitis in 9% of asymptomatic subjects, and duodenitis is also found commonly in patients with non-ulcer dyspepsia [48, 55]. The study by Jenkins *et al.* [64] suggests that the duodenitis in patients with ulcers or erosions of the bulb differs from that found in those without such lesions. The distinguishing features are a markedly increased neutrophil infiltrate, villous atrophy, decreased plasma cell infiltrate, and ulceration [64]. The etiology of inflammation in duodenitis is unknown: is it acid-induced, or a consequence of *H. pylori* infection, or a result of other undetermined factors?

As with gastric histology, the differences in duodenal mucosal secretory function between asymptomatic subjects and patients with

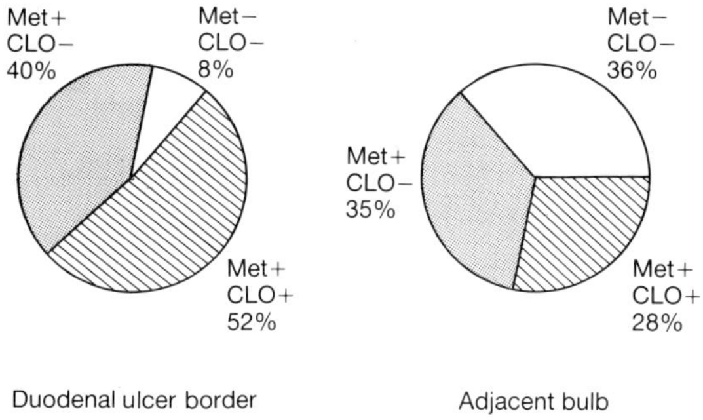

Fig. 11.2 Gastric metaplasia in 88 patients with duodenal ulcer. CLO, *Campylobacter*-like organism; Met, gastric metaplasia.

ulcers [65] do not correlate with differences in duodenal histology [66]. Does *H. pylori* affect duodenal mucosal function? Are there derangements of duodenal mucosal function that are permissive of ulceration?

The immune response

It is known that both systemic [67] and local [68] humoral immune responses are stimulated by *H. pylori*. It is also known that *H. pylori* stimulates a cellular immune response and increases expression of class II transplantation antigens [69]. It is not known whether there are differences in the immune response between infected subjects who develop ulcers and those who do not. This is an area that deserves closer scrutiny.

H. pylori and the natural history of duodenal ulcer

Currently, there is no proof that *H. pylori* infection actually causes ulceration. Animal models of the infection demonstrate that the bacterium causes histologic gastritis [70, 71]. More recently, gastric erosions have been observed in a germ-free rat model of the acute infection [72]. An animal model that incorporates the histologic findings of the human duodenum has not been developed. Therefore, much of the evidence suggesting a role for *H. pylori* in the pathogenesis of duodenal ulcer is based on empirical data. These data may be divided into three categories: (1) therapy of active disease; (2) effects on short-term recurrence rates; and (3) relationship to long-term outcome in duodenal ulcer disease.

Therapy of active disease

It is notable that clearance of *H. pylori* infection is not required for healing of the ulcer crater. For example, healing rates for colloidal bismuth subcitrate (CBS) are similar to those achieved with cimetidine [10, 73]. Clearance of the infection is not required for the healing effect of CBS [10, 15], although CBS may be less effective in the *H. pylori*-negative patient [74]. Antibiotic treatment of duodenal ulcer has been poorly studied and the data are equivocal [75–78]. Clearance of *H. pylori* infection may accelerate the rate of healing of the ulcer crater [15, 79], but this finding requires better definition.

It would be useful to know if CBS could heal *H. pylori*-negative (HP−) ulcers as well as *H. pylori*-positive (HP+) ulcers. HP− duodenal ulcers are rare, however, so the question can only be addressed in gastric ulcer where 30–40% of patients are HP− (see below).

Despite adequate therapy, a minority of ulcer craters fail to heal and are termed refractory [80]. Refractoriness is generally unpredictable, but appears to be associated with cigarette smoking, and poorly associated with acid hypersecretion [1]. Some of these patients respond to continued treatment with higher doses of H2 receptor antagonists [80]. A number of studies suggest that CBS is more effective than H2 receptor antagonists in these patients [81, 82]. Preliminary data suggest [83] that this effect of bismuth is related to its antibacterial effect. Further studies are needed in this interesting subset of patients.

Relationship of *H. pylori* to short-term recurrence rates

It has long been noted that recurrence of ulcer disease (at 12 months) in patients on no maintenance therapy, following treatment of the ulcer crater with CBS, is less than that seen in patients treated with H2 receptor antagonists [84–87]. Studies from a number of different institutions demonstrate [14, 15, 79, 88] that this effect of bismuth correlates closely with its antibacterial effect, such that the patient in whom *H. pylori* is cleared has almost no risk of developing recurrent disease in the 12 month follow-up period. If possible, these data should be confirmed in large double-blind placebo-controlled trials.

Despite the close correlation of recurrences with *H. pylori* status, it must be noted that sucralfate is reported to have lower recurrence rates than cimetidine in a 2 year follow-up study [89]. The sucralfate effect seems to be weaker, however, since large numbers of patients are necessary to demonstrate different relapse rates. In small studies where CBS and/or antibacterial drugs have been compared with H2 blockers, large, highly significant differences in relapse are the rule [15, 84]. Perhaps the effect of bismuth is the result of a non-specific cytoprotective effect, although the close association between infection and recurrence argues against this.

It should be noted also that recurrences are episodic and unpredictable [1]. Smoking is a significant predictor of duodenal ulcer recurrence [90]. However, none of these factors can predict the time of recurrence in the individual patient; the same is true for *H. pylori* infection, unless it can be shown that the activity of the infection or the host response to the infection varies with time. Little is known of the dynamics affecting recurrence rates.

H. pylori and long-term outcome in duodenal ulcer disease

There are few studies on the long-term outcome in duodenal ulcer disease. Studies of the natural history of ulcer disease in the community suggest [91, 92] that duodenal ulcer "burns out" over a period of 12–15 years. Correlation of this phenomenon with *H. pylori* status and gastric histology would be of interest. Is the "burn-out" related to proximal progression of the gastritis, with subsequent diminution of acid secretion? It is also of interest that some patients develop gastric ulcer during follow-up, and this is reported to be associated with proximal progression of the gastritis [40] (Fig. 11.3).

Summary

There is much evidence supporting a role for *H. pylori* infection in the pathogenesis of duodenal ulcer disease: *H. pylori* is found in almost every patient with duodenal ulcer; the associated gastric and duodenal histology may be unique, although this requires further study; there is some evidence that the infection may be more virulent in patients with duodenal

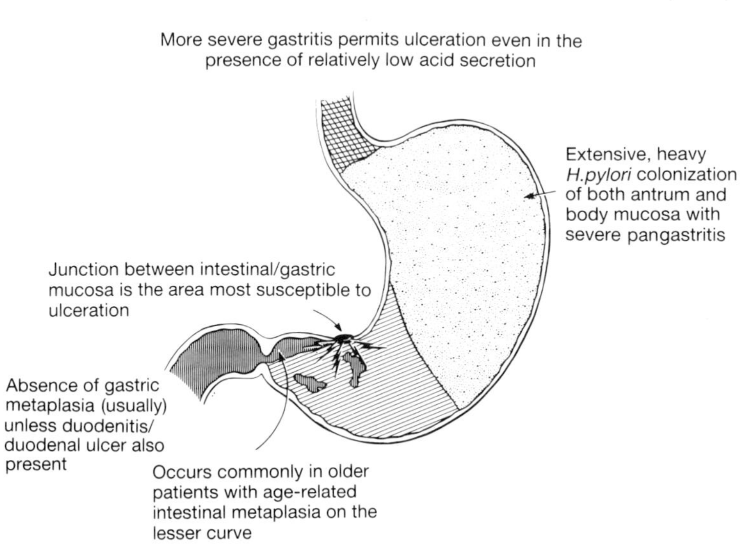

Fig. 11.3 Model of gastric ulcer disease.

ulcer; *H. pylori* may have a role in refractory ulcers; and, most importantly, *H. pylori* status is a major predictor of relapse.

This evidence has to be tempered by the realization that there are some contrary data: there are major discrepancies between the epidemiologies of duodenal ulcer and *H. pylori* infection; it is not known how *H. pylori* interacts with other factors known to be of significance in the pathogenesis of duodenal ulcer, such as acid secretion and cigarette smoking; most ulcers heal regardless of *H. pylori* status; and *H. pylori* alone does not explain the episodic nature of ulcer disease.

Conclusion

I believe that *H. pylori* infection, while not being a sufficient factor alone, is the major determinant of duodenal ulcer disease. This opinion is based on its universality in duodenal ulcer (unlike acid hypersecretion and smoking), and the consistent relationship (to date) with recurrence rates. It is reasonable, at this time, to offer the patient who suffers from frequent recurrences of duodenal ulcer a course of therapy aimed at eradicating the infection. Treatment of the infection is outlined in Chapter 13.

References

1 Soll, AH. Duodenal ulcer and drug therapy. In: Sleisenger, MH, & Fordtran, JS (eds), *Gastrointestinal Disease*, 4th edn. Philadelphia: WB Saunders, 1989, pp. 814–79.

2 Spiro, HM. Peptic ulcer is not a disease — only a sign. *J. Clin. Gastroenterol.* 1987;**9**:623–4.

3 Rotter, JI. Gastric and duodenal ulcers are each many different diseases. *Dig. Dis. Sci.* 1981;**26**: 154–60.

4 Kirk, RM. Are gastric and duodenal ulcers separate diseases or do they form a continuum? *Dig. Dis. Sci.* 1981;**26**:149–54.

5 Warren, JR, & Marshall, BJ. Unidentified curved bacillus on gastric epithelium in active chronic gastritis (letter). *Lancet* 1983;**i**:1273–5.

6 Rollason, TP, Stone, J, & Rhodes, JM. Spiral organisms in endoscopic biopsies of the human stomach. *J. Clin. Pathol.* 1984;**37**:23–6.

7 Marshall, BJ, & Warren, JR. Unidentified curved bacilli in the stomach of patients with gastritis and peptic ulceration. *Lancet* 1984;**i**:1311–5.

8 Rauws, EAJ, Langenberg, W, Houthoff, HJ, Zanen, HC, & Tytgat, GNJ. *Campylobacter pyloridis*-associated chronic active gastritis. A prospective study of its prevalence and the effects of antibacterial and antiulcer treatment. *Gastroenterology* 1988;**94**:33–40.

9 Steer, HW. The gastro-duodenal epithelium in peptic ulceration. *J. Pathol.* 1985;**146**:355–62.

10 Dooley, CP, McKenna, D, Humphreys, H, *et al.* Histological gastritis in duodenal ulcer: relationship to *Campylobacter pylori* and effect of ulcer therapy. *Am. J. Gastroenterol.* 1988;**83**: 278–82.

11 Marshall, BJ, McGechie, DB, Rogers, PA, & Glancy, RJ. Pyloric *Campylobacter* infection and gastroduodenal disease. *Med. J. Aust.* 1985;**142**: 439–44.

12 Price, AB, Levi, J, Dolby, JM, *et al. Campylobacter pyloridis* in peptic ulcer disease: microbiology, pathology, and scanning electron microscopy. *Gut* 1985;**26**:1183–8.

13 Pettross, CW, Appleman, MD, Cohen, H, Valenzuela, JE, Chandrasoma, P, & Laine, L. Prevalence of *Campylobacter pylori* and association with antral mucosal histology in subjects with and without upper gastrointestinal symptoms. *Dig. Dis. Sci.* 1988;**33**:649–53.

14 Coghlin, JG, Gilligan, D, Humphreys, H, *et al. Campylobacter pylori* and relapse of duodenal ulcers. *Lancet* 1987;**ii**:1109–11.

15 Marshall, BJ, Goodwin, CS, Warren, JR, *et al.* Prospective double-blind trial of duodenal ulcer relapse after eradication of *Campylobacter pylori*. *Lancet* 1988;**ii**:1437–42.

16 Megraud, F, Brassens-Rabbe, MP, Denis, F, Touhami, M, & Hoa, DQ. *Campylobacter pylori* infection — evidence for a worldwide distribution and a high prevalence in developing countries (abstract). *Gastroenterology* 1989;**96**:A338.

17 Klein, PD, The Gastrointestinal Physiology Working Group of Cayetano Haeredia and The Johns Hopkins Universities, Graham, DY, *et al.* High prevalence of *Campylobacter pylori* infection in poor and rich Peruvian children determined by ^{13}C urea breath test (abstract). *Gastroenterology* 1989;**96**:A260.

18 Dooley, CP, Fitzgibbons, PL, Cohen, H, Appleman, MD, Perez-Perez, GI, & Blaser, MJ. Prevalence and distribution of *Campylobacter pylori* in an asymptomatic population (abstract). *Gastroenterology* 1988;**94**:A102.

19 Siurala, M, Sipponen, P, & Kekki, M. *Campylobacter pylori* in a sample of Finnish population: relations to morphology and functions of the gastric mucosa. *Gut* 1988;**29**:909–15.

20 Drumm, B, Perez-Perez, G, Blaser, M, & Sherman, P. Intrafamilial clustering of *Campylobacter pylori* infection (abstract). *Gastroenterology* 1989;**96**:A130.

21 Rauws, EAJ, Langenberg, W, Oudbier, J, Mulder,

CJJ, & Tytgat, GNJ. Familial clustering of peptic ulcer disease colonized with *H. pylori* of the same DNA composition. *Gastroenterology* 1989;**96**: A409.
22 Kawai, K, Shirakawa, K, Misaki, F, Hayashi, K, & Watanabe, Y. Natural history and epidemiologic studies of peptic ulcer disease in Japan. *Gastroenterology* 1989;**96**:581–5.
23 Majewski, SIH, & Goodwin, CS. Restriction endonuclease analysis of the genome of *Campylobacter pylori* with a rapid extraction method: evidence for considerable genomic variation. *J. Infect. Dis.* 1988;**157**:465–71.
24 Eaton, KA, Morgan, DR, & Krakowka, S. Virulence factors for *Campylobacter pylori* in gnotobiotic piglets (abstract). In: *Program and Abstracts of the Vth International Workshop on Campylobacter Infections, Puerto Vallarta, Mexico,* February 1989. Mixcoac, Mexico: Obsidiana S.A. de C.V., p. 181.
25 Ferrero, RL, Hazell, SL, & Lee, A. The urease enzymes of *Campylobacter pylori* and a related bacterium. *J. Med. Microbiol.* 1988;**27**:33–40.
26 Slomiany, BL, Bilski, J, Sarosiek, J, *et al. Campylobacter pyloridis* degrades mucin and undermines gastric mucosal integrity. *Biochem. Biophys. Res. Commun.* 1987;**144**:307–14.
27 Sarosiek, J, Slomiany, A, van Horn, K, Zalesna, G, & Slomiany, BL. Lipoytic activity of *Campylobacter pylori*: effect of sofalcone (abstract). *Gastroenterology* 1988;**94**:A399.
28 Bode, G, Malferteiner, P, & Ditschuneit, H. Pathogenetic implications of ultrastructural findings in *Campylobacter pylori* related gastroduodenal disease. *Scand. J. Gastroenterol.* 1988;**23**(suppl 142):25–39.
29 Evans, DG, Evans, DJ Jr, Moulds, JJ, & Graham, DY. *N*-Acetylneuraminyllactose-binding fibrillar hemagglutinin of *Campylobacter pylori*: a putative colonization factor antigen. *Infect. Immun.* 1988;**56**:2896–906.
30 Guerrant, RL, Barrett, LJ, & Marshall, BJ. Cytotoxin production by *C. pylori* (abstract). In: *Program and Abstracts of the Vth International Conference on Campylobacter Infections, Puerto Vallarta, Mexico,* February 1989. Mixcoac, Mexico: Obsidiana S.A. de C.V., p. 188.
31 Leunk, RD, Johnson, PT, David, BC, Kraft, WG, & Morgan, DR. Cytotoxic activity in broth-culture filtrates of *Campylobacter pylori. J. Med. Microbiol.* 1988;**26**:93–9.
32 Cover, TL, Dooley, CP, & Blaser, MJ. Human serologic response to *Campylobacter pylori* cytotoxin-associated proteins (abstract). *Gastroenterology* 1989;**96**:A101.
33 Figura, N, Guglielmetti, P, Rossolini, A, *et al.* Cytotoxin production by *Campylobacter pylori* strains isolated from patients with peptic ulcers and from patients with chronic gastritis only. *J. Clin. Microbiol.* 1989;**27**:225–6.
34 Defize, J, Goldie, J, & Hunt, RH. Inhibition of acid production by *Campylobacter pylori* in isolated guinea pig parietal cells (abstract). *Gastroenterology* 1989;**96**:A114.
35 Cave, DR, & Vargas, M. *Campylobacter pylori* inhibits uptake of ^{14}C-aminopyrine by rabbit gastric epithelial cells (abstract). *Gastroenterology* 1989;**96**:A79.
36 Dooley, CP, & Cohen, H. The clinical significance of *Campylobacter pylori. Ann. Int. Med.* 1988;**108**:70–9.
37 Blaser, MJ. Gastric *Campylobacter*-like organisms, gastritis, and peptic ulcer disease. *Gastroenterology* 1987;**93**:371–83.
38 Barthel, JS, Westblom, TU, Havey, AD, Gonzalez, FJ, & Everett, ED. Gastritis and *Campylobacter pylori* in healthy asymptomatic volunteers. *Arch. Int. Med.* 1988;**148**:1149–51.
39 Dehesa, M, Dooley, CP, Cohen, H, Fitzgibbons, P, Perez-Perez, GI, & Blaser, MJ. High prevalence of *Campylobacter pylori* in an asymptomatic Hispanic population (abstract). *Gastroenterology* 1989;**96**:A115.
40 Tatsuta, M, Iishi, H, & Okuda, S. Location of peptic ulcers in relation to antral and fundal gastritis by chromoendoscopic follow-up examinations. *Dig. Dis. Sci.* 1986;**31**:7–11.
41 Schrager, J, Spink, R, & Mitra, S. The antrum in patients with duodenal and gastric ulcers. *Gut* 1967;**8**:497–508.
42 Kekki, M, Saukkonen, M, Sipponen, P, Varis, K, & Siurala, M. Dynamics of chronic gastritis in the remnant after partial gastrectomy for duodenal ulcer. *Scand. J. Gastroenterol.* 1980;**15**: 509–12.
43 Tarpila, S, Kekki, M, Samloff, IM, Sipponen, P, & Siurala, M. Morphology and dynamics of the gastric mucosa in duodenal ulcer patients and their first-degree relatives. *Acta Hepat. Gastroenterol.* 1983;**30**:198–201.
44 Siurala, M, Sipponen, P, & Kekki, M. Chronic gastritis: dynamic and clinical aspects. *Scand. J. Gastroenterol.* 1985;**20**(suppl 109):69–75.
45 Meikle, DD, Taylor, KB, Truelove, SC, & Whitehead, R. Gastritis, duodenitis, and circulating levels of gastrin in duodenal ulcer before and after vagotomy. *Gut* 1976;**17**:719–28.
46 Quierroz, DMM, Barbosa, AJA, Mendes, EN, *et al.* Distribution of *Campylobacter pylori* and gastritis in the stomach of patients with and without duodenal ulcer. *Am. J. Gastroenterol.* 1988;**83**:1368–70.
47 Peterson, WL, Lee, EL, & Feldman, M. Relationship between *Campylobacter pylori* and gastritis in healthy humans after administration of placebo or indomethacin. *Gastroenterology* 1988;**95**:1185–97.
48 Johnston, BJ, Reed, PI, & Ali, MH. Prevalence of

Campylobacter pylori in duodenal and gastric mucosa — relationship to inflammation. *Scand. J. Gastroenterol.* 1988;**23**(suppl 142):69–75.

49 Patrick, WJA, Denham, D, & Forrest, APM. Mucus change in the human duodenum: a light and electron microscopic study and correlation with disease and gastric acid secretion. *Gut* 1974; **15**:767–76.

50 Kreuning, J, Bosman, FT, Kuiper, G, van der Wal, AM, & Lindeman, J. Gastric and duodenal mucosa in "healthy" individuals. An endoscopic and histopathological study of 50 volunteers. *J. Clin. Pathol.* 1978;**31**:69–77.

51 Fitzgibbons, PL, Dooley, CP, Cohen, H, & Appleman, MD. Prevalence of gastric metaplasia, inflammation and *Campylobacter pylori* in the duodenum of a normal population. *Am. J. Clin. Pathol.* 1988;**90**:711–14.

52 James, AH. Gastric epithelium in the duodenum. *Gut* 1964;**5**:285–94.

53 Johansen, A, & Hansen, OH. Heterotopic gastric epithelium in the duodenum and its correlation to gastric disease and acid level (abstract). *Acta Pathol. Microbiol. Scand.* 1973;**81**:676–80.

54 Rhodes, J. Experimental production of gastric epithelium in the duodenum. *Gut* 1964;**5**:454–8.

55 Shousha, S, Spiller, RC, & Parkins, RA. The endoscopically abnormal duodenum in patients with dyspepsia: biopsy findings in 60 cases. *Histopathology* 1983;**7**:23–34.

56 Shousha, S, Parkins, RA, & Bull, TB. Chronic duodenitis with gastric metaplasia: electron microscopic study including comparison with normal. *Histopathology* 1983;**7**:873–85.

57 Antonius, JI, Gump, FE, Lattes, R, & Lepore, M. A study of certain microscopic features in regional enteritis and their possible prognostic significance. *Gastroenterology* 1960;**38**:889–905.

58 Moshal, MG, Gregory, MA, Pillay, C, & Spitaels, JM. Does the duodenal cell ever return to normal? A comparison between treatment with cimetidine and Denol. *Scand. J. Gastroenterol.* 1978;**13**(suppl 56):48–51.

59 Gregory, MA, Moshal, MG, & Spitaels, JM. The effect of tripotassium dicitrato-bismuthate on the duodenal mucosa during ulceration: an ultrastructural study. *S. Afr. Med. J.* 1982;**62**:52–5.

60 Hoedemaeker, PJ. Heterotopic gastric mucosa in the duodenum. *Digestion* 1970;**3**:165–73.

61 Lessells, AM, & Martin, DF. Heterotopic gastric mucosa in the duodenum. *J. Clin. Pathol.* 1982; **35**:591–5.

62 Ikeda, K, Sannohe, Y, Murayama, H, Ikeda, R, & Inutsuka, S. Heterotopic gastric mucosa in the duodenum — reaction to congo red under fiberoptic observation. *Endoscopy* 1982;**14**: 168–70.

63 Nawaz, K, Graham, DY, Fechner, RE, & Eiband, M. Gastric heterotopia in the ileum with ulceration and chronic bleeding. *Gastroenterology* 1974;**66**:113–7.

64 Jenkins, D, Goodall, A, Gillet, FR, & Scott, BB. Defining duodenitis: quantitative histological study of mucosal responses and their correlations. *J. Clin. Pathol.* 1985;**38**:1119–26.

65 Isenberg, JI, Selling, JA, Hogan, DL, & Koss, MA. Impaired proximal duodenal mucosal bicarbonate secretion in patients with duodenal ulcer. *N. Engl. J. Med.* 1987;**316**:374–9.

66 Basuk, PM, Hogan, DL, Marin, M, *et al.* Diminished duodenal mucosal bicarbonate secretion in duodenal ulcer is independent of mucosal histologic abnormalities; a prospective study (abstract). *Gastroenterology* 1989;**96**:A33.

67 Perez-Perez, GI, Dworkin, B, Chodos, J, & Blaser, MJ. *Campylobacter pylori*-specific antibodies in humans. *Ann. Int. Med.* 1988;**109**:11–17.

68 Wyatt, JI, Rathbone, BJ, & Heatley, RB. Local immune response to gastric *Campylobacter* in non-ulcer dyspepsia. *J. Clin. Pathol.* 1986;**39**: 863–70.

69 Engstrand, L, Scheynius, A, Pahlson, CL, Grimelius, L, Schwan, A, & Gustavsson, S. Association of *Campylobacter pylori* with induced expression of class II transplantation antigens on gastric epithelial cells. *Infect. Immun.* 1989;**57**:827–32.

70 Lambert, JR, Borromeo, M, Pinkard, KJ, Turner, H, Chapman, CB, & Smith, ML. Colonization of gnotobiotic piglets with *Campylobacter pyloridis* — an animal model (letter)? *J. Infect. Dis.* 1987;**155**:1344.

71 Krakowka, S, Morgan, DR, Kraft, WG, & Leunk, RD. Establishment of gastric *Campylobacter pylori* infection in the neonatal gnotobiotic piglet. *Infect. Immun.* 1987;**55**:2789–96.

72 Droy-Lefaix, MT, Bonneville, F, Moyen, EN, *et al. Campylobacter pylori* and gastritis: a new animal model in germ-free rats (abstract). *Gastroenterology* 1989;**96**:A130.

73 Vantrappen, G, Rutgeerts, P, Broeckaert, L, & Janssens, J. Randomized open controlled trial of colloidal bismuth subcitrate tablets and cimetidine in the treatment of duodenal ulcer. *Gut* 1980;**21**:329–33.

74 Humphreys, H, Bourke, S, Dooley, CP, *et al.* Effect of therapy on *Campylobacter pyloridis*: a randomized trial. *Gut* 1988;**29**:279–83.

75 Zheng, ZT, Wang, ZY, Chu, YX, *et al.* Double-blind short-term trial of furazolidone in peptic ulcer (letter). *Lancet* 1985;**i**:1048–9.

76 Zhao, HY, Li, G, Guo, J, *et al.* Furazolidone in peptic ulcer (letter). *Lancet* 1985;**ii**:276–7.

77 Shirokova, KI, Filomonov, RM, & Poliakova, LV. Metronidazole in the treatment of peptic ulcer. *Klin. Med. (Mosk.)* 1981;**59**:48–50.

78 Anand, BS, Kumar, N, & Nanda, R. *Campylobacter pyloridis* is not responsible for duodenal

ulcer formation: results of a controlled therapeutic trial (abstract). *Dig. Dis. Sci.* 1986;**31**:151S.

79 Graham, DY, Lew, GM, & Michaletz, PA. Randomized controlled trial of the effect of eradication of *C. pylori* on ulcer healing and relapse (abstract). *Gastroenterology* 1989;**96**:A181.

80 Bardhan, KD. Refractory duodenal ulcer. *Gut* 1984;**25**:711–7.

81 Bianchi-Porro, G, Parente, F, Lazzaroni, M, & Pace, F. Colloidal bismuth subcitrate and two different dosages of cimetidine in the treatment of resistant duodenal ulcer. Preliminary results. *Scand. J. Gastroenterol.* 1986;**21**(suppl 122): 39–41.

82 Lam, SK, Lee, NW, Koo, J, Hui, WM, Fok, KH, & Ng, M. Randomized crossover trial of tripotassium dicitrato-bismuthate versus high dose cimetidine for duodenal ulcers resistant to standard dose of cimetidine. *Gut* 1984;**25**:703–6.

83 Wagner, S, Bar, W, & Schmidt, FW. Bismuth therapy of H-2 blocker resistant peptic ulcers colonized by *Campylobacter pylori* (abstract). In: *Program and Abstracts of the Vth International Conference on Campylobacter Infections, Puerto Vallarta, Mexico,* February 1989. Mixcoac, Mexico: Obsidiana S.A. de C.V., p. 72.

84 Martin, DF, Hollanders, D, May, SJ, Ravenscroft, MM, Tweedle, DE, & Miller, JP. Difference in relapse rates of duodenal ulcer after healing with cimetidine or tripotassium dicitrato-bismuthate. *Lancet* 1981;**i**:7–10.

85 Bianchi-Porro, B, Lazzaroni, M, Parente, F, & Petrillo, M. The influence of colloidal bismuth subcitrate on duodenal ulcer relapse. *Scand. J. Gastroenterol.* 1986;**21**(suppl 122):35–8.

86 Lee, FI, Samloff, IM, & Hardman, M. Comparison of tripotassium dicitrato-bismuthate tablets with ranitidine in healing and relapse of duodenal ulcers. *Lancet* 1985;**i**:1299–302.

87 Hamilton, I, O'Connor, HJ, Wood, NC, Bradbury, I, & Axon, AT. Healing and recurrence of duodenal ulcer after treatment with tripotassium dicitrato-bismuthate tablets or cimetidine. *Gut* 1986;**27**:106–10.

88 Smith, AC, Price, AB, Borriello, P, & Levi, AJ. A comparison of ranitidine and tripotassium dicitrato bismuth in relapse rates of duodenal ulcer disease (abstract). *Gastroenterology* 1988; **94**:A431.

89 Lam, SK, Hui, WM, Lan, WY, *et al.* Sucralfate overcomes adverse effect of smoking on duodenal ulcer healing and prolongs subsequent remission. *Gastroenterology* 1987;**92**:1193–201.

90 van Deventer, GM, Elashoff, JD, Reedy, TJ, Schneidman, D, & Walsh, JH. A randomized study of maintenance therapy with ranitidine to prevent the recurrence of duodenal ulcer. *N. Engl. J. Med.* 1989;**320**:1113–9.

91 Fry, J. Peptic ulcer: a profile. *Br. Med. J.* 1964;**2**: 809–12.

92 Greibe, J, Bugge, P, Gjorup, T, *et al.* Long-term prognosis of duodenal ulcer: follow-up study and survey of doctors' estimates. *Br. Med. J.* 1977;**2**: 1572–4.

12: Practical diagnosis of Helicobacter pylori

B.J. MARSHALL

Introduction

The idea of antibiotic treatment for peptic ulcer disease was introduced in 1984 but execution of the concept proved difficult. Whereas therapy with H2 blockers could be instituted on the same day as the endoscopy, the final results of mucosal biopsies for *Helicobacter pylori* were available only after 2–3 days. Thus patient management could not be decided immediately, and an extra clinic visit was usually necessary. Although biopsy detection of *H. pylori* is still the "gold standard," accurate non-invasive tests promise to make diagnosis and treatment of the infection a simple event for most physicians. This chapter reviews currently available diagnostic methods, and outlines the role for each method in various types of practice. Algorithms used to diagnose *H. pylori* at the University of Virginia are shown in Figs. 12.1 and 12.2.

Where do you find *H. pylori*?

Early papers on *H. pylori* isolation stated that the bacterium was more prevalent in the antrum of the stomach than the body mucosa [1]. Subsequent reports indicate that, while larger numbers of *H. pylori* are present in the antrum, organisms are also present in body mucosa, and are easily detected in both regions of the stomach [2–5]. This issue has specifically been addressed by Bayerdorffer *et al.* [6]. In 50 patients undergoing endoscopy, 32 of which were *H. pylori*-positive (HP+), biopsies were taken from 10 locations to estimate the concordance between gastritis and *H. pylori* colonization throughout the stomach. Active gastritis (both acute and chronic inflammation) was present in 100% of 32 patients with *H. pylori*, but in none of the 18 patients without *H. pylori*. Although not every biopsy sample from HP+ patients contained *H. pylori*, multiple samples improved the sensitivity of histology to almost 100%, as shown in Fig. 12.3. It can also be seen that both the antrum and body mucosa were colonized in nearly all patients. Bayerdorffer concluded that the distribution of *H. pylori* usually exceeded the distribution of active gastritis, and that the bacterium could be found in most areas of the stomach.

Our experience is similar. In 130 consecutive HP+ patients biopsied at the University of Virginia, 128 had *H. pylori* in both the antrum and body mucosa (two specimens were usually taken from each site). As in Bayerdorffer *et al.*'s study, we found that an extremely patchy distribution of *H. pylori* occurred when intestinal metaplasia was present. As described below, this led us to use blind suction biopsy to obtain culture specimens from some patients in whom endoscopy was not otherwise indicated.

H. pylori distribution in gastric and duodenal ulcer

The distribution of *H. pylori* may vary depending on the disease state present. Since duodenal ulcers are associated with high or normal acid secretion [7], it is not surprising that in duodenal ulcer disease the body mucosa tends to be histologically normal with lower numbers of *H. pylori* present [2, 3, 5]. In gastric ulcer disease, the body mucosa is more severely affected by gastritis and acid secretion tends to be lower [8]. This trend suggests that in asymptomatic persons without acid–peptic disease or dyspepsia, acid secretion may be lower and colonization

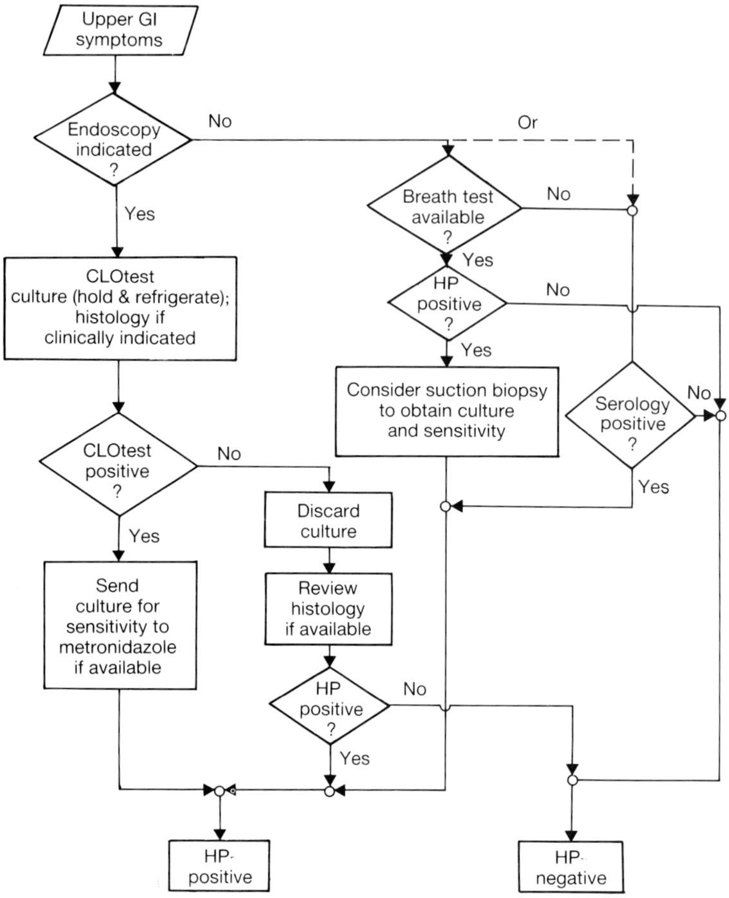

Fig. 12.1 Initial diagnosis of *H. pylori*. Note that when a CLOtest is taken, a specimen may be saved and refrigerated, so that a culture can be sent if the CLOtest is positive. This is cost effective in our hospital where the prevalence of *H. pylori* is only 40%, and most of the cultures would otherwise be negative.

with *H. pylori* may be very dense in all areas of the stomach.

The reasons for varying *H. pylori* distribution are unknown. Genetic (blood group, secretor status), environmental (diet, medications), and bacterial virulence factors (attachment, toxins) may be involved. No doubt the anatomy of the gastric mucosa is also an important factor. Antral mucosa consists of mucus-secreting epithelial cells folded into glandular structures, whereas in body mucosa the mucus-secreting cells are only on the flat surface and in the superficial portions of the gland necks. As a consequence, there is far more mucus-secreting surface present in the antrum, so a far greater bacterial load may find attachment.

H. pylori in dental plaque

Recently, *H. pylori* was found in dental plaque by Shames *et al.* [9]. The strain gave an identical restriction pattern to that seen in the stomach, suggesting that it may have seeded the gastric mucosa, or vice versa. Of concern is the consideration that, if *H. pylori* does arise in dental plaque, it is likely to be relatively infectious and be easily spread by kissing. In our 1982 study [1], I did not observe any association between poor dental hygiene and *H. pylori* infection, so at present I am skeptical that dental plaque is a major source of *H. pylori*. There is little doubt, however, that live organisms do reach the mouth in refluxed gastric juice, and could be infectious. A recent report by Majmudar *et al.* [10] described a very high isolation rate for an *H. pylori*-like organism (HPLO) from dental plaque. Urease was of course present in the dental plaques, possibly caused by the HPLO. The bacteria in question were identified as oxidase, catalase and urease positive spiral Gram-negative organisms but they await more exact identification by poly-

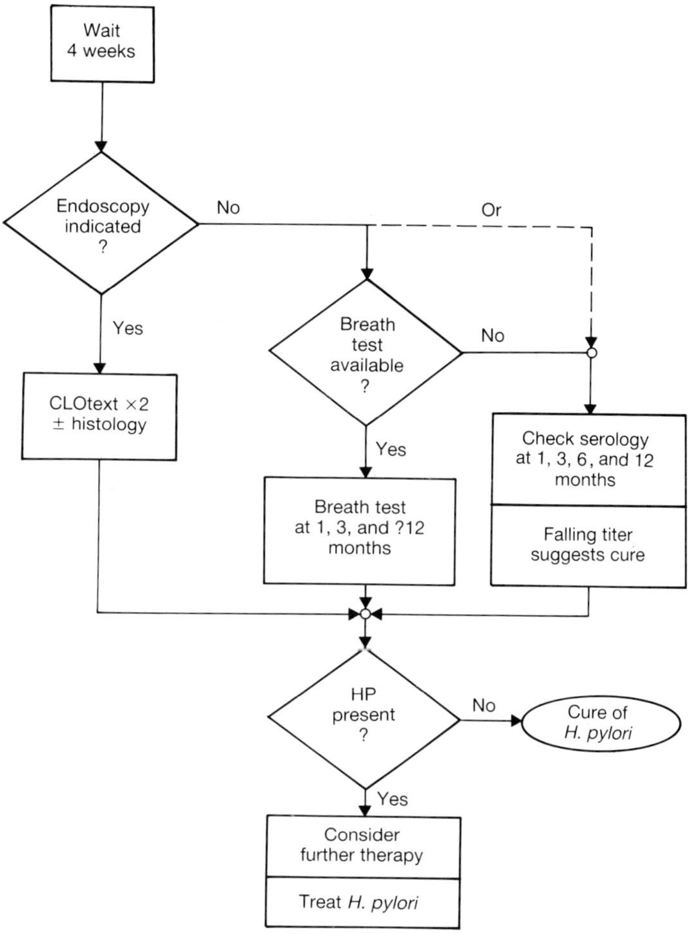

Fig. 12.2 Post-therapy diagnosis of *H. pylori*. After treatment, more care needs to be taken with detection of *H. pylori* and, if possible, serology should be replaced with a definitive test, i.e. breath test or biopsy.

acrylamide gel electrophoresis and restriction endonuclease.

H. pylori in the esophagus

The quantity of *H. pylori* in any mucosal site depends on the number of mucus-secreting epithelial cells present. Gastric mucosa, as part of Barrett's epithelium in the esophagus, may become colonized by *H. pylori*. Usually however, the amount of true gastric epithelium in Barrett's mucosa is small, the majority of the cells being of intestinal type. Usually therefore, only small numbers of *H. pylori* can be found in Barrett's epithelium, and inflammation is not associated with presence of the bacterium [11].

An exception to this may occur in Barrett's ulcers. Endoscopically, these may appear identical to gastric ulcers and are often difficult to heal. In some of these ulcers gastric mucus-secreting mucosa is the predominant type, in which case *H. pylori* and gastritis may play a pathogenic role as they do in the stomach. A child with Barrett's ulcer of the esophagus and associated *H. pylori* has been reported by De Giacomo *et al.* [12]. In this case large numbers of the bacteria were present and healing was achieved with a combination of acid-reducing therapy and amoxicillin.

H. pylori have recently been described adhering to the so-called "inlet patch," a small island of heterotopic gastric mucosa present in the esophagus at about the level of C6 in some persons [13]. Borhan-Manesh & Farnhum [14] noted that nine of 22 patients with *H. pylori* and gastric *H. pylori* infection also had infection of the upper esophageal gastric mucosa, some-

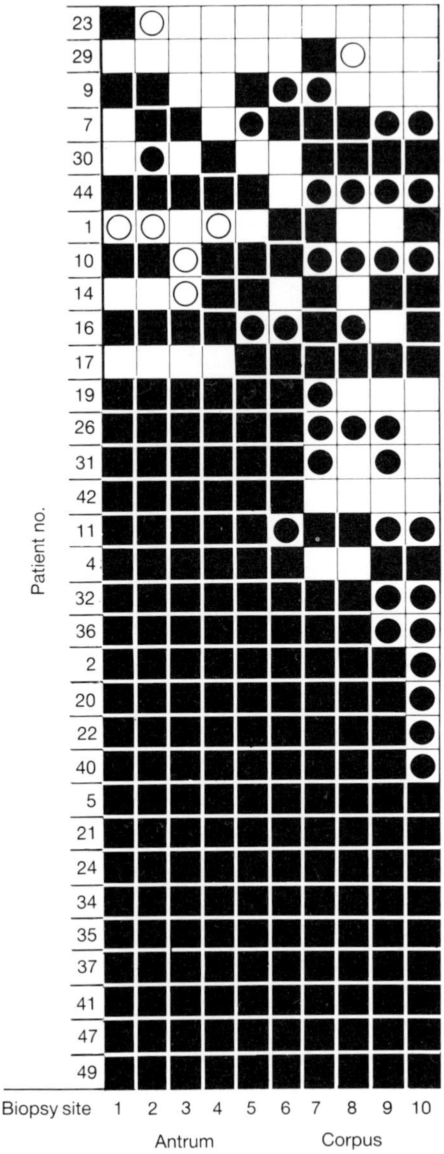

Fig. 12.3 Distribution of *H. pylori* and gastritis in the stomach of 32 patients with *H. pylori*. ■, biopsy sites with HP+ active chronic gastritis; ○, HP− active chronic gastritis; ●, HP+ sites with normal mucosa; □, neither gastritis nor *H. pylori* found. (From Bayerdorffer *et al.* [6].)

times in association with typical active gastritis. This may be a relevant factor in the design of therapy since an oral medication excreted in saliva would be needed to reach such an *H. pylori* colony and eradicate the organisms. Conversely, swallowed bismuth tablets might be less effective at *H. pylori* eradication in such patients.

H. pylori in the duodenum with metaplasia and heterotopia

H. pylori is often found in the duodenum, but almost always in association with gastric epithelium. Gastric tissue takes two forms in the duodenum. The most common form is an antral type of epithelium referred to as gastric metaplasia (as seen in Fig. 12.4). Gastric metaplasia is present in 92% of duodenal ulcer borders and is seen elsewhere in the duodenal bulb 50% of the time. When *H. pylori* is present in the antrum, associated gastric metaplasia in the duodenum will be colonized 50% of the time.

Since duodenal gastric metaplasia is patchy and cannot be identified through the endoscope, biopsy of the duodenal bulb has a very high sampling error, and may miss both gastric metaplasia and *H. pylori*. For this reason diagnosis of *H. pylori* cannot be excluded with a duodenal biopsy. In any case, whenever patchy *H. pylori* is present in the duodenum, bacteria are always present in the antrum and are more easily diagnosed by gastric biopsy.

At the University of Virginia, we have also found gastric metaplasia in 60% of patients with non-ulcer dyspepsia. In the study reported by Frierson *et al.* [15], two biopsies were taken from the proximal duodenal bulb in patients with non-ulcer dyspepsia. In addition, patients with a history of peptic ulcer disease were excluded from the study. Frierson found that gastric metaplasia was only associated with duodenitis when *H. pylori* was present, in the antrum if not in the duodenum. Gastric metaplasia was so prevalent that it was almost a normal finding, and was only associated with duodenitis when *H. pylori* infection coexisted. These findings support those of Wyatt *et al.* [16], who showed a near 1 : 1 relationship between duodenitis and *H. pylori*–gastric metaplasia. Frierson and others have also noted that *H. pylori* is never seen attached to duodenal epithelium unless gastric metaplasia is present.

A second form of gastric mucosa, gastric heterotopia, may also be present in the duodenum. Gastric heterotopia is true body-type

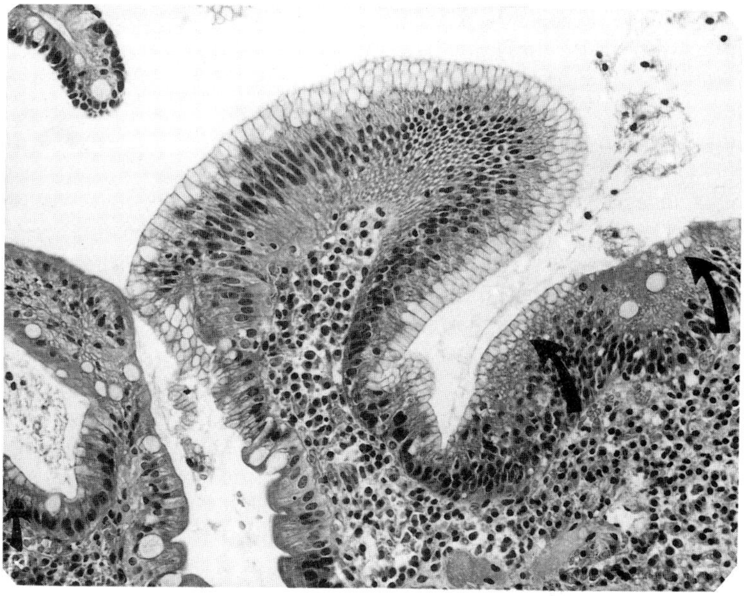

Fig. 12.4 Gastric metaplasia in the duodenal bulb. Most of the large villus is lined by gastric metaplasia, as readily seen in this H&E-stained section. Much smaller foci of gastric metaplasia are also present (arrows). H&E, × 250. (From Frierson *et al.* [15].)

acid-secreting mucosa, rather than mere mucus-secreting antral-type mucosa seen in gastric metaplasia. The role of gastric heterotopia in duodenal ulcer is unknown, but potentially important. According to Carrick *et al.* [17], islands of gastric heterotopia are found in 30% of biopsy samples taken adjacent to duodenal ulcers. If the bulb was sprayed with congo red and the patient was given pentagastrin prior to endoscopy, Carrick *et al.* could demonstrate functional acid-secreting tissue in over two-thirds of duodenal ulcer patients. So far the association between gastric heterotopia and duodenal ulcer has not been confirmed in other centers.

H. pylori in Meckel's diverticula and in the rectum

The remarkable affinity which *H. pylori* has for gastric epithelium is further demonstrated when gastric metaplasia or gastric heterotopia occurs in the gut distal to the duodenum. De Cothi *et al.* found gastric metaplasia in 13 Meckel's diverticula [18]; eight showed gastritis, and *H. pylori* were seen in half of these. Morris *et al.* have also reported *H. pylori* in Meckel's diverticula [19]. An even rarer finding of *H. pylori* in the rectum was reported by Dye *et al.* [20]. They described a woman with gastric heterotopia in a small reduplication cyst of the rectum. A *Campylobacter*-like organisms test (CLOtest) of the tissue was strongly positive, and histology revealed typical active chronic gastritis with CLO present on gastric body-type mucosa. Electron micrographs were compatible with *H. pylori* colonization.

Thus, the histology of *H. pylori* infection is the same, regardless of its location. In addition, *H. pylori*-associated disease (gastritis) may be expected in any location where gastric mucosa is found, i.e. throughout the gut. Finally, the stomach is the major reservoir of *H. pylori* only because gastric epithelial cells are concentrated there. The presence of *H. pylori* in the rectum is strong evidence that live *H. pylori* organisms are present in the feces, that *H. pylori* can easily compete with colonic flora for the juxtamucosal site, and that acid is not necessary for *H. pylori* to colonize gastric-type mucosa.

When to biopsy

Before taking a gastric mucosal biopsy, the risks and benefits need to be assessed. The only contraindication to a small pinch biopsy is a severe bleeding disorder. Usually patients can be safely biopsied if the prothrombin time is not more than 150% of normal (15 seconds). Since mucosal biopsies for *H. pylori* are usually taken away from any mucosal lesions, there is no need for concern, even in patients with bleeding ulcers. When significant bleeding occurs, it is most likely to be from a biopsied ulcer border or a rebleed from an existing lesion. It is my practice to include mention of a gastric biopsy in every endoscopy consent form, and to state the risk of hemorrhage or perforation from a biopsy as 1000 : 1, but the real risk is certainly much smaller, perhaps 50 000 : 1.

Obtaining a culture without doing endoscopy

Since *H. pylori* organisms are distributed throughout the gastric mucosa, blind biopsy of the gastric mucosa may be used to obtain a culture of *H. pylori* when endoscopy is not otherwise necessary. Contraindications to blind biopsy are the presence of a coagulopathy or presence of esophageal diverticula pouches, etc. For this procedure, the patient fasts overnight and attends the gastroenterology clinic at 9 am. The patient sits on the endoscopy table and the throat is sprayed with local anesthetic. After measuring the length of the patient from teeth to xiphoid, a "Quinton" suction biopsy tube and capsule (diameter 3.5 mm) is passed through the patient's mouth, and the location within the stomach is checked by injection of air and auscultation over the stomach. Usually a little resistance is felt at the esophagogastric junction, which is helped by a drink of water. In most cases some gagging and eye-watering occurs, but patients usually tolerate the tube for 10 minutes without excessive difficulty.

A negative pressure is then drawn on the tube, and after the tube becomes obstructed with gastric mucosa, a cable pulls a small guillotine within the biopsy capsule and (usually) a mucosal biopsy is obtained. The process may be repeated so that two or even three samples can be taken with one pass of the tube. The mucosa should be examined with a magnifying glass after removal from the device. Usually gastric mucosa is orange because of blood within it, and small dots (gastric pits) can be seen on its surface. Even though the hole in the biopsy capsule is only 2 mm wide, suction biopsies tend to be quite large and can be divided with a scalpel to provide specimens for culture and histology.

Using this method, we studied 13 consecutive patients attending the gastritis clinic in whom *H. pylori* status was known (nine HP+, four HP−), but in whom culture had not been performed. Tissue was sent primarily for culture, then for histology and CLOtest, depending on the amount obtained. The tube was successfully passed without sedation in all 13 patients, but in three patients no biopsy material was retrieved. Of the 10 patients successfully biopsied, tissue was obtained for culture and histology in every case, and for CLOtest in seven. In the nine HP+ patients, histology revealed *H. pylori* and gastritis in all nine (100%), and *H. pylori* was cultured in eight (89%). CLOtest was positive in all six HP+ patients tested (100%), but in the other three HP+ subjects insufficient tissue was obtained to do a CLOtest. According to the histology, biopsy samples were obtained from the antrum in three patients (33%) and from body mucosa in six (66%). In two patients who underwent endoscopy after the suction biopsy, suction marks were seen on the greater curve in the mid-body mucosa.

One week after the test, patients completed a mailed questionnaire to evaluate their impression of the procedure. Patient scores, representing grades from "no difficulty" to "great difficulty", ranged between 0 and 10, with an average score of 2.6. Of 10 patients who had undergone upper endoscopy in the past, seven preferred the suction biopsy. In most patients, therefore, suction biopsy can obtain sufficient material to perform culture and histology for *H. pylori*. In this small series the sensitivity of the test was 100% in persons from whom tissue was obtained. We suggest that this technique may be a useful way for non-endoscopists to easily obtain tissue and culture for *H. pylori* studies. Since the test appears quite sensitive (probably 90% for a single gastric mucosal biopsy), it may also be used to screen for the infection or follow up patients after treatment.

Staining of fresh tissue

Gram staining of a smeared gastric biopsy was the first rapid method used to diagnose *H. pylori* [21]. With a sensitivity of 80–90%, Gram staining added at least 60 minutes to the endoscopy session while the sections were stained and examined. Pinkard *et al.* [22] found that phase contrast microscopy of a squashed mucosal biopsy was a faster (5 minutes) and highly sensitive method (100% in 44 infected patients) of detecting the spiral organism. In ideal circumstances, the above tests were performed immediately, in the endoscopy room, by a trained technician. Whereas this was possible in a research setting, it was not practical for general use. Stains of fresh tissue have been superseded by the biopsy urease test.

Biopsy urease test

Langenberg *et al.* were the first to note the vigorous urease production of *H. pylori* [23], and Owen *et al.* reported that they could rapidly identify cultures of the new spiral organism by an immediate color change in urease detection agar (Christensen's medium) [24]. For weaker urease positive organisms (e.g. *Proteus*), the bacterium had to be cultured in the agar and a color change only occurred after many hours.

The idea of placing a gastric biopsy into such a medium was patented in 1985, and an enhanced urease test became available as the CLOtest in 1988 [25]. The rapid urease test is highly sensitive (90–95%) and very specific, as evidenced by the large number of publications on the subject (18 in 1989 alone) [26–34]. In most studies, a single biopsy sample for the urease test has been compared with a "gold standard" of multiple biopsies for histology and/or culture. The question of which is most sensitive, a single urease test or a single sample for histology, was addressed by Dye *et al.* [35]. They found that the rapid urease test (CLOtest) was more sensitive than histology or microbiology when these other modalities were only allowed a single biopsy sample. In addition, whereas histology and culture were expensive, labor intensive, and gave a result in 24–72 hours, the CLOtest could be read in the endoscopy room by the nurse, with 90% of positive results available before outpatients left the hospital.

Urease tests have been reviewed in Chapter 7. In brief, a faster urease test can be produced if occasional false-positive results are accepted. The CLOtest is buffered so that false-positive results are rare, but this limits its sensitivity to around 95% per biopsy.

Histological stains

Initial *H. pylori* studies used the Warthin–Starry silver stain, but many laboratories could not obtain consistent results with this difficult method. Instead, most changed to simpler stains such as the Giemsa [36], Gimenez [37] or acridine orange [38, 39]. All these are simple one-step stains which can be produced for minimal cost ($20 US) at the same time as routine hematoxylin and eosin (H&E) stained sections. They are almost as sensitive as a good silver stain.

A good pathologist will suspect *H. pylori* whenever the H&E section shows gastritis, and the bacteria are often easily visible in such sections at ×500 magnification. If the bacteria can be identified, further special stains are unnecessary. To save expense, an extra paraffin section can be cut during initial processing of the tissue, and only stained if there is doubt as to the presence or absence of *H. pylori*.

Culture of *H. pylori*

Transport of specimens

There is no need to culture the gastric biopsy immediately in the endoscopy room. At the University of Virginia in 1987 we compared isolation rates from immediate plating and gassing of biopsies with standard laboratory processing by a laboratory technician. We found that heavy contamination often occurred when the specimen was plated in the endoscopy room. Isolation rate was slightly better if the specimen was merely placed in a drop of saline, refrigerated and sent to the laboratory up to 2 hours later.

Achlorhydria

Endoscopists should be aware of the special problems with *H. pylori* culture. The normal stomach is sterile but patients with achlorhydria or gastric stasis, or who take omeprazole, may have heavy colonization of the stomach with aerobic and anaerobic flora. Because *H. pylori* grows slowly, it may be overrun by more vigorous bacteria and thus not be cultured. Therefore, when one of the above complications is suspected, selective culture plates should be used with antibiotics such as vancomycin, nalidixic acid, cefsulodin, and amphotericin present in the medium. A Skirrow's plate used for *Campylobacter* isolation is a reasonable alternative in most laboratories. In a research setting, sensitivity of 95–99% can be obtained using selective media for the isolation of *H. pylori* [29].

Several investigators have noted improved growth of *H. pylori* on fresh media rather than media from commercial sources [40], and most have emphasized the necessity for the atmosphere to be very humid. Finer points of culturing *H. pylori* are discussed in Chapter 7.

Radiographic findings in gastritis

According to de Lange *et al.* [41, 42], the radiographic features of gastritis vary, and the diagnosis is sometimes difficult to make because the findings may be subtle. However, to improve the detectability of the abnormalities, it is important that a state-of-the-art technique be used for the radiographic examination of the upper gastrointestinal tract. The biphasic contrast technique is considered the most sensitive method to detect abnormalities in the stomach, including gastritis. This radiographic examination consists of two techniques, a double-contrast and a single-contrast method combined in one study. It is important to use this technique for the evaluation of gastritis, because some features are only visible on double-contrast radiographs, whereas other findings are best seen on single-contrast films during compression of the stomach (Figs. 12.5, 12.6). For optimal results it is essential to use a medium-dense barium suspension, and glucagon (0.2 ml) is administered intravenously for gastric distension.

Radiographically, gastritis may be present when the following findings are demonstrated: erosions, nodules, polyps, transverse folds in the antrum, crenulation, antral spasm, S-shaped antrum, paucity of folds, and coarse areae gastricae (Figs. 12.5, 12.6). Not all of these findings may be present at the same time, and usually only one or two features are demonstrated. Erosions and coarse areae gastricae are

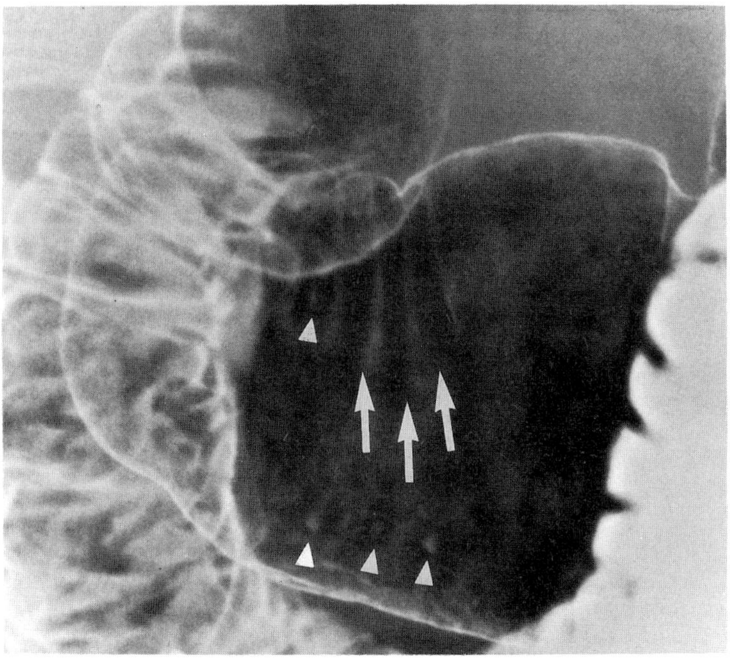

Fig. 12.5 There are multiple transverse antral folds perpendicular to the lesser curvature (⇧). Erosions are also present (arrowheads); some of the erosions are aligned along the folds. (From de Lange [41].)

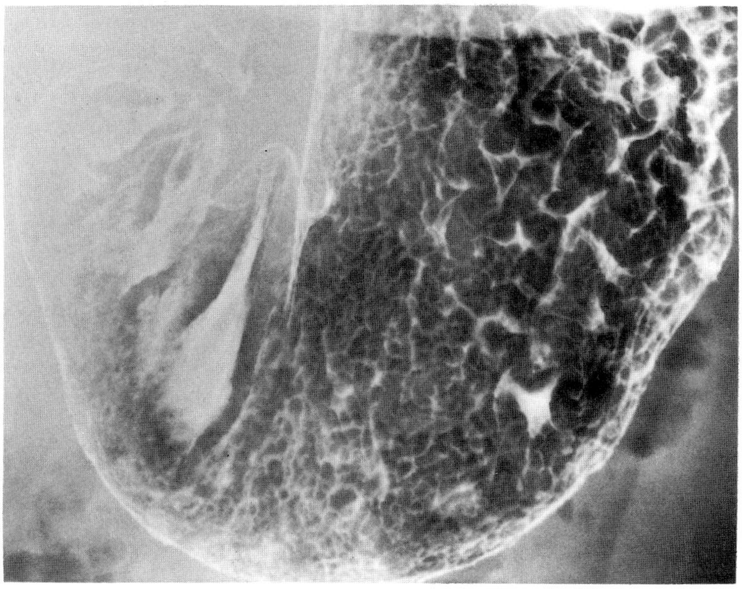

Fig. 12.6 Coarse areae gastricae. The individual mucosal units have an irregular shape and are pronounced. They measure 5–6 mm in diameter. Note the presence of transverse folds and thickened antral folds. (From de Lange [41].)

usually best seen during the double-contrast phase of the biphasic examination, whereas nodules and polyps are usually demonstrated during the single-contrast graded-compression phase. Transverse folds, S-shaped antrum, antral spasm, and crenulation are demonstrated on both single- and double-contrast films.

It is impossible to distinguish radiographically between acute and chronic gastritis, as both entities may present with similar findings. However, findings such as transverse folds, antral deformity, nodularity, and polyps are in favor of chronic gastritis. Erosions can be seen in both acute and chronic gastritis, but demonstration of transverse folds together with erosions (Fig. 12.5) is in favor of chronic disease.

When performed properly by a skillful and experienced radiologist, the biphasic contrast examination may be a sensitive, non-invasive test for the evaluation of the stomach for gastritis. As the findings may be subtle, careful and meticulous evaluation of the radiographs is necessary to detect the various features.

Immunologic detection of *H. pylori* in biopsy material

A rapid ELISA method was described by Engstrand *et al.* [43] for detecting *H. pylori* rapidly in fresh biopsy material. Biopsy specimens were smeared onto a glass slide which was incubated with an IgG mouse monoclonal antibody directed towards a 23 kDa *H. pylori* antigen. After washing, the presence of adherent mouse IgG was detected by staining with an anti-mouse antibody conjugated to fluorescein. The method was at least as sensitive as silver stain of multiple biopsy specimens, and could be performed in 1 hour.

Shadowen & Sciortino have used latex agglutination to detect *H. pylori* antigen in fresh biopsy specimens [44]. Briefly, latex beads are coated with monoclonal antibody to *H. pylori*, a biopsy or mucus sample is mixed with the latex suspension, and agglutination occurs if *H. pylori* antigens are present in the sample. The sensitivity of the method equals that of histology (95–100%).

A third method, which Cartun *et al.* [45] have found to be highly sensitive and specific for *H. pylori*, is to stain histologic sections with monoclonal antibody to *H. pylori*. The monoclonal antibody used is commercially available and the methodology is standard in most histology laboratories.

The advantage of immunologic methods is that they provide positive identification of *H. pylori* organisms without culture, and are unaffected by similar-looking commensal bacteria visible in some histology specimens. The sensitivity of immunologic methods on a single biopsy specimen is at least equal to careful examination of a silver-stained specimen, and in some hands exceeds histologic methods [45]. At present, however, immunologic detection of *H. pylori* in biopsy material is a research tool rather than a routine method of diagnosis.

Serologic tests for *H. pylori*

After 1984, many microbiologists developed serologic tests for *H. pylori*. The first of these, reported by Jones *et al.* [46], used a complement fixation test similar to those described for the detection of antibodies to *Campylobacter jejuni*. Antibodies to *H. pylori* were usually present in high titer and the sensitivity of the early tests easily reached 85%. In Western Australia we produced a passive hemagglutination test using a supernatant of sonicated *H. pylori* organisms to coat type O human red blood cells. After washing in phosphate-buffered saline and resuspending the cells in dilute calf serum, the cells survived for 5 days. The test only took 20 minutes to complete and gave a sensitivity of 90–95% and a specificity of 83% [47, 48].

After 1984, investigators detected *H. pylori* antibodies with enzyme-linked immunosorbent assays (ELISAs), using commercially available reagents and standard methodology [49, 50, 51]. The sensitivity of the ELISA can be increased by selecting the most antigenic *H. pylori* proteins to coat the wells. In the case of *H. pylori* these are flagella, surface-exposed urease, and attachment proteins such as the *N*-acetyl-neuraminyllactose-binding hemagglutinin (a lectin) described by Evans *et al.* [52]. ELISA tests can be made very sensitive (few false-negatives) or specific (few false-positives) by adjusting the upper limit of normal for HP− patients. Many commercial kits are in development and some of the technology is protected by patents in the United States. As yet these serologic tests have not been evaluated by independent investigators, so their sensitivity and specificity in various patient groups are poorly defined.

The role of serologic tests in management

Since serologic tests offer a cheap and rapid way to diagnose *H. pylori*, they will be widely used in the near future. Already *H. pylori* ELISA kits are available from commercial sources in the United States, United Kingdom, and Europe. Ideally, ELISA tests should be very sensitive, so that no HP+ patients are missed during a serologic screen. Strongly positive results in the correct clinical setting are sufficient evidence to initiate therapy, whereas borderline ELISA results should be confirmed with a breath test or biopsy before treatment (see Fig. 12.1).

Some physicians believe that a diagnosis of duodenal ulcer is reason enough to commence *H. pylori* therapy, without further diagnostic tests. I am skeptical of this practice, because in many patients the diagnosis of "duodenal ulcer" has never been proved or was made in the distant past. Often, so-called ulcer symptoms are due to esophageal reflux disease or residual dyspepsia, persisting long after *H. pylori* has disappeared. Suggested algorithms used to sort out such patients are shown in Fig. 12.1 and Chapter 13.

Serologic follow-up of *H. pylori* infections has been reported by a number of investigators [53–55]. Due to large individual variations in titer, however, absolute antibody levels are a poor indicator of cure. It is our experience that, in patients who fail therapy, antibody titer falls during treatment but rebounds 4 weeks later. This makes serologic follow-up impractical in the weeks immediately following treatment.

When immediate proof of eradication is not essential, a consistently falling antibody titer over 3–6 months is a useful indicator of bacteriologic cure. For best results, acute and convalescent sera should be tested in the same ELISA plate. As shown in Fig. 12.2, I recommend that convalescent sera be tested at 1, 3, 6, and 12 months after treatment to confirm long-term eradication of *H. pylori*, or recrudescence.

The urea breath test

The urea breath test is the most specific non-invasive way to detect *H. pylori*. Urease is not

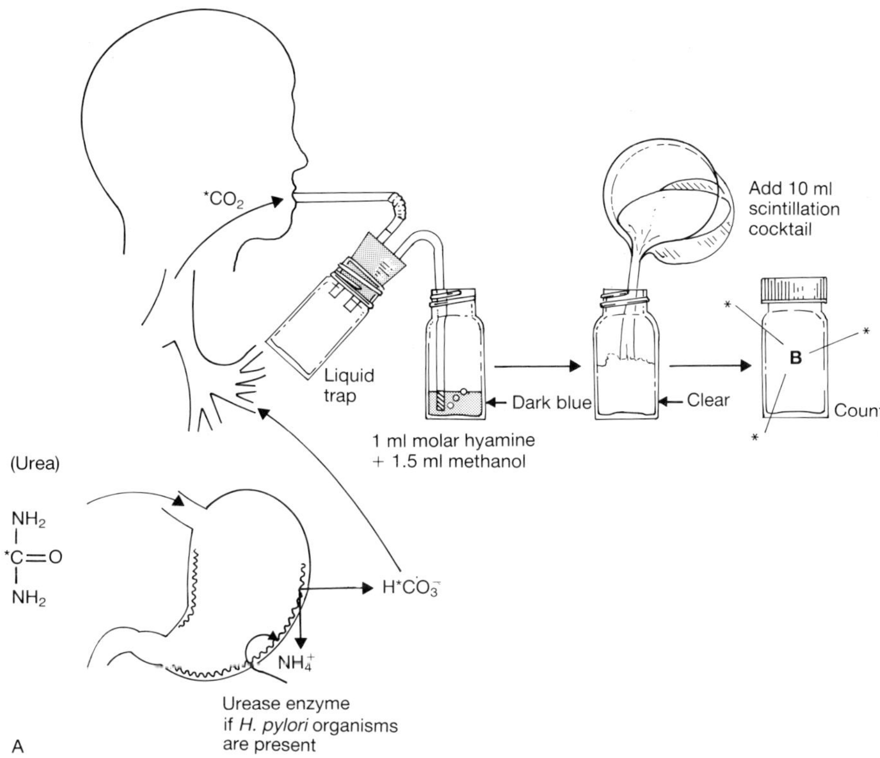

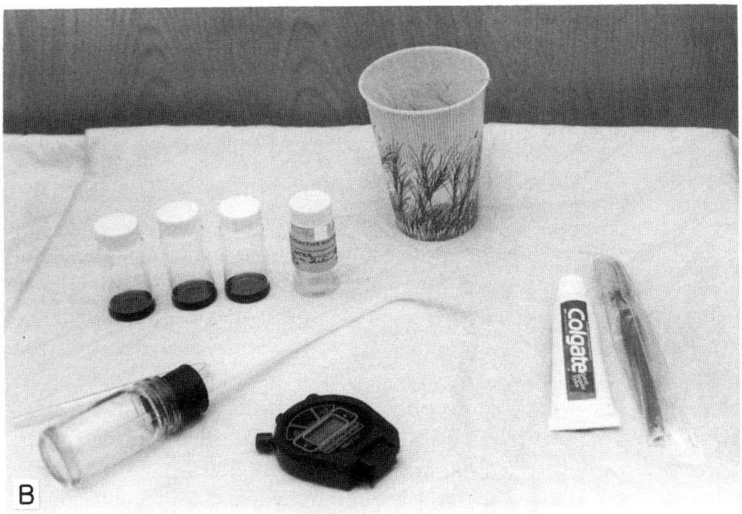

Fig. 12.7 A, if urease (*H. pylori*) is present in the gastric mucosa, isotope-labeled urea is hydrolyzed forming $^{14}CO_2$ which is expired in the breath. Patients blow through a disposable drinking straw attached to a liquid trap, into a 20 ml vial containing methanol, hyamine, and a pH indicator. The blue (alkaline) solution changes to colorless upon CO_2 saturation. Scintillation fluid (10 ml) is added to the sample, which is then counted for 5 minutes in a scintillation counter. Note: caution is required in handling hyamine solution, a strong base. (From Marshall *et al.* [65].) B, actual equipment needed for the UVA breath test (counterclockwise from right: toothbrush and toothpaste, cup, isotope, breath collection bottles containing hyamine/methanol and blue indicator, trap with drinking straw attached, stop watch).

present in mammalian cells, so the presence of urease enzyme in the stomach is proof that bacteria are present [56]. Swallowed urease from mouth bacteria is denatured below pH 4.0 [57], so it is quickly destroyed by gastric acid and cannot interfere with the test. When urease is produced beneath the gastric mucus layer, however, it is protected from luminal acid and remains fully active. The action of urease on urea in the extracellular fluid yields HCO_3^- and NH_4^+, both of which rapidly enter the blood on the mucosal side, and serve to further maintain an alkaline mucus layer on the luminal side of the mucus gel [58]. The principle of the breath test is shown in Fig. 12.7.

In order to detect gastric urease, urea labeled with a carbon isotope is swallowed by the patient. If urease (*H. pylori*) is present, urea is split into HCO_3^- and NH_4^+ at the interface between the gastric epithelium and lumen. Ammonium ion is sequestered in the gastric acid, but the CO_2 (from HCO_3^-) enters the bloodstream, where it is carried to the lungs and rapidly expired. About 50% of the urea is either absorbed through the mucosa unchanged, or leaves the stomach through the pylorus without being hydrolyzed [59, 60]. This intact urea is then excreted in the urine over the next 48 hours. In persons without *H. pylori*, very little of the isotope appears in the breath and most is excreted as unchanged urea in the urine.

^{13}C-urea breath test

The urea breath test was first described by Graham *et al.* [61]. Recognizing a need for a non-invasive means of detecting *H. pylori* in asymptomatic normal persons (for epidemiologic studies), they administered ^{13}C-urea orally and detected the $^{13}CO_2$ expired in the breath of patients who had *H. pylori* infection. About 1.1% of all carbon in nature is ^{13}C, and the ratio of ^{13}C to ^{12}C expired in the breath varies with diet and the level of physical activity [62]. This natural abundance of ^{13}C means that a relatively large dose of substrate is necessary to measurably increase $^{13}CO_2$ excretion. In practice, 2–5 mg kg^{-1} of urea (75–250 mg per patient) is used to obtain the necessary >0.6% increase in ^{13}C seen in infected patients [61, 63].

Aware of the above limitations, Graham *et al.* [61, 63] collected a baseline sample to control for intersubject expired-^{13}C variations, and then used a high-calorie liquid test meal (Sustacal) to hold the isotopic urea in the stomach. *H. pylori* urease enzyme has a K_m of around 1 mmol of urea [64], a concentration exceeded by the ^{13}C-urea test, so it was necessary to hold the reagents in the stomach for a time while the reaction proceeded. In addition, because the urea was diluted in 150 ml of liquid, mixing was required to bring the unchanged urea into contact with the gastric mucosa. Alveolar breath samples were collected in a balloon and transferred to glass test tubes for analysis in an automated isotope ratio mass spectrometer. Samples at 40–60 minutes were sensitive and specific indicators of *H. pylori* infection.

The meal-based ^{13}C-urea test has the ability to quantify accurately gastric mucosal urease, since the enzyme is saturated with substrate, and the reaction proceeds at a rate dependent on urease concentration rather than substrate concentration. By correcting for endogenous CO_2 production, the results can be expressed as the urea hydrolysis rate in μmol minute^{-1}. The disadvantage of the test is the relatively large investment in patient and technician time, the cost of the isotope, the number of samples required and, as a result, the expense.

^{14}C-urea breath test

In 1985 Ivor Surveyor and I devised a ^{14}C-urea test [59, 65] to follow up patients after antibiotic treatment of *H. pylori*. Unlike the ^{13}C-urea breath test, the ^{14}C-urea test used only a tiny amount of isotope (1 μg) dissolved in 20 ml of water, so hydrolysis occurred swiftly once the urea wetted the gastric mucosa. This made a meal unnecessary. In addition, the isotope was cheap and the collected breath could be counted in a scintillation counter which was available in our hospital. Since our initial description, the test has been further refined at the University of Virginia [66].

In order to observe the speed of urea hydrolysis and CO_2 excretion in the breath, we studied four patients with proved *H. pylori*, and two patients without *H. pylori*. After an overnight fast, a soft plastic tube was passed into the upper esophagus and 20 ml of water containing

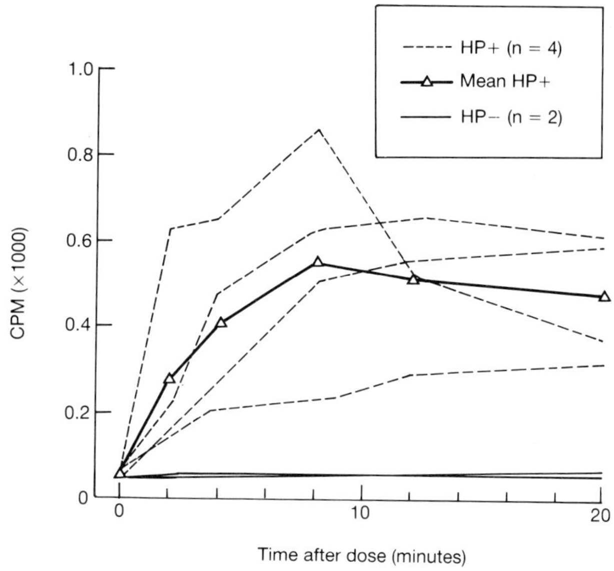

Fig. 12.8 When ^{14}C-urea is given directly into the esophagus, a gradual rise in $^{14}CO_2$ excretion is seen in HP+ subjects, easily detectable by 4 minutes (upper curve). In HP− subjects, only a very small rise in $^{14}CO_2$ excretion is seen (flat lines near bottom of graph). Dose = 37 kBq. (From Marshall *et al.* [66].)

37 kBq (1 μCi) of ^{14}C-urea was injected. HP+ patients gave diagnostic levels of $^{14}CO_2$ in breath within 4 minutes, whereas HP− patients showed no significant increase (Fig. 12.8). These results served to demonstrate that urease from bacteria in the esophagus was too weak to cause a positive breath test. In contrast, gastric urease (beneath the mucus layer) caused immediate release of $^{14}CO_2$ into the bloodstream.

Administration of labeled urea: with meals or not?

This is a controversial point among breath test experts. If urea solution is given in 20 ml water (as in our rapid test), some urea is hydrolyzed as it touches bacterial urease in the mouth. This effect of oral urease makes early readings (before 15 minutes) ambiguous. In contrast, if labeled urea is given with a high-calorie liquid meal, the isotope is very dilute as it passes through the mouth and oral urea hydrolysis is greatly reduced. The disadvantage of this method is that the breath test is usually much prolonged if a meal is given, and isotope is excreted very slowly in the breath, making it necessary to count samples for a very long time, or use a larger isotope dose [67].

When very quick results are preferred, oral contamination needs to be minimized, so that early breath samples (5–15 minutes) can discriminate between HP+ and HP− patients. To obtain a very early rise, the isotope should be given in enough water to ensure that it can be easily swallowed and reaches the stomach. A small volume of water (<20 ml) wets the gastric mucosa and pools in the antrum. Larger volumes (>20 ml) empty through the pylorus and waste the ^{14}C-urea. The disadvantage of using a small volume is that it exposes a higher proportion of labeled urea to the oropharynx, and so causes greater levels of oral urease contamination. This can be circumvented by collecting breath samples in a plastic bag and pumping them through hyamine solution, rather than having the patient blow bubbles in the solution. In the latter case, breath passes through the patient's mouth very slowly and is heavily contaminated with the products of oral urea hydrolysis. With the bag, patients blow out quickly and contamination from the oral mucosa (CO_2 being slowly released) is minimized.

Table 12.1 details the various methods used for both ^{13}C-urea and ^{14}C-urea breath tests. All are highly sensitive (85–95%) and specific (90–98%) depending on where the investigator decides to place his upper limit of normal value for HP− patients. Fig. 12.9 gives a graphical comparison of each. All ^{14}C-urea breath tests

Table 12.1 Breath tests published in the reviewed literature

Author	Isotope dose	Type of meal	Isotope given in	Collection time (minutes)
Graham [61]	^{13}C 5 mg kg^{-1}	Sustacal liquid 120 ml	Water	60
Marshall [59]	^{14}C 370 kBq	None	Water 20 ml	20
Bell [77]	^{14}C 400 kBq	Liquid 350 ml	Water 20 ml	60–120
Ormand [67]	^{14}C 370 kBq	Sustacal liquid 120 ml	Water 25 ml	20–60
Veldhuyzen van Zanten [68]	^{14}C 185 kBq	Sustacal liquid 120 ml	Water + 50 mg cold urea	60–120
Rauws [78]	^{14}C 111 kBq	Sustacal liquid 120 ml	Water	40
Eggers [60]	^{13}C 75 mg	0.1 M Citrate 200 ml	Citrate 5 ml	30–60

37 kBq = 1 μCi.

have been corrected to show counts per minute (CPM) mmol^{-1} 10 μCi^{-1} of expired CO_2. It can be seen that the highest excretion occurs when the isotope is dissolved in 20 ml of water and given without a meal [59, 65]. Similar values may be obtained by placing the urea within a quick-dissolving capsule of lactose, a method which also prevents oral urease contamination. Note that all methods which use a meal have a longer collection time although, according to Ormand *et al.* [67], a 20-minute collection will still diagnose most patients, even in meal-based tests.

Using a modified ^{13}C-urea breath test, Eggers *et al.* [60] claimed that a 20-minute collection could be used with a meal-based test. Eggers *et al.* gave 75 mg of ^{13}C-urea in 200 ml of 0.1 M citric acid solution. They also measured $^{13}CO_2$ breath collections after ingestion of labeled $NaH^{13}CO_3$ and compared the results with the ^{13}C-urea breath test. They revealed that with this method, most of the ^{13}C-urea was emptied from the stomach before hydrolysis could occur, and only 21% of the isotope was recovered as CO_2 in breath during 30 minutes' collection. Although this methodology makes comparisons difficult, it appears that retention of the isotope in the stomach is only partly achieved with the liquid meals used in the ^{13}C-urea breath test.

With ^{14}C-urea, a tiny amount of substrate and a fast reaction time (4–10 minutes) mean that prolonged retention in the stomach is not essential for diagnosis. On the other hand, if ^{14}C-urea is being used to accurately quantitate gastric urease, maximum reproducibility can be obtained if the isotope is given within a liquid meal. Veldhuyzen van Zanten *et al.* [68] have even added 50 mg of unlabeled urea to their

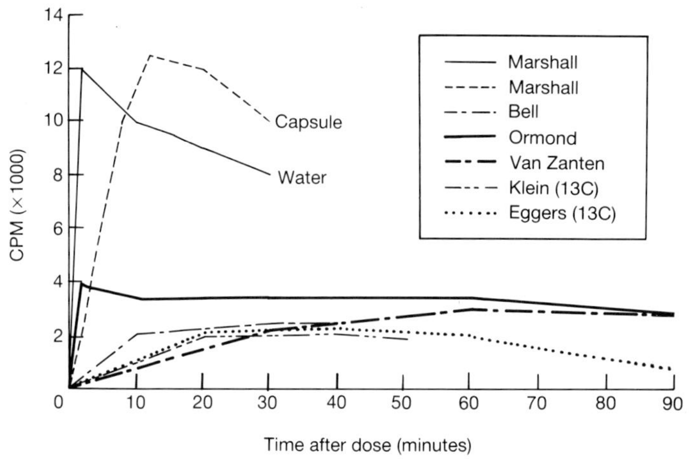

Fig. 12.9 Comparison of various breath test methods showing CO_2 excretion curves. All ^{14}C-urea tests have been adjusted to reflect a 10 μCi dose. (Further information is provided in Table 12.1.) References: [59], [66], [77], [67], [68], [63], [60].

meal-based ^{14}C-urea test to slow the reaction even further and ensure "zero order kinetics." This means that, as in the ^{13}C-urea test, the enzyme is saturated with urea and the reaction proceeds at a constant rate, proportional to the concentration of urease present.

University of Virginia method for a rapid ^{14}C-urea breath test

Lyophilized ^{14}C-urea is obtained in a 9250 kBq (250 μCi) ampule, and is reconstituted with 25 ml of sterile water; 185 kBq (0.5 ml) of the solution is pipetted into a 20 ml vial with an additional 2.0 ml of sterile water. A 0.01 ml sample of this solution is used as a batch standard. Each 2.5 ml dose is frozen at −20 °C until use. Immediately before use, the solution is thawed to room temperature and 17.5 ml of tap water is added.

Breath samples are collected in the following manner (Fig. 12.7). Patients blow through a disposable drinking straw attached to a liquid trap, into a 20 ml glass scintillation vial containing 2.5 ml of methanol, in which 1 mmol of hyamine (methylbenzethonium hydroxide) is dissolved, and to which thymolphthalein pH indicator has been added. The blue (alkaline) solution changes to colorless upon CO_2 saturation, at which time a constant amount (≈1.0 mmol) of CO_2 has been collected.

Ten milliliters of liquid scintillant (Ready-Safe; Beckman catalog #158735) is added to each vial and each sample is counted in a liquid scintillation counter (Rackbeta; Pharmacia LKB), using a quenching correction with the output expressed as CPM. A standard provided by the manufacturer indicates the counting efficiency of our machine is 93.6%. Disintegrations per minute (DPM) may thus be derived by multiplying CPM by 1.068 (100 ÷ 93.6).

A sample of 153 patients, (77 females, 76 males) took the breath test during the week of their endoscopy. After they had fasted for at least 6 hours, a baseline breath sample was collected to familiarize the patient with the technique. Each patient then removed false teeth (if present), cleansed his or her mouth with toothpaste, and was then given 185 kBq (5 μCi) of ^{14}C-labeled urea dissolved in 20 ml of water. The radioisotope was taken in a single swallow in an attempt to prevent the solution from coating the inside of the mouth. The mouth was then cleansed a second time by rinsing with water, and the patient remained seated during the remainder of the test. A breath sample was taken at 2 minutes in order to quantify urea hydrolysis in the oropharynx, and further samples were taken at 15, 20, 25, and 30 minutes.

Of the 154 patients, 104 were HP+ as determined by biopsy studies. Breath tests from the 49 HP− patients were used to define the negative (normal) range. For any time point, "normal" was a breath CPM value below the mean + 3SD obtained for the HP− group. A positive test was thus defined as a $^{14}CO_2$ excretion above this range.

In patients with *H. pylori*, the $^{14}CO_2$ excretion peaked about 10 minutes after ingestion of the isotope, then fell in an almost linear fashion. There was a 10-fold difference between HP+ and HP− patients (300 CPM vs 3000 CPM) (Fig. 12.10). At 15 and 20 minutes, the upper limits of normal for negative patients (mean + 3SD) were 1422 and 928 CPM, respectively. A scattergram of 20-minute samples from the 153 patients is shown in Fig. 12.11.

Improvements and theoretical limitations of the ^{14}C-urea breath test

Using a 5 μCi dose of ^{14}C-urea, we obtain CPM of less than 930 in HP− patients. To define a sample as 930 CPM ± 2.5% requires a maximum counting time of only 8 minutes. If the patient dose was decreased to 1 μCi, the upper limit of normal would be 200 CPM, which would require a counting time of up to 33 minutes for a borderline sample [69], but most samples could be defined as HP+ or HP− in less than 10 minutes. Collection of more than 1 mmol of breath CO_2 would allow further reduction of the isotope dose (more CPM collected), but we believe this is impractical insofar as it requires quite a prolonged breath collection.

Microdose version of the ^{14}C-urea breath test

Although 5 μCi ^{14}C-urea breath tests produce trivial radiation doses, a lower isotope dose is

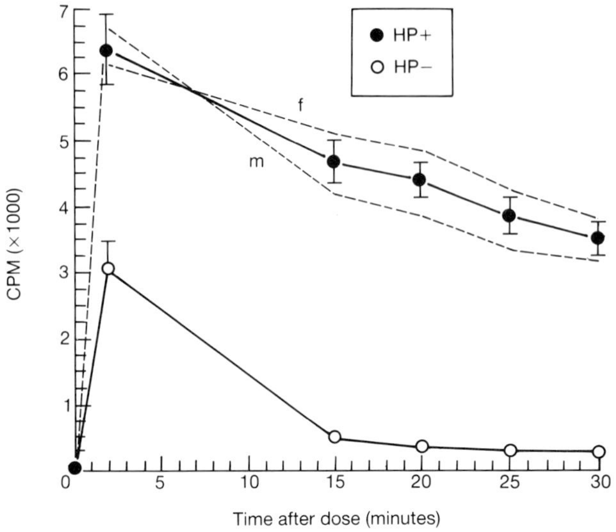

Fig. 12.10 Graph displaying the mean ^{14}C excretion between 2 and 30 minutes for the University of Virginia rapid 5 μCi breath test. In HP+ patients, females (f) gave slightly higher counts. At 15 and 20 minutes, upper limits of normal for negative patients (mean+3SD) were 1422 and 928 CPM, respectively. m, male patients.

desirable and theoretically possible. By supplying the isotope in a capsule form, ^{14}C-urea is not exposed to mouth urease. We have done preliminary evaluation of a microdose capsule-based breath-test methodology, with the aim of achieving optimal safety, speed, accuracy, and cost.

Individual 1 μCi doses of ^{14}C-urea were mixed with lactose and loaded into gelatin capsules. In preliminary studies ($n = 5$), dummy lactose capsules were given prior to routine endoscopy and observed endoscopically 5 minutes after ingestion. Thirteen patients biopsied for HP (seven HP+) fasted for 6 hours, then swallowed a capsule with 20 ml of water. Breath was collected in bags at 2, 4, 8, 12, 20, and 30 minutes. Samples were pumped through hyamine solution and read in a scintillation counter to an accuracy of ±2.5%. To assess reproducibility, HP+ patients repeated the test the following day.

Capsules viewed at endoscopy had all disintegrated on the corpus mucosa. In the breath test, HP+ patients averaged 1926 ± 578 CPM at 12 minutes, whereas HP− patients averaged 47 ± 11 CPM. Fig. 12.12 shows excretion curves for the HP+ group. At 12 minutes the test easily differentiated between patients as either HP+ or HP−. Correlation between first and second tests was also high ($r = 0.78$). Total radiation exposure was equal to environmental background received in 24 hours. Our initial assessment is that the microdose capsule-based ^{14}C-urea breath test is safe, fast, as accurate as earlier variations of the test, simple to perform, and environmentally benign (very little scintillation fluid is needed because patients may be diagnosed with a single breath sample taken at 15–20 minutes).

Safety of ^{14}C-urea

Biologic and physical half-life of ^{14}C

In the ^{14}C-urea breath test, ^{14}C-urea is either hydrolyzed and expired as $^{14}CO_2$, or excreted unchanged as urea in urine. Because the biologic half-life is so short (hours–days), the total cumulative radiation dose received from each breath test is small, and far below variations in natural radiation received within the United States. Concern with ^{14}C usually arises because of its long half-life, but this is immaterial for compounds such as CO_2 and urea, which are rapidly excreted.

Dose equivalence (DE)

To allow radiation sources to be compared, emissions of various origins are expressed in "dose equivalence (DE) units." The DE for ^{14}C takes into account the fraction of isotope

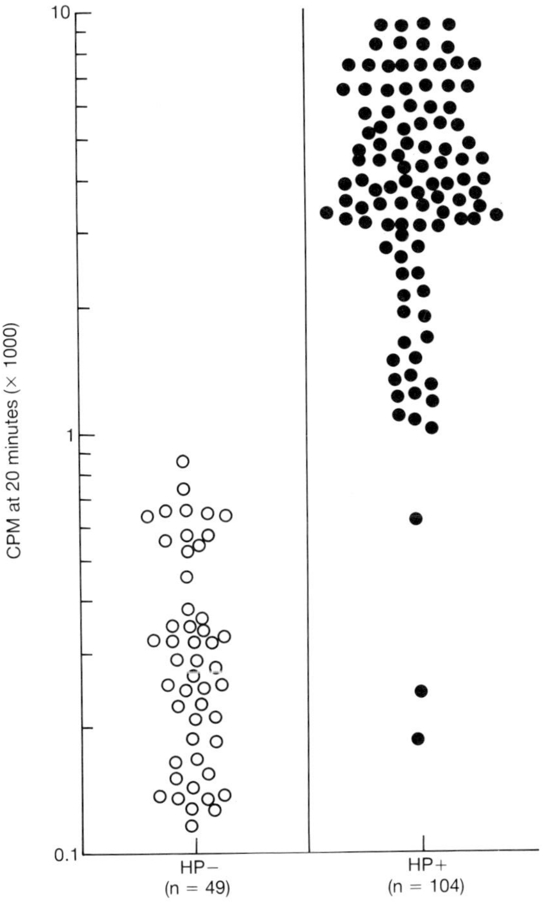

Fig. 12.11 ^{14}C-urea breath tests from 153 patients. With the logarithmic Y axis, large differences between HP− and HP+ are less apparent. (From Marshall *et al.* [66].)

sequestered in each organ, the biological half-life of the isotope in that tissue, the effective energy of β particles compared with standard ionizing radiation (a 200 kV X-ray source), and the administered dose. The long half-life of ^{14}C simplifies calculations, because the activity of the administered isotope can be regarded as constant for the time it is present in the body. DE is expressed in Sieverts (1 Sievert [Sv] = 100 rem, 10^{-5} Sv = 1 mrem).

Environmental sources of radiation

The average DE from cosmic radiation, terrestrial radiation, and endogenous naturally occurring radioisotopes in the United States is a minimum of 88 mrem year^{-1} [70]. In addition, the population is exposed to approximately 50 mrem year^{-1} of radiation due to diagnostic X-rays [71]. Therefore, DE for the average American is 2–3 mrem week^{-1} (much higher if recent observations of natural radon exposure in the United States are taken into account). Natural radiation is doubled for persons living in Colorado, and may also be increased by air travel at the rate of 0.3 mrem hour^{-1}. Because most people in the United States do not concern themselves with the risk of radiation from air travel or living in Colorado, radiation doses of less than 10 mrem year^{-1} are generally regarded as trivial. In addition, it should be noted that a normal person already carries ~0.1 μCi (3.7 kBq) of naturally occurring ^{14}C within body tissues.

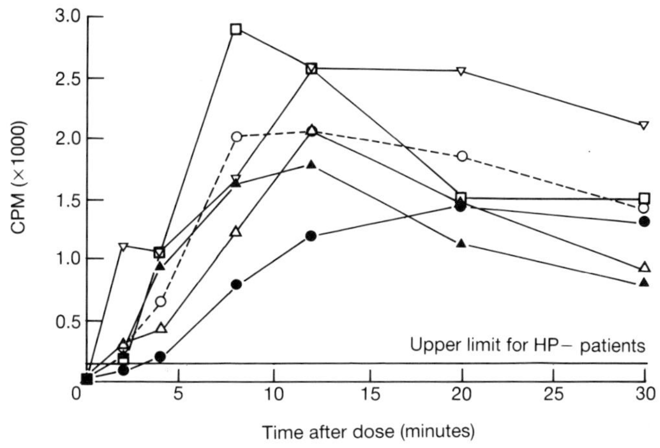

Fig. 12.12 Microdose capsule ^{14}C-urea breath test. Dose = 37 kBq.

Table 12.2 The ^{14}C-urea breath test compared with other common sources of radiation exposure

	185 kBq (5 μCi) ^{14}C-urea (mrem**)	Chest X-ray (mrem)	Upper GI series (mrem)	Natural sources* (2 weeks) (mrem)	Round trip by air, L.A.–N.Y. (mrem)
Bone	14.2	—	—	5.0	3.0
Breasts	3.5	14.0	53.0	5.0	3.0
Lungs	0.5	4.0	476.0	5.0–40.0***	3.0
Thyroid	0.3	6.5	7.0	5.0	3.0
Marrow	0.3	3.0	114.0	5.0	3.0
Testes	0.3	<0.01	0.4	5.0	3.0
Ovaries	0.3	0.06	45.0	5.0	3.0

Data from references [62, 70–76].
* Highest in Colorado (9 mrem); lowest in Louisiana (3 mrem).
** 1 mrem = 10^{-5} Sievert (Sv).
*** Lung doses much higher in high radon areas.

Calculations for ^{14}C-urea from existing data

The maximum radiation dose received from the ^{14}C-urea breath test occurs, in a theoretical subject, when 100% of the ingested urea is broken down by gastric urease and all the CO_2 enters the blood bicarbonate pool. From ^{14}C-labeled bicarbonate studies [72], it is known that in the first 5 hours, 75% is expired in the breath. The remaining 25% of the ^{14}C is taken up by metabolic processes with an excretion half-life of 10–12 days in soft tissues. Of this sequestered isotope, 10% (2.5% of the administered dose or 0.125 μCi in our test) enters bone and is excreted with a half-life of 40 days. Taking all deposited ^{14}C into account, the cumulative gonadal dose is a maximum of 0.06 mrem for every 1 μCi ^{14}C administered; i.e. 0.3 mrem in a 5 μCi breath test.

There is some concern about the DNA transmutation effect of ^{14}C. In brief, ^{14}C changes to nitrogen when it decomposes, an event which may cause mutation if it takes place within a DNA base pair. In experimental studies this effect is difficult to demonstrate, so that the transmutation effect of ^{14}C is not significantly more than the DE received from an equivalent γ-ray source [73]. A very conservative approach suggested by Totter *et al.* [74] is to double the effective DE for ^{14}C in order to account for any transmutation effects. It can be seen from Table 12.2 that natural radiation in 2 days gives more exposure to marrow and gonads than the 5 μCi ^{14}C-urea breath test [75], and 100 breath tests give less marrow exposure than a single upper gastrointestinal series (barium meal) [76].

Restrictions on use of the ^{14}C-urea breath test

The test should be used with similar guidelines to radiologic procedures. For example, ^{14}C-urea should not be given to women of child-bearing potential. It is our practice to observe the 10-day rule and obtain a pregnancy test if there is doubt about the possibility of pregnancy.

References

1 Marshall, BJ, & Warren, JR. Unidentified curved bacilli in the stomach of patients with gastritis and peptic ulceration. *Lancet* 1984;**i**:1311–15.
2 Hazell, SL, Borody, TJ, Gal, A, & Lee, A. *Campylobacter pyloridis* gastritis I: detection of urease as a marker of bacterial colonization and gastritis. *Am. J. Gastroenterol.* 1987;**82**:292–6.
3 Hazell, SL, Hennessy, WB, Borody, TJ, *et al.* *Campylobacter pyloridis* gastritis II: distribution of bacteria and associated inflammation in the gastroduodenal environment. *Am. J. Gastroenterol.* 1987;**82**:297–301.
4 Cohen, H, Gramisu, M, Fitzgibbons, P, Appleman, M, Skoglund, M, & Valenzuela, JE. *Campylobacter pylori*: associations with antral and fundic mucosal histology and diagnosis by serology in patients with upper gastrointestinal symptoms. *Am. J. Gastroenterol.* 1989;**84**: 367–71.
5 Queiroz, DM, Barbosa, AJ, Mendes, EN, *et al.* Distribution of *Campylobacter pylori* and gas-

tritis in the stomach of patients with and without duodenal ulcer. *Am. J. Gastroenterol.* 1988;**83**: 1368–70.

6 Bayerdorffer, E, Oertel, H, Lehn, N, *et al.* Topographic association between active gastritis and *Campylobacter pylori* colonisation. *J. Clin. Pathol.* 1989;**42**:834–9.

7 Royston, CM, Polak, J, Bloom, SR, *et al.* G cell population of the gastric antrum, plasma gastrin, and gastric acid secretion in patients with and without duodenal ulcer. *Gut* 1978;**19**:689–98.

8 Schrager, J, Spink, R, & Mitra, S. The antrum in patients with duodenal and gastric ulcers. *Gut* 1967;**8**:497–508.

9 Shames, B, Krajden, S, Fuksa, M, Babida, C, & Penner, JL. Evidence for the occurrence of the same strain of *Campylobacter pylori* in the stomach and dental plaque. *J. Clin. Microbiol.* 1989;**27**:2849–50.

10 Majmudar, P, Shah, SM, Dhunjibhoy, KR, & Desai, HG. Isolation of *Helicobacter pylori* from dental plaques in healthy volunteers. *Indian J. Gastroenterol.* 1990;**9**(4):271–2.

11 Talley, NJ, Cameron, AJ, Shorter, RG, Zinsmeister, AR, & Phillips, SF. *Campylobacter pylori* and Barrett's esophagus. *Mayo Clin. Proc.* 1988;**63**: 1176–80.

12 De Giacomo, C, Fiocca, R, Villani, L, Bertolotti, L, & Maggiore, G. Barrett's ulcer and *Campylobacter*-like organisms infection in a child. *J. Pediatr. Gastroenterol. Nutr.* 1988;**7**:766–8.

13 Taylor, AL. The epithelial heterotopias of the alimentary tract. *J. Pathol. Bact.* 1927;**30**:415–49.

14 Borhan-Manesh, F, & Farnhum, JB. Does *Campylobacter pylori* infect the heterotopic gastric mucosa (HGM) at the upper esophageal sphincter (UES)? *Gastroenterology* 1990;**98**(5, suppl 2):A23.

15 Frierson, HF, Caldwell, SH, & Marshall, BJ. Duodenal bulb biopsy findings for patients with non-ulcer dyspepsia with or without *Campylobacter pylori* gastritis. *Modern Pathology* 1990; **3**:271–6.

16 Wyatt, JI, Rathbone, BJ, Dixon, MF, & Heatley, RV. *Campylobacter pyloridis* and acid induced gastric metaplasia in the pathogenesis of duodenitis. *J. Clin. Pathol.* 1987;**40**:841–8.

17 Carrick, J, Lee, A, Hazell, S, Ralston, M, & Daskalopoulos, G. *Campylobacter pylori*, duodenal ulcer, and gastric metaplasia: possible role of functional heterotopic tissue in ulcerogenesis. *Gut* 1989;**30**:790–97.

18 de Cothi, GA, Newbold, KM, & O'Connor, HJ. *Campylobacter*-like organisms and heterotopic gastric mucosa in Meckel's diverticula. *J. Clin. Pathol.* 1989;**42**:132–4.

19 Morris, A, Nicholson, G, Zwi, J, & Vanderwee, M. *Campylobacter pylori* infection in Meckel's diverticula containing gastric mucosa. *Gut* 1989; **30**:1233–5.

20 Dye, KR, Marshall, BJ, Frierson, HF Jr, Pambianco, DJ, & McCallum, RW. *Campylobacter pylori* colonizing heterotopic gastric tissue in the rectum. *Am. J. Clin. Pathol.* 1990;**93**:144–7.

21 Marshall, BJ, McGechie, DB, Rogers, PA, & Glancy, RJ. Pyloric *Campylobacter* infection and gastroduodenal disease. *Med. J. Aust.* 1985;**142**: 439–44.

22 Pinkard, KJ, Harrison, B, Capstick, JA, Medley, G, & Lambert, JR. Detection of *Campylobacter pyloridis* in gastric mucosa by phase contrast microscopy. *J. Clin. Pathol.* 1986;**39**:112–3.

23 Langenberg, ML, Tytgat, GN, Schipper, ME, Rietra, PJ, & Zanen, HJ. *Campylobacter*-like organisms in the stomach of patients and healthy individuals (letter). *Lancet* 1984;**i**:1348–9.

24 Owen, RJ, Martin, SR, & Borman, P. Rapid urea hydrolysis by gastric campylobacters (letter). *Lancet* 1985;**i**:111.

25 Marshall, BJ, Warren, JR, Francis, GJ, Langton, SR, Goodwin, CS, & Blincow, ED. Rapid urease test in the management of *Campylobacter pyloridis*-associated gastritis. *Am. J. Gastroenterol.* 1987;**82**:200–210.

26 Barthel, JS, & Everett, ED. Diagnosis of *Campylobacter pylori* infections: the "gold standard" and the alternatives. *Rev. Infect. Dis.* 1990;**12**: S107–S114.

27 Santogade, PJ, Bokkenheuser, VD, Faisal, MA, Kotler, DP, Scholes, JV, & Holt, PR. Evaluation of methods for identification of *Campylobacter pyloridis* infection. *N. Y. State. J. Med.* 1990;**90**: 4–7.

28 Gad, A. Rapid diagnosis of *Campylobacter pylori* by brush cytology. *Scand. J. Gastroenterol.* 1989; **167**(suppl):101–103.

29 McNulty, CA, Dent, JC, Uff, JS, Gear, MW, & Wilkinson, SP. Detection of *Campylobacter pylori* by the biopsy urease test: an assessment in 1445 patients. *Gut* 1989;**30**:1058–62.

30 Morris, A, Ali, MR, Brown, P, Lane, M, & Patton, K. *Campylobacter pylori* infection in biopsy specimens of gastric antrum: laboratory diagnosis and estimation of sampling error. *J. Clin. Pathol.* 1989;**42**:727–32.

31 Schubert, TT, & Schnell, GA. Prevalence of *Campylobacter pylori* in patients undergoing upper endoscopy. *Am. J. Gastroenterol.* 1989;**84**: 637–42.

32 Schnell, GA, & Schubert, TT. Usefulness of culture, histology, and urease testing in the detection of *Campylobacter pylori*. *Am. J. Gastroenterol.* 1989;**84**:133–7.

33 Deltenre, M, Glupczynski, Y, De Prez, C, *et al.* The reliability of urease tests, histology and culture in the diagnosis of *Campylobacter pylori*

infection. *Scand. J. Gastroenterol.* 1989;**160** (suppl):19–24.
34 Nanivadekar, SA, Bhat, PP, Sawant, PD, *et al.* Rapid diagnostic test of *Campylobacter pylori* infection in patients of gastritis, duodenal ulcer and gastric ulcer. A study of 100 cases. *J. Assoc. Physicians India* 1989;**37**:307–10.
35 Dye, KR, Marshall, BJ, Frierson, HF, Barrett, LJ, Guerrant, RL, & McCallum, RW. Is CLOtest alone adequate to diagnose *Campylobacter pylori* (abstract)? *Am. J. Gastroenterol.* 1988;**83**:1032.
36 Borsch, G, Adamek, R, Sandmann, M, *et al.* Comparison of biopsy urease test and histologic examination for detection of *Campylobacter pylori* in duodenal, antral and fundic biopsies. *Hepatogastroenterology* 1987;**34**:236–41.
37 Parsonnet, J, Welch, K, Compton, C, *et al.* Simple microbiologic detection of *Campylobacter pylori. J. Clin. Microbiol.* 1988;**26**:948–9.
38 Walters, LL, Budin, RE, & Paull, G. Acridine-orange to identify *Campylobacter pyloridis* in formalin-fixed, paraffin-embedded gastric biopsies (letter). *Lancet* 1986;**i**:42.
39 Chodos, JE, Dworkin, BM, Smith, F, Van Horn, K, Weiss, L, & Rosenthal, WS. *Campylobacter pylori* and gastroduodenal disease: a prospective endoscopic study and comparison of diagnostic tests. *Am. J. Gastroenterol.* 1988;**83**:1226–30.
40 Coudron, PE, & Kirby, DF. Comparison of rapid urease tests, staining techniques, and growth on different solid media for detection of *Campylobacter pylori. J. Clin. Microbiol.* 1989;**27**:1527–30.
41 de Lange, EE. Radiographic features of gastritis using the biphasic contrast technique. *Curr. Probl. Diagn. Radiol.* 1987;**16**:276–319.
42 de Lange, EE, Shaffer, HA, & Croft, BY. Radiographic examination of the stomach and duodenum: comparison of single-, double-, and biphasic-contrast methods. *Eur. J. Radiol.* 1990;**10**:167–74.
43 Engstrand, L, Pahlson, C, Schwan, A, & Gustavsson, S. Monoclonal antibodies for detection of *Campylobacter pylori* in biopsy smears and frozen sections. *Scand. J. Gastroenterol.* 1988;**142**(suppl):50–52.
44 Shadowen, RD, & Sciortino, CV. Rapid identification of *Campylobacter pylori* using monoclonal antibodies directed against outer membrane proteins. *Virginia Medical 1989;* **116**:512.
45 Cartun, RW, Pedersen, CA, Krzymowski, A, & Berman, MM. Immunocytochemical detection of *Helicobacter pylori* in formalin fixed tissue biopsy specimens (letter). *J. Clin. Pathol.* 1990;**43**:518.
46 Jones, DM, Lessells, AM, & Eldridge, J. *Campylobacter*-like organisms on the gastric mucosa: culture, histological, and serological studies. *J. Clin. Pathol.* 1984;**37**:1002–6.
47 Marshall, BJ, McGechie, DB, Francis, GJ, & Utley, PJ. Pyloric campylobacter serology (letter). *Lancet* 1984;**ii**:281.
48 Marshall, BJ, Whisson, M, Francis, G, & McGechie, DB. Correlation between symptoms of dyspepsia and *Campylobacter pyloridis* serology in Western Australian blood donors. In: Pearson, AD, Skirrow, MB, Lior, H, & Rowe, B, (eds), *Campylobacter III. Proceedings of the Third International Workshop on Campylobacter Infections.* London: Public Health Laboratory Service, 1985, pp. 188–9.
49 Goodwin, CS, Blincow, E, Peterson, G, *et al.* Enzyme-linked immunosorbent assay for *Campylobacter pyloridis*: correlation with presence of *C. pyloridis* in the gastric mucosa. *J. Infect. Dis.* 1987;**155**:488–94.
50 von Wulffen, H, & Grote, HJ. Enzyme-linked immunosorbent assay for detection of immunoglobulin A and G antibodies to *Campylobacter pylori. Eur. J. Clin. Microbiol. Infect. Dis.* 1988;**7**:559–65.
51 Mitchell, HM, Lee, A, Berkowicz, J, & Borody, T. The use of serology to diagnose active *Campylobacter pylori* infection. *Med. J. Aust.* 1988;**149**:604–9.
52 Evans, DJ Jr, Evans, DG, Smith, KE, & Graham, DY. Serum antibody responses to the *N*-acetylneuraminyllactose-binding hemagglutinin of *Campylobacter pylori. Infect. Immun.* 1989;**57**:664–7.
53 Vaira, D, Holton, J, Osborn, J, *et al.* Endoscopy in dyspeptic patients: is gastric mucosal biopsy useful. *Am. J. Gastroenterol.* 1990;**85**:701–4.
54 Oderda, G, Vaira, D, Holton, J, Dowsett, JF, & Ansaldi, N. Serum pepsinogen I and IgG antibody to *Campylobacter pylori* in non-specific abdominal pain in childhood. *Gut* 1989;**30**:912–16.
55 Newell, DG, & Stacey, A. Antigens for the serodiagnosis of *Campylobacter pylori* infections. *Gastroenterol. Clin. Biol.* 1989;**13**:37B–41B.
56 Delluva, AM, Markley, K, & Davies, RE. The absence of gastric urease in germ-free animals. *Biochim. Biophys. Acta* 1968;**151**:646–50.
57 Mobley, HT, Cortesa, MJ, Rosenthal, LE, & Jones, BD, Characterization of urease from *Campylobacter pylori. J. Clin. Microbiol.* 1988:**26**:831–6.
58 Marshall, BJ, Barrett, L, Prakash, C, McCallum, RW, & Guerrant, RL. Urea protects *Helicobacter (Campylobacter) pylori* from the bactericidal effect of acid. *Gastroenterology* 1990;**99**:697–702.
59 Marshall, BJ, & Surveyor, I. ^{14}Carbon urea breath test for the diagnosis of *Campylobacter pylori* associated gastritis. *J. Nucl. Med.* 1988;**29**:11–16.
60 Eggers, RH, Kulp, A, Ludtke, FE, & Bauer, FE. Characterization of the ^{13}C urea breath test for diagnosis of *Campylobacter pylori* infections.

In: Chapman, TE, Berger, R, Reijngoud, DJ, & Okken, A (eds), *Stable Isotopes in Paediatric Nutritional and Metabolic Research*. Andover: Intercept, 1990, pp. 295–301.

61 Graham, DY, Klein, PD, Evans, DJ Jr, *et al.* *Campylobacter pylori* detected noninvasively by the ^{13}C-urea breath test. *Lancet* 1987;**i**:1174–7.

62 Schoeller, DA, Schneider, JF, Solomons, NW, Watkins, JB, & Klein, PD. Clinical diagnosis with the stable isotope ^{13}C in CO_2 breath tests: methodology and fundamental considerations. *J. Lab. Clin. Med.* 1977;**90**:412–21.

63 Klein, PD, & Graham, DY. Detection of *Campylobacter pylori* by the ^{13}C-urea breath test. In: Rathbone, BJ, & Heatley, RV (eds), *Campylobacter pylori and Gastroduodenal Disease*. Oxford: Blackwell Scientific Publications, 1989, pp. 94–105.

64 Mobley, HT, Cortesa, MJ, Rosenthal, LE, & Jones, BD. Characterization of urease from *Campylobacter pylori*. *J. Clin. Microbiol.* 1988;**26**:831–6.

65 Surveyor, I, Goodwin, CS, Mullan, BP, Geelhoed, E, Warren, JR, Murray, RN, Waters, TE, & Sanderson, CR. The ^{14}C-urea breath-test for the detection of gastric *Campylobacter pylori* infection. *Med. J. Aust.* 1989;**151**:435–9.

66 Marshall, BJ, Plankey, MW, Hoffman, SR, *et al.* A 20-minute breath test for the diagnosis of *H. pylori*. *Am. J. Gastroenterol.* 1991;**86**:438–45.

67 Ormand, JE, Talley, NJ, Carpenter, HA, *et al.* ^{14}C-urea breath test for the diagnosis of *Helicobacter pylori*. *Dig. Dis. Sci.* 1990;**35**:879–84.

68 Veldhuyzen van Zanten, SJ, Tytgat, KM, Hollingsworth, J, *et al.* ^{14}C-urea breath test for the detection of *Helicobacter pylori*. *Am. J. Gastroenterol.* 1990;**85**:399–403.

69 Kessler, MJ. Statistics in liquid scintillation counting. In: *Liquid Scintillation Analysis, Science and Technology*. Downers Grove, Illinois Packard Instrument Co. 1990; 5.1–5.5

70 Oakley, DT. Natural radiation exposure in the United States. Washington, D.C: U.S. Environmental Protection Agency, Office of Radiation Programs, Surveillance and Inspection Division, 1972.

71 Last, JM. *Public Health and Preventive Medicine*. Norwalk, Connecticut: Appleton-Century-Crofts, pp. 753.

72 Yap, SH, Hafkenscheid, JCM, Goossens, CMIC, Buys, WCAM, Binkhorst, RA, & Van Tongeren, JHM. Estimation of radiation dosage and transmutation effect of ^{14}C involved in measuring the rate of albumin synthesis with ^{14}C bicarbonate. *J. Nucl. Med.* 1974;**16**:642–8.

73 National Council on Radiation Protection and Measurements. Task group 11 on genetic risk. II Title III. Genetic effects from internally deposited radionuclides. *National Council on Radiation Protection and Measurements report No. 89*:**4**, 21–25, 1987.

74 Totter, JR, Zelle, MR, & Hollister, H. Hazard to man of ^{14}carbon. *Science* 1958;**128**:1490–95.

75 Kathryn, RL. *Radioactivity in the Environment: Sources, Distribution, and Surveillance*. New York: Harwood Academic, 1985; pp. 78–90.

76 Keriakes, J, & Rosenstein, M (eds). *The Handbook of Radiation Doses*. Boca Raton: CRC Press Inc., 1980.

77 Bell, GD, Weil, J, Harrison, G, Morden, A, Jones, PH, Gant, PW, Trowell, JE, Yoong, AK, Daneshmend, TK, & Logan, RF. ^{14}C-urea breath analysis, a non-invasive test for *Campylobacter pylori* in the stomach (letter). *Lancet* 1987;**i**: 1367–8.

78 Rauws, EAJ, Royen, EAV, Langenberg, W, Woensel, JV, Vrij, AA, & Tytgat, GN. ^{14}C-urea breath test in *C. pylori* gastritis. *Gut* 1989;**30**: 798–803.

13: Treatment of Helicobacter pylori

B.J. MARSHALL

Introduction

Historical notes

Even before the discovery of spiral gastric bacteria, bismuth therapy was commonly prescribed for gastrointestinal complaints and, as such, was probably the first therapy used for *Helicobacter pylori*. Kussmaul advocated bismuth subcarbonate for gastric ulcer [1], Ogle treated non-ulcer dyspepsia with bismuth subcitrate [2], and Osler sometimes offered bismuth subnitrate lozenges for acute and chronic gastritis [3]. In 1901, the forerunner of "Pepto-Bismol" (bismuth subsalicylate) was advocated for the treatment of infantile cholera, a disorder which in retrospect may have actually been *C. jejuni* gastroenteritis. The anti-spirochetal action of bismuth was subsequently proven by Robert & Sauton in 1916 [4], after which it was used extensively as an anti-spirochetal agent in human syphilis.

The first attempt to actually treat *H. pylori* infection was made by myself and Robin Warren in 1981. An elderly man, with suspected abdominal angina but normal endoscopy, was found to have *Campylobacter*-like organisms (CLO) and gastritis on biopsy. After 14 days' treatment with 500 mg q.i.d. of tetracycline syrup, the histology had improved, CLO could not be demonstrated, and the patient was asymptomatic.

The idea that *H. pylori* could be treated with bismuth arose in 1983, following the observation by Martin *et al.* [5] that duodenal ulcers healed with colloidal bismuth subcitrate (CBS) did not relapse as often as those treated with cimetidine. Investigating the cause of this effect, Gregory *et al.* [6] had studied duodenal ulcer borders and had shown circular profiles of CLO in pretreatment electron micrographs. I noted that the bacteria had disappeared in post-treatment illustrations. To see if CBS inhibited the bacteria, a disc was dipped in liquid "DeNol" and placed onto a culture plate of *H. pylori*, and 3 days later a large zone of inhibition was seen (Fig. 13.1).

As a result of that experiment, a controlled trial of duodenal ulcer therapy with either cimetidine or CBS was undertaken, with gastric biopsy to observe changes in gastritis and CLO. After treating 10 patients in each group, it became evident that CLO were suppressed, but not usually eradicated, by CBS therapy [7].

The first bismuth/antibiotic combination therapy for *H. pylori* was tried in 1983. A gastritis patient, treated with an 8-week course of CBS chewing tablets ("DeNol"), relapsed clinically and histologically 1 month later. On the second occasion, amoxicillin, 500 mg q.i.d., was added to the bismuth therapy causing eradication of the organism [8]. *H. pylori*, although not an anaerobe, is usually susceptible to bismuth/nitroimidazole combination therapy. I noted this when a patient developed a sore mouth while taking CBS. Suspecting periodontitis, I added metronidazole to his therapy. Long-term follow-up confirmed eradication of CLO and healing of gastritis. Experience in a large series of patients revealed a failure rate of 20–50% with both these regimens, causing Borody *et al.* to develop the present triple therapy regimens for *H. pylori* during 1986–87 in Sydney, Australia [9].

Table 13.1 lists *H. pylori* cure rates and minimal inhibitory concentrations (MICs) for most commonly used antibiotics. Data for Table 13.1 were derived from the references

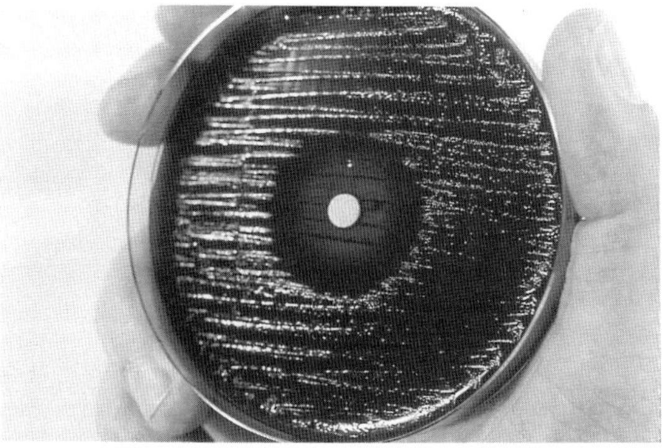

Fig. 13.1 Three-day-old culture of *H. pylori* inhibited by colloidal bismuth subcitrate ("DeNol"). The disc contains 50 μg of bismuth subcitrate.

cited in the text, and updated at the 1990 World Congress of Gastroenterology. More detailed information is available in papers by Bayerdorffer & Ottenjann [10], Glupczynski *et al.* [11], and McNulty *et al.* [12, 13]. It should be noted that only combination drug therapy has produced useful eradication rates.

Rules for assessing *H. pylori* therapies

In an early study [7], we noted the disappearance of *H. pylori* with therapy, but reappearance of the bacterium in 85% of patients 6 weeks later. Restriction endonuclease analysis of relapsing patients by Langenberg *et al.* [14] demonstrated that apparent reinfection in their patients was usually bacteriologic relapse with the original

Table 13.1 Antibiotics used in the treatment of *H. pylori*

			Eradication (%)	
	Notes	MIC ($mg\ l^{-1}$)	Single agent	Combination therapy
Bismuth subcitrate	abck	4–30	0–40	70–90
Bismuth subsalicylate	abck	4–30	0–10	70–90
Metronidazole	degk	1–4	5	70
Tinidazole	degk	1–4	5	70
Amoxicillin	abdk	<1	10–20	30–40
Ampicillin	abdfhk	<1	20	?50
Penicillin	ai	0.01–0.1	?0	—
Tetracycline	abcfk	0.5–2	10–20	70–90
Minocycline	acf	0.5	?0	—
Doxycycline	abcdi	0.1–3	5	5
Erythromycin	adgk	0.01–1	10	40–60
Clindamycin	ag	2–8	?10	?
Gentamicin	afg	0.1–1	?	—
Furazolidone	abcg	2–12	20–40	30
Nitrofurantoin	abcg	2–12	15–30	30
Rifampicin	afh	0.2–4	?	—
Ofloxacin	bdfgh	0.1–2	13	30
Ciprofloxacin	dfgh	0.1–8	0	—
Cefalexin	abfh	0.5–8	0	—
Cefoxitin	afh	0.1–0.5	?	—
Imipenem	afh	0.12–2	?	—
Thiamphenicol	ai	2–8	0	—
Sulfonamides	j	—	—	—
Vancomycin	j	—	—	—

a, *H. pylori* is (almost) always sensitive *in vitro*; b, monotherapy may be effective in some patients; c, seems to act by a topical effect; d, seems to act by a topical and/or a systemic effect; e, resistant organisms very common in some countries; f, not evaluated fully *in vivo*; g, *H. pylori* quickly develops resistance *in vivo*; h, potentially a useful agent; i, very poor eradication results *in vivo*; j, *H. pylori* is not inhibited *in vitro*; k, effective in double or triple therapy (see text).

strain. This implied that the infections had been inadequately treated, and that a negative biopsy immediately after therapy was useless as an indicator of bacteriologic cure. The explanation for this phenomenon is that reappearance of the organism may be in a patchy fashion, so that biopsy sampling of mucosa results in false-negative specimens in the first month post-treatment.

In a double-blind trial of cimetidine versus bismuth/tinidazole therapy for duodenal ulcer [15], we observed disappearance of *H. pylori* in 29 patients biopsied 2 weeks after completing therapy. During a 12 month follow-up period, relapse of infection occurred in two (14%), and apparent reinfection occurred in one. This suggested that biopsy 2 weeks after therapy was also too soon, since false-negative biopsy results still occurred in 14% of patients. Rauws *et al.* [16] studied patients treated by several different therapies, and found that a negative biopsy 1 month after completing therapy was proof of cure. Reappearance of the bacterium after 1 month was due to reinfection.

For the above reasons, discussion of eradication of *H. pylori* must be based only on studies in which follow-up biopsy was performed more than 28 days after completing therapy. In these studies, the test used to prove eradication should be sensitive, and should detect a component of the bacterium rather than an immunologic response. Currently, biopsy of the gastric mucosa for histology is still the most sensitive means of detecting *H. pylori*. At least two biopsy specimens should be tested by staining, urease tests, immunologic methods, or culture (see Chapter 12). Alternatively, the urea breath test may be used [17]. If the above methods are unavailable, serial antibody titers [18], which show falling titers 1 and 6 months after treatment, are circumstantial evidence of cure (Fig. 13.2).

Agents used in the treatment of *H. pylori*

Bismuth

Pharmacology of bismuth salts

Bismuth is the heaviest non-radioactive element, with an atomic number of 83, and an atomic weight of 209. It is chemically related to phosphorus, arsenic, and antimony, which occur in the same group of the periodic table.

The primary bismuth salt, bismuth nitrate, is produced by the action of concentrated nitric acid on bismuth metal. This may be hydrolyzed to bismuth subnitrate in boiling water. Bismuth nitrate will react in solution with soluble basic salts such as carbonates, salicylates, and citrates to form bismuth subcarbonate, bismuth subgallate, bismuth subsalicylate (BSS) or bismuth subcitrate. With the addition of ammonia, bismuth subcitrate forms a colloidal solution in which the trivalent bismuth atom links to trivalent citrate moieties to produce large complexes in a viscous solution. This solution is now spray-dried to form the current CBS formulation called "swallowable tablets," which are undergoing evaluation in the United States.

Bismuth salts are poorly soluble in water, and in hydrochloric acid they convert to bismuth oxide [Bi_2O_3], bismuth hydroxide [$Bi(OH)_3$], and bismuth oxychloride [$BiOCl$], which are very insoluble. As a result, most bismuth salts form a precipitate of BiOCl in the stomach. In the upper small intestine they may be converted back to the subcarbonate; but this too is in-

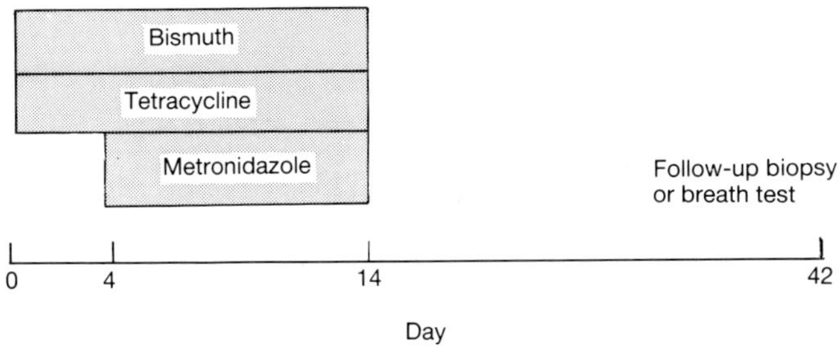

Fig. 13.2 Timeline of therapy for *H. pylori*.

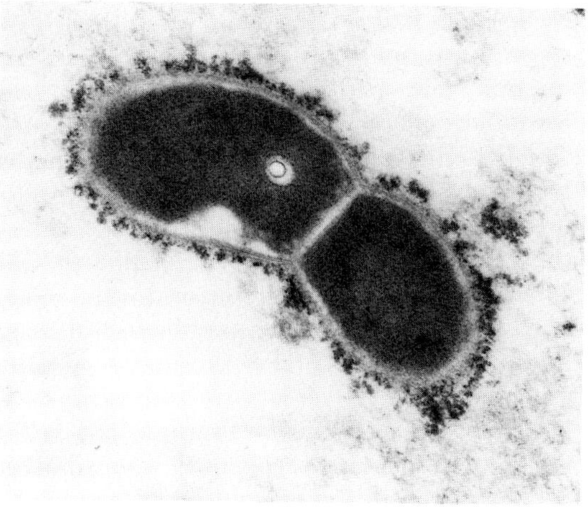

Fig. 13.3 *H. pylori* organism surrounded by dense bismuth granules. The bacterium has detached from the mucosa and is starting to lyse. (Electron micrograph taken 60 minutes after dosing with 120 mg bismuth subcitrate.)

soluble. Only trace amounts of bismuth (1–2% of an oral dose) are absorbed, probably via localization on the brush border glycocalyx of intestinal enterocytes and subsequent phagocytosis by the cells [19, 20].

Bismuth is excreted by the kidneys. The half-life of bismuth in blood is 5 days, but the half-life in cerebrospinal fluid (CSF), a more important factor in estimating toxicity, is 15 days. In the colon, bismuth salts are converted to black bismuth sulfide by the action of H_2S produced by bacteria. This causes the dark stools and tongue staining seen in patients regularly taking bismuth.

Action of bismuth on H. pylori

Bismuth salts probably work as topical antibacterial agents against *H. pylori* in the gastric mucosa. The exact mechanism of bacterial killing is unknown, but may be similar to that of the arsenical antibacterial agents, which are also trivalent cations which bind reversibly to sulfhydryl groups in proteins [21]. The most well-known example of such interaction is the inhibition of glycolytic enzymes by arsenic [22].

In electron microscope studies of gastric mucosa 60 minutes after dosing, bismuth granules are seen encircling non-viable, detached *H. pylori* organisms [7] (Fig. 13.3). The mechanism for this is unknown, but *in vitro*, bismuth salts inhibit *H. pylori* enzymes, particularly urease [23] and phospholipases [24].

Graham *et al.* [25] and Weil & Bell [26] have both noted disappearance of breath test urease activity soon after patients ingested bismuth, suggesting rapid killing of the organism or inactivation of its urease. Lanza *et al.* [27] observed that *in vivo*, clearance of *H. pylori* from gastric mucosa occurred in 80% of patients within 14 days, and that further therapy did not seem to increase the clearance rate. The half-life of bismuth in the gastric mucus may be too short to ensure inhibition of *H. pylori* for more than 4 hours after a dose (see Chapter 15), so more frequent dosing (e.g. 3-hourly) may be worthwhile.

The major advantage of bismuth salts for the treatment of *H. pylori* lies in their very low incidence of major side effects. In the absence of renal failure, there is virtually no toxicity of bismuth when given for 14 days in the doses recommended here.

Bismuth subsalicylate

In the United States, bismuth is readily available over the counter as "Pepto-Bismol" or similar generic formulations. "Pepto-Bismol" is a suspension of bismuth subsalicylate (BSS), 171 mg 10 ml^{-1}, in a vehicle containing magnesium aluminum silicate (montmorillonite clay), methylcellulose, methyl salicylate, and pink food coloring. The tablets contain 262 mg BSS plus 350 mg of calcium carbonate. The usual dose for diarrhea prophylaxis is 30 ml or two tablets, four to eight times daily. Each dose contains salicylate equivalent to 258 mg of salicylic acid [28]. Maximum strength "Pepto-Bismol" liquid contains double the above amount of BSS. Several other generic brands are also available in drug stores.

Early studies with BSS demonstrated that it healed gastritis and suppressed *H. pylori* infection [27, 29], but our observation is that suppression is only temporary. In a double-blind placebo-controlled study in which patients received 21 days' therapy with BSS [30], *H. pylori* was eradicated in only 6% (one in 17). For this reason, BSS is usually used in combination with another antibacterial agent. Only 14 days are required in such courses, so there is no concern about chronic toxicity.

Colloidal bismuth subcitrate

In Europe, Great Britain, and Australia, colloidal bismuth subcitrate (CBS, "DeNol"), is used for the treatment of gastric and duodenal ulcers. In its original form, called "liquid DeNol" or tripotassium dicitrato-bismuthate, it was noted to prevent duodenal ulcer relapse [5], but its antibacterial properties *in vivo* were never tested. It was superseded by a spray-dried tablet form called "chewable tablets," which was also proved to lower duodenal ulcer relapse [31], and which eradicated *H. pylori* in about 30% of patients [15, 32].

More recently, the chewable tablets were replaced by swallowable tablets. The new formulation is probably equivalent to BSS in its antibacterial properties, since it does not eradicate *H. pylori* by itself, but must be used in combination with another antibacterial agent [33]. The dose used is four tablets daily, equivalent to 480 mg of bismuth. Ulcer regimens have used this dose of CBS for up to 8 weeks with only minor elevation of serum bismuth levels [34]. Transient (1 hour) elevations of serum bismuth were noted with swallowable tablets by Nwokolo *et al.* [35].

Alternative formulations of bismuth

In the United States, two other bismuth products can be obtained. Bismuth subgallate is sold as a stool deodorizer for colostomy patients. The 200 mg tablets are available as "Devrom*". The efficacy of the formulation is unknown, but we have used 4–8 tablets per day in patients who say they are allergic to salicylate or "pink dye."

Bismuth subcitrate suspension may be obtained by mail order as "Bismagel**". The suspension comes as 120 mg per 5 ml in a 1 liter bottle. Patients take one teaspoonful four to eight times daily. The stability and shelf-life of the mixture makes it unsuitable for mass production, but patients can obtain the fresh formulation by mail order at reasonable cost. In two patients tested while on this medicine, we have seen complete suppression of *H. pylori* urease on ^{14}C-urea breath test, so we believe the efficacy is similar to that of BSS or CBS. The medicine has a slight aniseed taste and, as with bismuth subgallate, may be useful in patients who cannot take the usual bismuth preparations.

Other less-well-known formulations which we have not used are bismuth subcarbonate, 260 mg per 30 ml, with kaolin and pectin ("K-C†"), and bismuth subgallate, 300 mg per 30 ml, with kaolin ("Dia-Eze††").

In Germany, several bismuth salts were components of over-the-counter antacid medications, allowing them to be quickly revived as *H. pylori* therapy with the discovery of their antibacterial action. Small clinical studies with most of these have demonstrated an ability to suppress *H. pylori* infection, but not to eradicate the organism without the aid of supplementary antibiotics. The names and dosages of these salts are: bismuth subnitrate 350 mg, two tablets t.i.d. ("Ulkowis," Temmler Pharma); bismuth subnitrate 150 mg, and bismuth aluminate 50 mg, two tablets b.i.d. ("Angass," Medice-Iserlohn); bismuth subgallate 50 mg, and bismuth subnitrate 100 mg, two tablets t.i.d. ("Bismofalk," Falk); bismuth aluminate 200 mg, two tablets t.i.d. ("Campylotec," Pfizer; "Ultin," DrRentschler). In addition, the more-well-known bismuth salts are available, such as CBS ("Telen," Byk-Gulden) and BSS ("Jatrox," Rohm-Pharma).

In evaluating potential *H. pylori* therapeutic agents, shrewd pharmaceutical companies still prefer to measure efficacy as *H. pylori* "clearance" immediately after therapy. This allows publication of suppression results, rather than the exhibition of very much weaker cure data from biopsy samples taken 1 month later.

* The Parthenon Co Inc, 3311 West 2400 South, Salt Lake City, Utah 84119 (1-800-453-8898).

** Clark Pharmacy, 15615 Bel-Red Road, Bellevue, Washington, 98008 (206-881-0222).

† Century Pharmaceuticals, 10377 Hague Road, Indianapolis 46256 (317-849-4210).

†† Central Pharmaceuticals, 120 E. 3rd St., PO Box 328, Seymour, Indiana 47274-9985 (812-522-3915).

Safety of bismuth salts

In the French epidemic of bismuth encephalopathy, patients often consumed 10–20 g of bismuth subnitrate or subgallate per day [36]. Recent reports of toxicity include the following cases:

1 The administration of high doses of BSS to a terminal AIDS patient with diarrhea due to extensive mucosal ulceration of the bowel [37] resulted in apparent bismuth encephalopathy, even though the serum bismuth level was only 200 $\mu g\,l^{-1}$. The patient died from other causes.

2 A 68-year-old man with chronic renal failure and a creatinine clearance of only 15 ml $minute^{-1}$ consumed twice the recommended amount of liquid "DeNol" (CBS) for 8 weeks [38]. He developed encephalopathy with a serum bismuth level of 880 $\mu g\,l^{-1}$. The syndrome was completely reversible over 50 days, in which time the EEG returned to normal and serum bismuth fell to below 50 $\mu g\,l^{-1}$. This formulation of bismuth is no longer available.

3 Acute renal failure developed 10 days after a 27-year-old man took 100 "DeNol" tablets in a suicide attempt [39]. The colon was found to be still loaded with bismuth. Encephalopathy was not present, even though the serum bismuth level was only slightly elevated at 260 $\mu g\,l^{-1}$. With purgation and hemodialysis he completely recovered in 5 days.

4 A 76-year-old man took 80 "DeNol" tablets in a suicide attempt [40]. He died eventually from a perforated duodenal ulcer, but developed encephalopathy and renal failure with a serum bismuth level of 1600 $\mu g\,l^{-1}$.

In the doses recommended here I have never seen a side-effect related to bismuth accumulation. I do not keep patients on bismuth salts longer than 2 months and, if repeated courses are required, the patients take the drug for only 2 months in every 4 months. In patients who have taken more than 4 months' bismuth therapy in 1 year, I estimate the plasma bismuth level before prescribing more. Done by atomic absorption spectrometry at an experienced laboratory, levels less than 5 $\mu g\,l^{-1}$ can be detected. A bismuth concentration of 100 $\mu g\,l^{-1}$ (100 ppb or 480 $nmol\,l^{-1}$) is the upper limit of the safe range, although most patients with encephalopathy have blood levels in the 200–2000 $\mu g\,l^{-1}$ range.

In patients with renal failure, bismuth is best avoided since the potential for toxicity is high. On the other hand, absorption is unlikely to be a problem if a single 14-day course is used. If BSS is given, the chance of salicylate toxicity also needs to be considered.

Metronidazole and tinidazole

Nitroimidazoles are used mainly for the treatment of anaerobic infections and parasites such as *Giardia* and *Trichomonas*. They are secreted in saliva and differ from each other only in dosage and half-life. Tinidazole is usually given as a single daily dose of 1 g, whereas metronidazole is given as 250–500 mg t.i.d.

In developed countries, about 75% of *H. pylori* isolates are sensitive to nitroimidazoles [12]. Goodwin *et al.* observed that the bacterium immediately became resistant to nitroimidazoles if they were used as single antibacterial agents [41]. This phenomenon meant that eradication of *H. pylori* was seen in only one of 29 patients (4%) given a cimetidine/tinidazole combination.

Similarly, any person previously exposed to nitroimidazoles, whether for *H. pylori* therapy or for other reasons, is likely to have a resistant *H. pylori* organism. Since women are more commonly treated with these drugs, their carriage of resistant *H. pylori* is slightly greater than men. In areas where parasitic infections are commonly treated with metronidazole, resistant isolates are far more common, so much so that Glupczynski *et al.* [42] do not recommend the use of metronidazole in Africa.

Resistance to nitroimidazoles does not usually develop if a second antimicrobial drug is given concurrently. This was first observed with tinidazole/bismuth therapy, but appears to hold true if the bismuth is replaced with amoxicillin or tetracycline. The reason for this was studied by Goodwin *et al.* [41], who were able to select out resistant *H. pylori* isolates from broth cultures of organisms which on initial assessment appeared to be inhibited by nitroimidazoles. It is suspected that the large pool of gastric *H. pylori* present in infected persons ($\approx 10^{10}$ organisms) usually contains a few with inherent nitroimidazole resistance.

Exposure to the agent selects out the resistant organism, which becomes the predominant strain. After initial suppression of infection, gastritis redevelops in a week or so as the resistant isolate recolonizes the stomach.

If *H. pylori* is attacked initially with bismuth or amoxicillin, only a few organisms remain viable and the chances are that a nitroimidazole-resistant strain will not emerge. The bismuth salt or antibiotic used is not critical for this effect, as long as "sterilization" of the mucosa is achieved before the nitroimidazole reaches the gastric mucosa. Failure of sensitive organisms to be eradicated by bismuth/nitroimidazole combinations might be due to incomplete coating of the gastric mucosa with the bismuth drug. Both Lanza *et al.* [29] and McNulty *et al.* [28] found that 20% of patients still have detectable organisms while on bismuth. In such patients the bismuth therapy would not be expected to protect against development of resistance. Our own experience is that when *H. pylori* is sensitive, 90% of patients are cured during dual therapy with bismuth and metronidazole [43, 44]. Whenever failure occurs with this therapy, a resistant isolate has emerged.

The optimal duration of *H. pylori* therapy has not been decided. Several investigators have reported success using 5- or 7-day therapies, but no direct comparison with 14-day or 28-day therapy has been performed. At the World Congress of Gastroenterology, held in Sydney, Australia, in 1990, the working party on *H. pylori* recommended a 14-day therapy of bismuth (CBS), one tablet q.i.d., in combination with metronidazole 1 g day^{-1} and tetracycline 2 g day^{-1}. Presently, we continue to use a 14-day therapy, with 10 days of metronidazole commencing on the 4th day. The dose of metronidazole is 20 mg kg^{-1} day^{-1} (1–1.5 g day^{-1} as a t.i.d. dose). Doses less than 1 g day^{-1} may be less effective (C. O'Morain, personal communication).

Side-effects with nitroimidazoles are common, but usually of little consequence. The drugs are known to give a positive result with the "Ames Test," a sensitive bacteriologic indicator of genetic damage. Nitroimidazoles are therefore potentially teratogenic and carcinogenic, and should be avoided in women who might be pregnant. Chronic use can cause a reversible peripheral neuropathy, but has not been seen in any of our patients treated for only 10 days. The drugs also have a disulfiram-like effect, so alcohol should be avoided while taking them. High doses cause a metallic taste in the mouth and may alter the bacterial flora, causing a temporary (1–2 weeks) furry coat on the tongue. Diarrhea occurs in around 20%, but in our experience is limited to the duration of therapy. Since nitroimidazoles are always given in combination with other agents, the cause of the side-effects is often uncertain, and could equally be due to bismuth or the other agent.

Amoxicillin

Amoxicillin is the most widely reported penicillin used in the treatment of *H. pylori*. Amoxicillin and ampicillin are acid-stable and are absorbed from the stomach as well as the intestine. Although all isolates of *H. pylori* are sensitive to amoxicillin *in vitro*, treatment results *in vivo* have been disappointing. For example, Rauws *et al.* found only a 10–20% cure rate using the drug as monotherapy [16]. The failure of amoxicillin monotherapy to eradicate *H. pylori* has not been adequately explained. McNulty *et al.* [13] studied mucosal levels of pivampicillin (an ampicillin pro-drug) and amoxicillin. They observed levels 2–10 times the serum level of antibiotic, easily exceeding the *in vitro* MIC for *H. pylori*. In contrast, Cooreman *et al.* [45] reported levels of only 0.2 mg l^{-1} in the antrum, and levels were even lower than this in corpus mucosa.

Eradication rates for penicillins which are not soluble in gastric acid (e.g. phenoxymethyl penicillin) have not been published, but are believed to be negligible. This suggests that gastric absorption of penicillins is important and luminal activity is responsible for eradication.

After some initial success in individuals, Goodwin *et al.* [41] treated patients with 14 days of CBS plus amoxicillin 2 g day^{-1} for either 7 or 14 days. Cure rates were around 40% for both regimens. At the University of Virginia, we have achieved cure rates of only 30% using amoxicillin/BSS combinations, so we do not use it as first-line therapy. In four of our patients, doses of amoxicillin up to 4 g daily for 14 days did not eradicate *H. pylori*, and in one patient pseudomembranous colitis developed.

Amoxicillin has been used as a supplementary antibiotic in combination with metronidazole or tinidazole. In this role it appears to act similarly to bismuth, perhaps sterilizing the gastric mucosa with a topical action and preventing the emergence of nitroimidazole resistance. In children, amoxicillin/tinidazole therapy eradicated 75% of infections during a 6-week course [18]. The dose of tinidazole was 20 mg kg^{-1} day^{-1} and of amoxicillin was 50 mg kg^{-1} day^{-1}.

Of interest is the observation that amoxicillin cure rates can be increased by adding omeprazole. In a controlled study, Unge *et al.* [46] observed eradication in 60–70% of patients given combination therapy with the two drugs. This suggests that *H. pylori* is protected by acid in the gastric lumen or in the parietal cell glands, and becomes adequately exposed to amoxicillin only when omeprazole is given. Lamouliatte *et al.* have had less success than the Swedish investigators, and only found a 40% cure rate using a dose of omeprazole 20 mg day^{-1} in combination with amoxicillin 2 g day^{-1} [47].

Triple therapy regimens have also benefited from the inclusion of amoxicillin. Coelho *et al.* [48] have reported 83% eradication of *H. pylori* in six patients treated with a regimen of furazolidone 100 mg, amoxicillin 500 mg, and metronidazole 250 mg, all given t.i.d. for 5 days. Note that the value of furazolidone remains unproved in this successful triple therapy regimen, since high cure rates are also obtained with amoxicillin and metronidazole dual therapy [18].

Since side-effects are related to duration of therapy, there are many advantages to using a short, rapidly-bactericidal therapy, but controlled trials comparing these short intensive therapies with bismuth combination therapies have not been performed.

Side-effects with amoxicillin are penicillin allergy, candidiasis, and diarrhea. We have not seen *C. difficile* colitis in patients given metronidazole/amoxicillin combinations, but two patients given amoxicillin/bismuth have developed it. We do not usually pursue the diagnosis if diarrhea is mild, proctoscopy is normal, stool is guaiac-negative and fecal leukocytes are absent.

Tetracyclines

H. pylori is always very sensitive *in vitro* to tetracyclines, and several have been studied as agents for *H. pylori* therapy. They vary in their half-life and acid stability, causing McNulty *et al.* [13] to suggest that tetracycline, which is active at low pH, would be the best agent to use. Tetracyclines chelate with bismuth salts, preventing absorption of the antibiotic [49]. This is not a problem in practice, since both bismuth and tetracycline may be acting topically in the stomach rather than depending on absorption for their action. Tetracycline, a less-well-absorbed drug than doxycycline, appears to be more effective for *H. pylori*, again pointing to a topical rather than a systemic antibacterial action. Minocycline, also poorly absorbed, may be an alternative. There are no data to suggest that spacing of tetracycline away from bismuth doses makes any difference to efficacy. Neither are there data to show that relationship to meals is important in *H. pylori* eradication.

Doxycycline has been studied by several investigators and found to be ineffective at eradicating *H. pylori*. At the University of Virginia, we did not see eradication in any of 15 patients treated with a doxycycline/BSS combination. Morris & Nicholson [50] and Unge & Gnarpe [51] have had similar experience. Unge found that doxycycline levels in mucosa were less than serum levels, perhaps explaining his poor results. Tetracyclines are concentrated in bile, so they may be useful in the post-gastrectomy stomach. Meshkinpour *et al.* [52] noted an excellent and reproducible clinical response in some individuals given doxycycline for "bile gastritis."

My own practice is to use doxycycline only as a "holding action" in patients who are acutely ill (with vomiting), who do not tolerate other medications. Suppression of *H. pylori* does occur, and the small once-daily dose (100–200 mg) is easy for nauseated patients to take. When the acute symptoms subside, more effective curative combinations can be started.

Erythromycin and other macrolides

Erythromycin

Erythromycin is available as erythromycin base, erythromycin stearate, erythromycin ethylsuccinate, and erythromycin estolate. The acid-stable forms of the drug were developed because erythromycin base, the active form, was quickly destroyed in gastric acid. Some of the gastric side-effects of erythromycin may be induced by acid metabolites [53] rather than erythromycin itself, so the acid-stable pro-drug forms are also better tolerated by patients. Erythromycin also increases gut motility by stimulating motilin receptors in the stomach. Abdominal cramping, gnawing, nausea, and diarrhea are all common with erythromycin therapy, often limiting its use. Erythromycin is secreted in bile, so may have more useful action in patients with free bile reflux.

Erythromycin stearate (ES), and erythromycin ethylsuccinate (EES), although acid-stable, are less active than erythromycin base and must be metabolized to the active drug after absorption. This may result in less activity for gastric infections. McNulty *et al.* [28] found that EES by itself eradicated less than 20% of *H. pylori* infections, suggesting that serum activity was ineffective at clearing the gastric mucosa. This poor *in vivo* effect is in striking contrast to the very low MIC seen for *H. pylori* with erythromycin *in vitro*. When mucosal levels of erythromycin were studied, McNulty *et al.* found 1–5 mg l^{-1}, about twice the serum level, to be present, but this still exceeded the MIC (0.1–1.0 mg l^{-1}).

Alternatives to locally inactive acid-stable formulations are enteric-coated erythromycin base delivered as small granules within a capsule ("Eryc," Park-Davis), and erythromycin base film-coated tablets ("Erythromycin base filmtabs," Abbott). The "Eryc" granules do not normally decompose until 90 minutes after they reach the neutral pH of the intestine, so they have fewer gastric side-effects and attain higher blood levels than the other forms of the drug. To achieve gastric dissolution and local action of the enteric-coated granules, the stomach should be rendered neutral with either high-dose H2 receptor antagonists or omeprazole, and the drug should be given with food.

Film-coated erythromycin base tablets can be expected to decompose in the stomach and supply active erythromycin to the mucosa, if the gastric pH can be kept neutral. I usually ask patients to take as much as they can tolerate of the 250 mg tablets by dosing every 3 hours. This ensures good absorption (a.c. doses) and prolonged gastric retention (p.c. doses). Therapy with high-dose H2 receptor antagonists (famotidine, 40 mg b.i.d.) or omeprazole, 40 mg day^{-1}, has given a cure rate of 70% in 30 patients we have treated with combination therapy B (see Fig. 13.4).

Erythromycin and bismuth appear to be synergistic *in vivo*. Goodwin *et al.* [41] observed that "DeNol" chewing tablets q.i.d., in combination with erythromycin ("Eryc"), achieved a 60% cure as assessed 14 days after treatment. These good results were in contrast to those reported by McNulty *et al.* [28] using EES alone. The improved clearance seen with combination therapy suggests that, whereas luminal and acid-exposed organisms are easily cleared by the bismuth, organisms in neutral pH areas such as antral mucus glands are attacked by erythromycin, either via the gastric lumen or systemically.

Our current practice at the University of Virginia is to use erythromycin combinations as second-line therapy for persons with metronidazole-resistant organisms. We always give the drug with acid reduction therapy (e.g. famotidine, 40 mg b.i.d., or omeprazole, 40 mg day^{-1}), to increase its gastric luminal activity and to decrease side-effects.

Other macrolides (clindamycin, azithromycin)

Clindamycin has been studied both as monotherapy, and in combination with BSS (U. Westblom, personal communication). Low eradication rates were achieved, suggesting that this is not a useful therapy. Theoretically, clindamycin should have been effective, since it is acid-stable and achieves very high intracellular levels in gastric mucosa and polymorphs, and is excreted in the bile [54].

Azithromycin, an acid-stable macrolide with a very long half-life, was also found to be

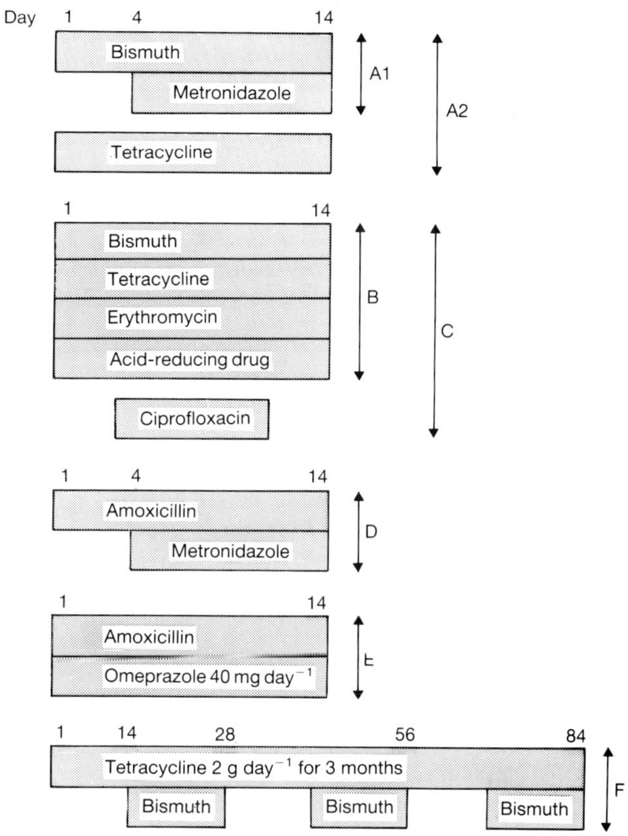

Fig. 13.4 Useful proven (A1, A2, B, D, E) and experimental (C, F) *H. pylori* therapies (see also Table 13.2).

ineffective for treating *H. pylori*. Glupczynski & Burette [55] found that 10 of 12 patients had persistent *H. pylori* during 7 days of azithromycin monotherapy, and that the infection relapsed in the remaining two. In most cases a resistant strain developed, tolerant also to erythromycin, clindamycin, and other macrolides. Similar poor results were seen with josamycin [56], which has been found to cause resistant *H. pylori* strains to emerge *in vitro* [57]. As with metronidazole and quinolones, a small proportion of *H. pylori* organisms seem to carry inherent macrolide resistance and emerge as the dominant strain when exposed to the drug. Thus, macrolides are best used in combination therapy rather than alone.

Rifampicin

Rifampicin has not been studied *in vivo* for the treatment of *H. pylori*, but may have some use. Experience with other organisms suggests that it should be used in combination therapy rather than alone, because resistant mutant bacteria usually emerge [54]. The MIC suggests that *H. pylori* is moderately sensitive to the drug and that mucosal levels will be adequate. The dose is 600–1000 mg day^{-1} (10–20 mg kg^{-1} day^{-1}), and the drug is available as 150 or 300 mg tablets. Absorption is not affected by food. Useful levels are found in saliva, and bile levels are 100 times those found in serum. Because of biliary excretion, lower doses are recommended in persons with liver disease.

Rifampicin is lipid-soluble and reaches high concentrations inside phagocytic cells, thus killing intracellular organisms. Mandell has shown it to be useful against *Staphylococcus aureus* in chronic granulomatous diseases caused by defective intracellular killing mechanisms [58]. A parallel exists in that *H. pylori* is chronic, phagocytosis occurs, immune mechanisms cannot eradicate the bacterium, and *H. pylori* is a strong catalase producer like *S.*

aureus. Catalase enzyme is known to protect phagocytosed bacteria from superoxide, the usual mechanism neutrophils use to kill ingested organisms [59].

Although I have no experience with rifampicin, I plan to try the drug in triple therapy regimens for patients with resistant organisms.

Quinolones (ciprofloxacin, norfloxacin, ofloxacin)

Quinolones inhibit *H. pylori in vitro* but have had limited success when used *in vivo*. Bayerdorffer *et al.* [60] reported that ofloxacin enhanced duodenal ulcer healing when used in addition to ranitidine. This effect was noted even though *H. pylori* could not be eradicated by the combination. When persistent *H. pylori* isolates were examined *in vitro* after therapy, they were found to be resistant to all quinolone drugs. Thus, quinolones cannot be used as monotherapy.

The failure of quinolones to eradicate *H. pylori* is paradoxical, because they achieve very high levels (2–10 × serum concentration) in the gastric mucosa [13]. Their use in combination regimens has not been evaluated, but they may have an adjuvant role in patients with resistant infections. Ciprofloxacin (which is less effective for *H. pylori*) is secreted in bile at 5–10 times the serum concentration [54]. Ofloxacin is secreted in saliva at concentrations equal to that in serum. We have used ciprofloxacin 1–1.5 g day^{-1} as a supplementary agent to triple therapy in a few patients (see Table 13.1), but it is very expensive and currently unproved. I recommend that, if it is available, ofloxacin, 300 mg day^{-1} be used instead of ciprofloxacin, since it has been proved to have some action *in vivo* against *H. pylori* [60].

Nitrofurantoin and furazolidone

The first reports suggesting activity for these drugs came from China, where Zheng *et al.* reported gastric and duodenal ulcer healing with low relapse after treatment with furazolidone [61]. The ulcer-healing action of the drug had been observed in China even before the discovery of *H. pylori*. Later reports by Morgan *et al.* [62] and by Borsch *et al.* [63] have shown that both furazolidone and nitrofurantoin are relatively ineffective as single agents in doses as high as 400 mg day^{-1}. In addition, gastric side-effects made clinical response difficult to assess. Morgan *et al.* found that *H. pylori* was usually suppressed, but eradicated in only 20–40% of the patients they could follow up [62].

Furazolidone is poorly absorbed and has been used in the United States as therapy for traveler's diarrhea. It is available as a 25 mg ml^{-1} suspension ("Furoxone," Norwich-Eaton) and as 100 mg tablets. The adult dose is 400 mg day^{-1} [60]. The drug has many gastrointestinal side-effects and sometimes causes a disulfiram-type reaction with alcohol. Nitrofurantoin has similar activity against *H. pylori*, although it is well absorbed and is usually used for urinary tract infections. The drug is available in a suspension (25 mg per 5 ml) and in 50 mg tablets ("Macrodantin," Norwich-Eaton). The daily dose is 200–400 mg. If used for *H. pylori*, frequent small doses may be most effective (see below).

Nitrofurans retain their *in vitro* activity towards *H. pylori* and may have some use as topical agents for the gastric mucosa. Graham *et al.* [25] have demonstrated that frequent low-dose furazolidone suspension (7 mg, seven times daily) suppresses *H. pylori* in most patients as assessed by ^{13}C-urea breath test. This suggests that it may be used as a gastric luminal antibacterial agent, supplementing the actions of bismuth, tetracycline, and amoxicillin. Against this are data from Borsch *et al.* [63], who did not observe any extra benefit if furazolidone was combined with BSS.

Triple therapy

Triple therapy (antibiotic/metronidazole/bismuth) gives far better *H. pylori* eradication than single drug therapy, but direct comparisons with dual therapy (metronidazole/bismuth) have not been performed. Borody *et al.* [64, 65] achieved 90–95% eradication using DeNol chewing tablets q.i.d. (28 days), tetracycline, 500 mg q.i.d. (28 days) and metronidazole, 200 mg q.i.d. (10 days). Most of the patients were suffering from duodenal ulcer in Borody *et al.*'s study. McNulty *et al.* [66] used this regimen in patients with non-ulcer dyspepsia, but only achieved a 65% eradication. Our experience is that triple therapy does not eradicate metronidazole-resistant organisms present in 10–25% of patients. Direct comparison studies have not been performed.

Triple therapies have the advantage of luminal activity and systemic activity. Luminally-active agents are bismuth, tetracycline, amoxicillin/ampicillin, and perhaps furazolidone [67]. Combining two luminally-active agents causes marked suppression of *H. pylori* and may have an inherent cure rate of 10–40%. In addition, these agents do not appear to cause resistance, so they may be used in repeated courses and in various combinations.

The luminally-active component of triple therapy usually includes bismuth because it is cheap and has very few side-effects. Tetracycline/bismuth, amoxicillin/bismuth, and tetracycline/amoxicillin are all effective, but the last two combinations may give more side-effects due to the broad-spectrum antibacterial suppression they produce. It is our experience that bismuth is very well tolerated except for patients allergic to the salicylate in BSS. With multiple antibiotic therapies, many patients develop vaginal or oral candidiasis or diarrhea. Usually we provide a prescription for topical antifungal therapy to be taken if needed.

Systemic action is achieved primarily with metronidazole or tinidazole. The dose of metronidazole is $20\,mg\,kg^{-1}\,day^{-1}$, which results in 1–1.5 g total daily dose. Borody *et al.* have achieved success using $800\,mg\,day^{-1}$ [64], although O'Morain has had less success with this lower dose, and now uses at least $1\,g\,day^{-1}$ (personal communication). If *H. pylori* is known to be resistant to nitroimidazoles, or if the patient has previously failed therapy with metronidazole, then metronidazole should be replaced with erythromycin, 500 mg q.i.d. Whenever erythromycin is used, omeprazole, $40\,mg\,day^{-1}$, or famotidine, 40 mg b.i.d., should be given to reduce gastric acidity.

Several regimens used successfully at the University of Virginia are described in Fig. 13.4 and Table 13.2.

Patients with severe gastric symptoms

In patients who are very unwell, and intolerant of high-dose antibiotic therapy (for example, with nausea and vomiting), triple therapy should be introduced cautiously. Commence treatment with bismuth (usually BSS, "Pepto-Bismol") as one tablet every 3 hours, supplemented with antiemetic and H2 blocker medication if necessary. When symptoms have settled somewhat, add tetracycline 250 mg every 3 hours, and finally metronidazole, 500 mg b.i.d. or t.i.d., can be commenced. If triple therapy can be continued at full dose for 5 days, cure should be expected. Patients in whom *H. pylori* is the only identifiable pathologic process will usually settle over 2–4 weeks. Continued symptoms may reflect delayed gastric emptying and should be treated concurrently with prokinetic agents (e.g. metoclopramide, or cisapride).

If a culture is available and the organism is found to be sentitive to metronidazole, therapy can be started with bismuth and supplemented with a quick course of metronidazole (oral or by suppository). This will result in the lowest possible incidence of side-effects and will give a very high cure rate. After therapy, symptomatic treatment is all that is necessary and symptoms settle over 2–4 weeks.

Duration of therapy

The optimal duration of therapy for *H. pylori* eradication is not known, but treatment courses as short as 5 days have been successful. Shorter therapy may have better compliance and fewer side-effects, as well as being less expensive. Since comparative studies have not been performed, we still recommend 14 days' treatment as routine. Longer therapy is not necessary, except when long-term suppression of a resistant *H. pylori* organism is planned (e.g. with bismuth or tetracycline).

There is a theoretical advantage to starting bismuth/tetracycline therapy 1–4 days prior to metronidazole. The broad-spectrum combination should cause marked suppression of *H. pylori* in this time, preventing the emergence of a resistant strain of *H. pylori* once the patient is exposed to metronidazole. In practice this may be of marginal benefit, since sensitive isolates had an 85% cure rate with dual therapy in the study reported by Marshall *et al.* [68], and the excellent results achieved by Borody *et al.* [64] reflect contemporaneous institution of triple therapy.

Table 13.2 Examples of triple therapy treatment of *H. pylori*

A1 90% cure in metronidazole-sensitive isolates, 70% cure if given blind (United States), depending on level of metronidazole resistance in the population	BSS ("Pepto-Bismol"), 1 tablet every 3 hours for 14 days (preferred); *or* 2 tablets q.i.d. for 14 days; *or* CBS ("DeNol"), 1 tablet q.i.d. (120 mg) for 14 days *AND* Metronidazole, 250 mg four to six times daily (20 mg kg^{-1} day^{-1}) for 10 days; *or* tinidazole 1 g day^{-1} for 10 days
A2 75–90% cure if given blind, depending on level of metronidazole resistance in the population. Good results in Sydney and Houston (duodenal ulcer patients), only 65% cure in United Kingdom (non-ulcer dyspepsia patients)	To A1, add tetracycline, 2 g day^{-1} for 14 days
B 60–80% cure in metronidazole-resistant organisms at University of Virginia. Side-effects of erythromycin limit its use in some patients.	BSS ("Pepto-Bismol"), 1 tablet every 3 hours for 14 days (preferred); *or* 2 tablets q.i.d. for 14 days; *or* CBS ("DeNol"), 1 tablet q.i.d. for 14 days *AND* Tetracycline, 250 mg eight times daily for 14 days *AND* Erythromycin, 250 mg eight times daily for 14 days *AND* Famotidine, 80 mg; *or* ranitidine, 600 mg; *or* omeprazole, 40 mg, daily for 14 days
C 40% of patients who fail therapy B obtain cure with regimen C ($n = 5$). The quinolones can only be used once because of antibiotic resistance. Instead of ciprofloxacin, try ofloxacin if it is available	Supplement B with ciprofloxacin, 500 mg b.i.d. or t.i.d. for 7 days. Use omeprazole as acid-reducing agent if possible
D 70% cure in several studies	In A1, bismuth and/or tetracycline can be replaced with amoxicillin, 1500–2000 mg day^{-1}
E ? 50% cure. Small numbers of patients treated but a very simple therapy	Amoxicillin, 250 mg every 3 hours for 14 days *AND* Omeprazole, 40 mg day^{-1} for 14 days
F ? 40–50% cure. Small numbers treated. A cheap regimen suitable for patients who have failed many other therapies and require suppression	Tetracycline, 500 mg q.i.d. for 3 months *AND* Any bismuth salt every 3 hours in 14-day pulses every month
G ? 40–50% cure. A modification of F incorporating breath test monitoring	Start bismuth salt as in A1, check breath test after 1 week. If breath test is still positive, increase the dose and add tetracycline, 250 mg every 3 hours. Repeat breath test. Escalate therapy with further suppressive agents (furazolidone, nitrofurantoin, amoxicillin) until breath test is negative, then add bactericidal drug(s) (erythromycin, amoxicillin, ?ciprofloxacin, rifampicin) for 14 days

Management of patients with *H. pylori*

Screening for *H. pylori*: is culture necessary?

At all endoscopies, the presence or absence of *H. pylori* should be ascertained by biopsy of the antrum. If the endoscopist is merely screening for the presence of the organism and the endoscopy is normal, then a rapid urease test such as the CLOtest is sufficient. If culture and sensitivity can be done, a second biopsy should be taken for microbiological studies because this extra information is a useful guide to therapy. It is our practice to discard this biopsy if the CLOtest is negative. If the CLOtest indicates presence of *H. pylori*, then the extra expense of culture is justified and the refrigerated culture specimen is processed. At the University of Virginia our endoscopy population has an *H. pylori* prevalence of 35%. Allowing a sensitivity of 95% for the CLOtest, we correctly determine the *H. pylori* status in 98 out of every 100 patients we screen, and HP– patients do not bear the expense of culture.

In CLOtest-positive patients, culture and antibiotic sensitivity testing of *H. pylori* takes about 10 days. While waiting for results, the patient should be treated with conventional ulcer therapy. If antibiotic sensitivity cannot be performed, then "blind" triple therapy for *H. pylori* may be commenced immediately, concurrently with acid-reducing ulcer therapy if indicated.

If the patient is very unwell, commence H2 receptor antagonists (H2RAs) and other appropriate symptomatic therapy, add bismuth as tolerated, then add the other antibiotics when the patient can tolerate them. Any treatment which suppresses *H. pylori* will provide maximal clinical improvement, so the drug used initially for this purpose is not critical. In this scenario it is my practice to use BSS ("Pepto-Bismol"), one tablet four to eight times daily, because it has the lowest potential for side-effects. *H. pylori* gastritis and associated ulcers should heal very quickly on any antibiotic/H2RA regimen and related symptoms should improve in 3–7 days.

When antibiotic sensitivity results are available, our usual practice is to mail the patient a prescription for the optimal combination. For organisms sensitive to metronidazole, we prescribe a 14-day course of BSS, one tablet eight times daily for 14 days, with the addition of metronidazole, 250 mg four to six times daily, from day 4 to day 14. At the end of therapy, patients who are well may take ulcer medication on a p.r.n. basis (as necessary), since nearly all ulcers will have healed after 1 month of *H. pylori*/H2RA therapy [59].

Metronidazole failure and persistence

In patients with metronidazole-resistant organisms, metronidazole or tinidazole add nothing to the efficacy of triple therapy [42]. After treating the acute ulcer and its symptoms as described above, second-line triple therapy may be commenced using bismuth–tetracycline–erythromycin. The duration of therapy should be 14 days, with erythromycin being given from day 1 to day 14. As described above, erythromycin in the required dose (2 g daily) has many side-effects which may benefit from acid-reducing therapy. Omeprazole, 40 mg daily, ranitidine, 300 mg b.i.d., or famotidine, 40 mg b.i.d., is usually added. Before starting second-line therapy, patients should be warned that they have a resistant organism which will be hard to treat, and that the cure rate for each course of therapy may be no more than 50%.

After therapy, patients should avoid all antibacterial drugs until follow-up study 1 month later. This may be endoscopy with biopsy, or breath test. If these tests indicate continuing infection, therapy should be repeated with an alternative antibiotic combination.

Treatment failures

Antibacterial therapy for *H. pylori* is ultimately limited by the occurrence of side-effects. Although these are rarely serious, patients in clinical remission with a persistent *H. pylori* infection will eventually decide to return to maintenance therapy of some kind, rather than continue with antibacterial regimens which have a progressively lower cure rate. Some patients experience marked improvement in their symptoms each time a suppressive therapy is given, and thus may request continued antibacterial therapy of some sort. Options at this

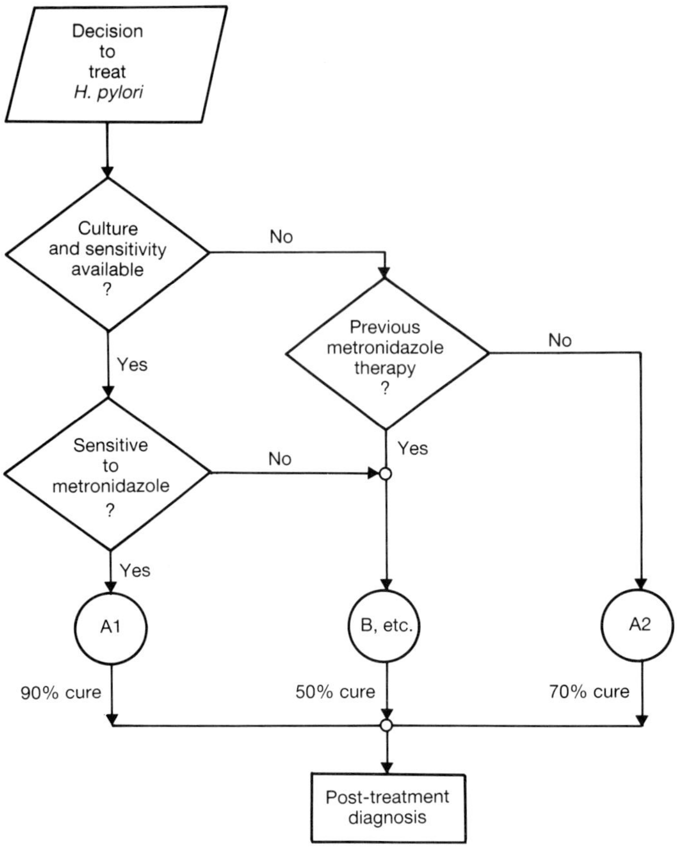

Fig. 13.5 Flow chart for antibiotic treatment of *H. pylori*.

stage include intermittent bismuth therapy (BSS, CBS), or antibiotics such as tetracycline, doxycycline, or amoxicillin. Since a topical suppressive effect is needed, I recommend that patients disperse the drug in water and take it morning and night on an empty stomach.

In patients who fail the usual therapy, an increased dose or different bismuth formulation may be successful. In occasional patients we have commenced treatment with BSS and monitored its efficacy 1 week later with a ^{14}C-urea breath test. If urease is still present, the dose is doubled for a further week and the breath test repeated. In this fashion, antibacterial agents can be added in a stepwise fashion until suppression of *H. pylori* has been achieved. Once the breath test is negative, the combination can either be continued for 4–6 weeks, or an additional agent can be added for a short burst of intensive therapy. An example would be the addition of erythromycin/omeprazole, amoxicillin/omeprazole, or ciprofloxacin/erythromycin/omeprazole. No doubt all these combinations are likely to cause side-effects, but they will be requested by well-motivated patients whose symptoms obviously respond to antibacterial therapy.

Using the flow chart in Fig. 13.5, 80–90% of patients will respond to an initial course of triple therapy or metronidazole/bismuth dual therapy. Of the remaining 10–20%, half will be cured with one of the alternative regimens, given as either the initial therapy (if sensitivities were obtained) or as a second therapy. Thus, after one or two treatments, 90% of all patients will have been cured of *H. pylori*. The remaining 10% will have the option of continuing therapy, trying long-term suppression, or abandoning attempts to eradicate *H. pylori*. At the University of Virginia, where all gastritis clinic patients are offered *H. pylori* therapy, we have eradicated the organism from 100 patients,

15 patients decided not to be treated, and in 15 patients treatment was abandoned after several unsuccessful attempts. Poor compliance is a factor in some of these treatment failures. They commonly occur in patients with limited financial resources who cannot afford the expense of therapy.

Reinfection

Reinfection is uncommon in Western countries. At the University of Virginia we have seen apparent reinfection in three patients (3%) followed for 1 year. In Australia the reinfection rate is similar, about 5% [15, 65]. In most reinfected patients a family source can be identified. Langenberg *et al.* report that in 0.1–1.0% of patients, reinfection occurs during endoscopy [69]. For this reason, I recommend that a dose of bismuth subsalicylate be given after follow-up endoscopy of HP− patients.

Should infected spouses be treated?

It is our practice to screen patients' spouses with the ^{14}C-urea breath test. Infected symptomatic spouses will usually request therapy, and so no dilemma exists in this group. Infected asymptomatic spouses need not be treated, because reinfection of the patient is the exception rather than the rule. If the patient's first course of therapy was effective, then it is simple enough to treat the spouse with the same thing and follow up with a breath test. If infection persists in the spouse, I do not usually attempt further therapy unless a clinical indication develops or the patient becomes reinfected.

Duodenal ulcer

As shown in the accompanying flow chart (Fig. 13.6), therapy for duodenal ulcer disease should be a two-pronged attack aiming both at the ulcer and the underlying gastritis. H2RAs do not appear to impair *H. pylori* eradication attempts, so may be used prior to, or concurrently with, antibacterial regimens. The patient should be given a proven ulcer-healing agent for at least 4 weeks. In the United States this will be H2RA, sucralfate, or perhaps omeprazole. In Europe and Britain, CBS ("DeNol") may be used for the ulcer-healing agent, and also as a component of the antibacterial therapy.

H2RAs are usually continued in full dose for 1 month, but in patients who are asymptomatic at the end of antibacterial therapy I allow p.r.n. therapy. Breath test or biopsy is repeated 4 weeks after completing antibacterial therapy. If HP−, patients may be reassured that ulcer relapse is unlikely. Depending on the age of the patient and the presence of other associated lesions, symptoms may persist after eradication of *H. pylori*. It is worthwhile to repeat endoscopy in these cases.

In most patients, symptoms will totally resolve after eradication of *H. pylori*, in which case patients should be provided with p.r.n. H2RAs and reviewed 3 months later. At the 3-month visit a non-invasive test such as a breath test should be performed to confirm long-term eradication of *H. pylori*. Patients who are HP− at 3 months, and who are asymptomatic, will benefit from a further endoscopy at this time. The absence of any identifiable lesion indicates a very good long-term prognosis and probable cure of the disease.

In a proportion of patients, symptoms continue to some degree. These are commonly related to persisting erosive duodenitis, particularly in older persons with very long-standing ulcer disease. Therapy with H2RAs or sucralfate should be given, but need only be continued while symptoms persist. Endoscopic lesions do not usually progress to frank ulceration once *H. pylori* has been eradicated, but patients with persisting gastroduodenal erythema and/or erosive changes remain very susceptible to non-steroidal antiinflammatory drug (NSAID)-induced damage.

Scarring and pyloric stenosis

The duodenal mucosa usually appears normal after eradication of *H. pylori*, but scarring and duodenal deformity may still worry the endoscopist. According to George *et al.* [65], these changes also gradually resolve over 1–4 years. While they persist, however, patients may have symptoms of bloating and post-prandial discomfort, particularly with undigestible dietary fiber and salads. Metoclopramide may help these symptoms.

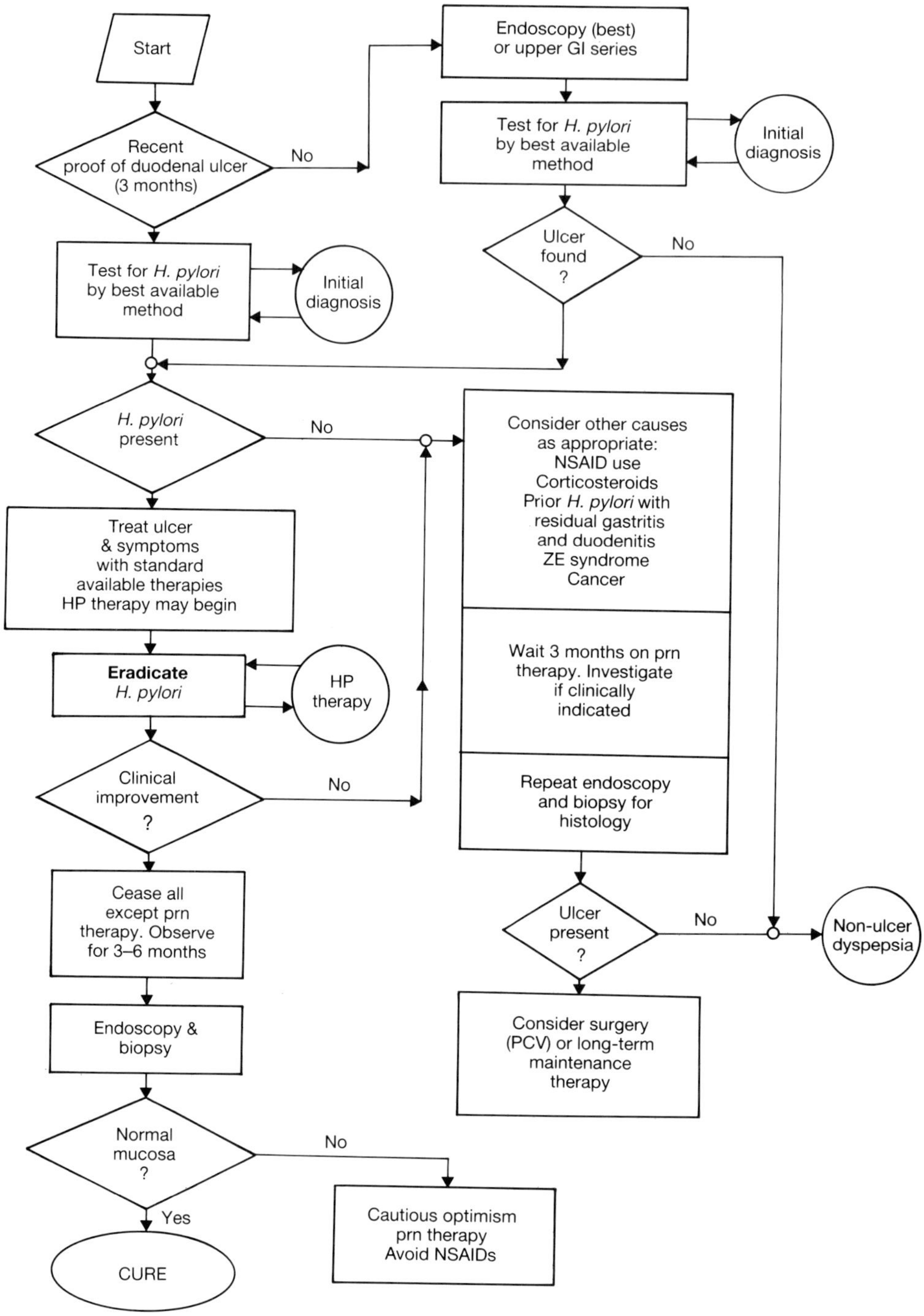

Fig. 13.6 Flow chart for the management of duodenal ulcer. PCV, parietal cell vagotomy; ZE, Zollinger–Ellison (syndrome).

Pyloric stenosis subsequent to duodenal ulcer may be a troublesome persistent component of the disease. Often, the high acid secretory state and delay in gastric emptying combine to cause erosive changes in the esophagus, which may be the major cause of persisting symptoms. When the esophagus is involved, treatment of gastric hyperacidity should be more intensive, and high-dose H2RAs or omeprazole should be given during and after antibacterial regimens. Breath tests may give weak false-positive results in patients rendered achlorhydric, so follow-up is best performed with endoscopy and biopsy.

At initial and subsequent endoscopies, balloon dilatation of any stricture should be performed. If the endoscope (9 mm) can pass the stricture, then the patient should be able to tolerate a low-residue soft diet. Once *H. pylori* has been eradicated, gradual improvement will occur except in patients with very hard pyloric fibrosis. These patients will still benefit from eradication of *H. pylori*, since at least the lesion will not progress. If they require surgical correction of the problem, a post-gastrectomy syndrome will be less likely if *H. pylori* and gastritis are no longer present. At this stage the surgeon may not have to address a continuing ulcer diathesis, and so should be encouraged to perform a conservative operation. Parietal cell vagotomy with pyloroplasty may suffice, rather than the usual Billroth II. Patients with large dilated stomachs should be assessed thoroughly prior to surgical intervention, since they may have hypomotility which would be worsened by vagotomy.

Gastric ulcer

In general, the management of gastric ulcer is similar to that of duodenal ulcer (Fig. 13.6), although gastric ulcer tends to be harder to treat and is more often related to factors other than *H. pylori*. The two main causes of gastric ulcer are *H. pylori* (~70%) and NSAIDs (~30%). As some ulcers are malignant, all gastric ulcers should be biopsied. Extra biopsies for *H. pylori* diagnosis should be taken away from the gastric ulcer, on the antral greater curve. If intestinal metaplasia is widespread, false-negative biopsies may occur, so when *H. pylori* is not detected on such a biopsy, idiopathic gastric ulcer should be investigated further with either serology or breath test to ensure that *H. pylori* has not been missed.

NSAID ingestion is the cause of ulcers which occur in histologically normal gastric mucosa. If the patient is known to be taking NSAID, *H. pylori* should still be excluded. Normal histology implies that the NSAID is the sole cause of the ulcer and that the patient will heal quickly once the offending agent is withdrawn. When the mucosa shows active and/or chronic gastritis (with or without intestinal metaplasia), *H. pylori* is equally likely to be the primary cause [70].

For patients in whom the NSAID is an essential medication, it makes sense to eradicate *H. pylori* in the hope that the mucosal defect will diminish and the NSAID will be able to be continued. It is my experience that about 50% of patients will be able to resume taking NSAID after the ulcer has healed and the *H. pylori* has been eradicated. Asymptomatic ulcer relapses are common in NSAID users, so endoscopic follow-up is advised for 3–6 months after *H. pylori* eradication.

Uncomplicated *H. pylori*-associated gastric ulcer should be treated similarly to duodenal ulcer, but with different expectations. Gastric ulcer patients usually have severe widespread histologic gastritis, and acid secretion may be normal or even decreased. In addition, gastric ulcer patients are usually older and may have had lifelong *H. pylori*. Thus the mucosal lesion is more severe than in duodenal ulcer, and may not revert to normal after treatment.

There are no clinical trials confirming the benefit of *H. pylori* therapy in gastric ulcer, but my own experience is that most patients are cured after the organism has been eradicated. Young patients with prepyloric ulceration, which has a natural history similar to that of duodenal ulcer, do very well. In older persons, the gastric mucosa often appears abnormal for many months after ulcer healing. If these endoscopic lesions, for example patchy erosive gastritis, are asymptomatic, I do not treat them. Nevertheless, it is my practice to follow them endoscopically for 1–2 years. Major ulceration sometimes occurs in patients who subsequently take NSAID.

In a minority of patients, ulceration redevelops at the original ulcer site, even when the histology shows that the gastritis has healed. After eradication of *H. pylori*, there is no further need for antibacterial therapy, and even the use of cytoprotective bismuth salts such as CBS is of doubtful benefit. Recurrence of an idiopathic gastric ulcer after eradication of *H. pylori* should be treated conventionally with H2RAs and/or sucralfate. It is reasonable to hope for improvement in the tendency to relapse for 12 months after treating *H. pylori*, but subsequent problems imply a permanent mucosal defect and indicate the need for long-term maintenance ulcer therapy. In such patients surgery may be an attractive option. Once the main component of the ulcer diathesis has been treated, however, more conservative surgical procedures may be possible, rather than the usual Billroth II. Since the mucosal defect may be localized to the area of recurrent ulceration, the surgeon should consider a local ulcer resection with parietal cell vagotomy.

Gastroesophageal reflux disease (GERD)

No link has been demonstrated between GERD and *H. pylori*-associated gastritis. Nevertheless, in one small study of therapy for esophagitis, the combination of bismuth–cimetidine was superior to cimetidine alone [71].

Many investigators have reported a 30% prevalence of reflux esophagitis in patients with duodenal ulcer [72, 73]. The reason for this is not clear. Duodenal ulcer patients may secrete more acid, or the gastric juice may be more toxic to the esophageal mucosa due to ammonia and other *H. pylori* toxins. Alternatively, long-standing pyloroduodenal disease, nausea and vomiting, belching, and associated alterations of motility, might compromise the esophageal sphincter.

It is my current practice to treat *H. pylori* gastritis when it is present in association with GERD. When taking the history, the presence of nausea indicates that the lesion is not solely due to esophageal acid reflux. In many patients, symptoms of reflux and of gastritis cannot be separated and, whereas GERD requires long-term acid suppression therapy, gastritis symptoms might be cured with a short course of triple therapy. Remember that patients with *H. pylori* gastritis sometimes have relative hypochlorhydria due to ammonia and toxin production. In a few patients, acidic dyspepsia worsens immediately after commencing antibacterial therapy. This responds well to acid reduction and is usually only a temporary phenomenon.

Antireflux surgery, a less frequent occurrence since the advent of H2RAs and omeprazole, is often complicated by the "gas bloat syndrome." In some patients this is aggravated by continuing *H. pylori* gastritis and/or a motility disturbance. The cause of the syndrome is in doubt, but appears to be secondary to both air trapping and gastric generation of gas. Since *H. pylori* may produce CO_2 by hydrolysis of urea in the stomach, the potential exists for the organism to aggravate this syndrome.

In two patients, both with *H. pylori*, I have seen gastric ulcers develop high on the lesser curve immediately adjacent to or beneath the esophageal wrap. I therefore attempt to eradicate *H. pylori* before referring patients for antireflux surgery. After such surgery patients cannot easily vomit, so they fare badly if nausea from *H. pylori* goes untreated.

Non-ulcer dyspepsia

What is non-ulcer dyspepsia?

Non-ulcer dyspepsia (NUD) exists in those patients with symptoms suggestive of ulcer disease who do not have an ulcer found at endoscopy. The proportion of these who have *H. pylori*-associated disease is between 40% and 70%, depending on geographic location, ethnic and socioeconomic factors. Italian series have a high prevalence of *H. pylori*, whereas only 38% of patients at the University of Virginia have it [74]. In general, the amount of *H. pylori*-associated NUD is at least equal to the amount of ulcer disease.

Can H. pylori gastritis cause NUD?

Gastritis is common in asymptomatic persons and the prevalence of gastritis in age-matched endoscopy patients is often very similar to this background prevalence. At the University of

Virginia, where *H. pylori* is uncommon (8% rising to 25% in elderly patients), the overall prevalence of dyspepsia in the population is 20% in normal persons and 55% in those persons with serologic evidence of *H. pylori* [75]. Thus the presence of *H. pylori* is associated with a 2.5 times increased risk of dyspepsia.

Logic dictates that NUD must be more common in patients with *H. pylori*. Non-ulcer dyspepsia includes many persons who have had ulcer disease in the past, and some others who will develop peptic ulcer disease if observed for long enough. Patients with new ulcer disease often give a long history of dyspepsia, in which various searches for an ulcer crater were negative. In between ulcer episodes, patients with duodenal ulcers often have continuing low-grade ulcer-type symptoms. In patients with well-documented ulcer disease, recurrence of severe ulcer symptoms often occurs in the absence of an ulcer crater. These patients have etiologies other than an ulcer crater for their pain, and in most cases only duodenitis or gastritis will be found.

Current thought is that factors such as gastric metaplasia in the duodenal bulb, level of acid secretion, and toxin production by *H. pylori*, will determine the expression of ulcer disease (see Chapter 11). Many believe that lesser degrees of ulcerogenesis result in symptoms but no macroscopic ulcer crater. This disease state is equal to the "Moynihan's disease" (chronic gastroduodenitis) referred to by Spiro [76]. These patients have minimal or no endoscopic abnormality, but may have severe histologic damage with subsequent ingress of hydrogen ion into the mucosa.

There are several controlled studies showing improvement of clinical symptoms with bismuth therapy for *H. pylori* in NUD patients. With the old formulation CBS ("DeNol") chewable tablets, Rokkas *et al.* [77] noted benefit after 3–5 weeks, as did Lambert *et al.* [78], Borody *et al.* [9], and Kang *et al.* [79]. More recently, Loffeld *et al.* [80] reported only marginal clinical benefit (nausea improved) using a q.i.d. dosage of the new formulation CBS 'swallowable' "DeNol" tablets, although the gastritis did improve histologically during therapy. Our observation [81], and data reported by McNulty *et al.* [28], indicate that short-term (3-weeks') suppression of *H. pylori* with BSS does greatly affect symptoms of NUD.

The discordant results of the above studies may have been due to the different formulations of bismuth they used, the variable degree of *H. pylori* suppression achieved, the inability of the medication to eradicate *H. pylori* when used as a single agent, the short time allowed to show improvement, and the very wide variety of possible etiologies present in any group of patients with NUD. To settle the issue, a 100-patient study is needed in which *H. pylori* is eradicated by therapy and 3-month follow-up is available. There is hardly any need to include HP− patients in such a study, because all the above investigators have failed to notice any difference between HP− NUD patients treated with bismuth, and those treated with placebo.

At the University of Virginia we have preliminary results from a follow-up survey of all patients seen at my clinic between 1987 and 1990 [82]. In patients with *H. pylori*, there was no change in symptoms if the bacterium remained and only conventional therapies were used (H2RAs, etc.). If the bacterium was eradicated, however, 50% of patients were markedly improved or cured, 25% were somewhat improved, and only 25% were unchanged. In patients who did not have *H. pylori* (HP− dyspepsia), a less remarkable but definite improvement also occurred, so that 25% were markedly improved, 50% were somewhat improved, and about 25% were unchanged during a 2-year follow-up. Of interest was the observation that the HP− group still required medication for their symptoms, whereas many of the treated *H. pylori* patients no longer required medication.

Symptoms which were improved after eradication of *H. pylori* were: bloating, burping, gnawing sensations, vomiting, intolerance to spicy food, bad taste in the mouth, acid reflux, heartburn, swelling, nausea, loss of appetite, flatulence, and constipation.

Approach to the patient with NUD

When first seeing patients with apparent NUD, the physician should be aware that a real diagnosis will be made in less than half, and that

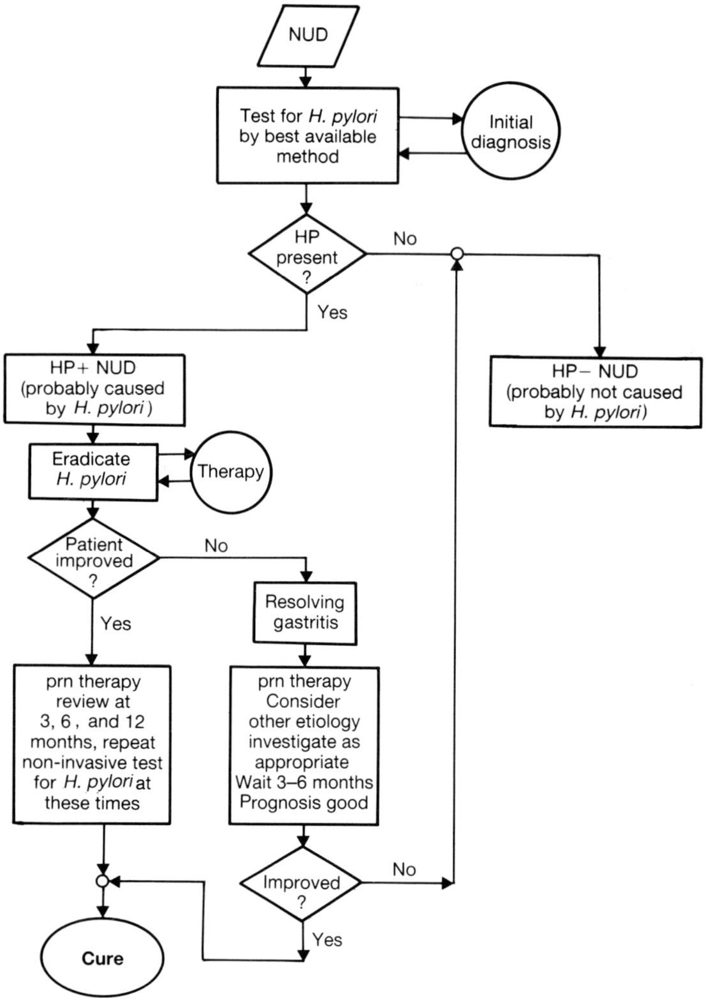

Fig. 13.7 Flow chart of management for non-ulcer dyspepsia (NUD) (see also Table 13.3).

curative therapy will be possible in very few. By the time a patient reaches a specialist gastroenterologist, he or she has usually already been investigated and common causes of dyspepsia have been ruled out. Often, asymptomatic gallstones will have been removed! Since *H. pylori* does not feature in most texts as a cause of abdominal symptoms, some patients with gastritis may have slipped through a diagnostic screen.

The physician should take a careful history, including a family history with enquiries about children and also the spouse's family. Travel may be important, especially to Third World countries and Latin America. Occupation is relevant, since *H. pylori* may be transmitted by the fecal–oral route and persons such as plumbers and sewerage engineers could acquire *H. pylori* in their occupation. Doctors (particularly senior gastroenterologists) are likely to pick up *H. pylori* from patients, as are nurses in medical and surgical wards and geriatric units, and perhaps persons in institutions for the mentally retarded.

Psychosomatic factors have been overemphasized in the past as causes for NUD. Talley *et al.* have published several studies in which major life events and/or abnormal personality traits were no more common in NUD patients than in any other group with chronic gastrointestinal diseases [83, 84]. Whereas "stress' can certainly aggravate an underlying medical condition, it rarely causes abdominal pain *de novo*. Most patients recognize that the diagnosis of "stress-induced" disease really means that the physician has been unable to find any organic cause for their symptoms. I prefer not to raise their hopes of an organic diagnosis in the first place, and to admit that there are many patients in whom the cause of abdominal pain cannot be determined with the current technology.

Usually the physical examination will be normal. Follow this with a set of laboratory tests to screen for overt organic disease (blood count, differential, erythrocyte sedimentation rate, urea and electrolytes, metabolic screen, amylase, and liver function tests). Have stool examined for leukocytes, ova, and parasites if diarrhea is present. Obtain a plain abdominal X-ray film if bowel sounds seem abnormal or abdominal distension is present.

If the above process fails to identify any abnormality, perform a test to exclude *H. pylori*. Usually this is a breath test (result immediately available in my clinic) or an antibody titer. If an endoscopy is indicated (see flow chart, Fig. 13.7), then accurate biopsy diagnosis is possible, followed by culture and sensitivity result if positive (see Chapter 12). If *H. pylori* is not detected, then the diagnosis of HP− dyspepsia is made. At this stage a positive serologic test may indicate recent *H. pylori*, and therefore a tendency to improve with time (residual gastritis). Otherwise, the investigation and treatment are quite conventional. Numerous articles have been written on the subject, but none really pretends to give a diagnosis or effective therapy in more than 50% of patients with HP−NUD [85, 86]. A detailed review of non-ulcer dyspepsia is available as a working party report chaired by Colin–Jones [86, 87]. The subject is also discussed in Chapter 3.

As shown in Table 13.3, the best approach is an attempt to pigeon-hole patients into one of five categories. These are briefly discussed below.

Esophageal-type. Atypical cardiac symptoms can mimic esophageal disease, so a cardiology opinion is often indicated before proceeding. Radiology, endoscopy, and motility studies have a role, depending on their availability. The Bernstein test may reproduce the pain, and can be done at the same time as the motility study. Twenty-four hour ambulatory pH monitoring may prove that acid reflux exists, although a therapeutic trial of omeprazole (see below) may replace this nowadays. After such a work-up, the treatment will usually be H2RAs or omeprazole, or calcium channel blockers. In general, esophageal disease requires much higher doses of acid-reduction therapy than does peptic ulcer disease.

Ulcer-like. Ulcer- and acidic-type symptoms centered in the epigastrium usually respond to acid-reduction therapy, and may be treated the same as peptic ulcer disease. In a gastroenterology practice, however, patients referred with these symptoms will have already tried H2RAs and responded poorly. Investigation should include endoscopy and biopsy of the gastric mucosa. In some patients with burning epigastric pain, I have seen widespread intestinal metaplasia of the gastric body with few parietal cells present. These persons, even if peak gastric acid secretion is quite low, may respond to omeprazole. Pancreatic and biliary disease need to be ruled out and endoscopic retrograde cholangiopancreatographic (ERCP) examination performed if any related investigations are abnormal. There may be a role for biliary manometry in persons with post-cholecystectomy syndromes.

Patients who do not respond to empiric trials of therapy should be investigated further, often coming to computed tomography (CT) scan and colonoscopy or barium enema. At least at the end of the work-up the physician should be able to confidently assure the patient that a malignancy is not present.

Dysmotility/hypomotility-type. Dysmotility-type dyspepsia includes a group with organic disease (scleroderma, diabetic neuropathy, previous peptic ulcer, or partial gastrectomy) which has caused hypomotility of the stomach. The symptoms are related to poor gastric emptying, which can be detected by a solid phase gastric emptying study. Results of gastric emptying studies vary in patients from day to day, and so a normal study does not absolutely exclude hypomotility. If the gastric anatomy

Table 13.3 Diagnosis of *H. pylori*-negative non-ulcer dyspepsia

Symptoms	Investigations
Type 1: esophageal-type dyspepsia Chest pain, dysphagia, heartburn, belching, reflux, bad taste in the mouth, worse after food and bedtime	Exclude cardiac causes; endoscopy, esophageal biopsy, barium swallow/upper GI series (fluoroscopy), esophageal motility study, 24-hour esophageal pH monitoring, Bernstein test, gastric analysis, trial of therapy with Ca^{2+} antagonists or nitroglycerin (esophageal spasm), omeprazole or H2RAs (reflux)
Type 2: ulcer-like (acidic) dyspepsia Burning epigastric pain, gnawing sensations, nausea, aching pain, epigastric tenderness, usually relieved by food or antacids	Endoscopy and biopsy of duodenum, antrum and body mucosa; upper GI series, ultrasound, computed tomography (CT) scan, gastric analysis, serum gastrin. Usually responds to H2RAs and/or omeprazole. Common in persons with a recent past history of *H. pylori*. *H. pylori* serology may be borderline-positive, and mild chronic gastritis may be present
Type 3: dysmotility/hypomotility-type dyspepsia Belching and bloating, gnawing/hunger, early satiety during meals, distension, nausea and vomiting (± undigested food), intolerance to salads and fiber, foul eructations, halitosis, ± reflux symptoms	Exclude *Giardia*; endoscopy and biopsy of duodenum, antrum and body mucosa; gastric emptying study, plus electrogastrogram (if available), upper GI series, ultrasound, CT scan. Trial of metoclopramide or other prokinetic agents (cisapride, clebopride, domperidone, ?erythromycin)
Type 4: irritable bowel-type dyspepsia Subsets of the above syndromes, associated with intermittent altered bowel habit (usually diarrhea) and lower GI pains associated with meals and upper GI symptoms	Upper GI endoscopy, biopsies, upper GI series, lactose tolerance test, small bowel series (?terminal ileal disease), lower GI series, colonoscopy and biopsy
Type 5: abdominal pain syndromes Right upper quadrant pains (usually after cholecystectomy), liver pain, colonic pain; left upper quadrant pain, splenic flexure pain, gastric/esophageal pain, diaphragmatic pain; central and other sharp pains, usually in post-surgical abdomen	Plain abdominal film during exacerbations, ESR, upper and lower GI series, upper GI endoscopy and biopsy, ultrasound, colonoscopy, CT scan, laparoscopy

and histology are normal, and there is no known predisposing condition, then gastric stasis is idiopathic and has an unpredictable course. If *H. pylori* has been recently treated, eradication of the bacterium will result in improvement of the patient's nausea over several months, although the actual motor disturbance may remain. Often such patients undergo apparent relapses, but these are usually short-lived and become less common with time. If *H. pylori* has not recurred then reassurance and symptomatic therapy are all that is required.

Often patients with past gastric disease, pyloric scarring, etc. cannot tolerate a high fiber diet, and improve if fiber is removed from the diet for a few weeks, after which various vegetables and fiber sources are selectively reintroduced. In many cases these patients have been deliberately increasing their dietary fiber to treat an "irritable bowel" syndrome. Prokinetic agents have a role in NUD, and in Europe, cisapride is already an accepted therapy. Gastric stasis and vomiting are reviewed in Chapter 14.

Irritable bowel-type. Irritable bowel syndromes are often part of an "irritable gut" and consist of a combination of upper and lower gastrointestinal symptoms. Women seem prone to a syndrome of colicky upper gastrointestinal discomfort, coming on unpredictably after meals, relieved by vomiting and associated with diarrhea. Sometimes these respond very well to anticholinergic drugs such as IV or sublingual scopolamine. Dicyclomine hydrochloride is standard therapy (20–40 mg q.i.d.) if attacks occur frequently. An alternative is hyoscyamine sulfate, available in oral or sublingual formulations. If all else fails, antidepressant drugs with their anticholinergic effect are useful, especially in patients with severe pain, anxiety, and sleep disturbance.

Abdominal pain syndromes. A few patients, usually middle-aged women, have undiagnosed abdominal pains. Associated findings may be fatty liver, cholecystectomy, previous multiple surgeries, or previous peptic ulcer disease, but no proven organic cause for the pain can be found. Often these patients have been diagnosed as "irritable bowel" for want of a better diagnosis. I categorize pain syndromes by their location, and direct investigations at the possible underlying organs. My experience with left and right upper quadrant pains is that they do not resolve. Occasional patients report improvement with antibiotics, but this is inconsistent. Laparoscopy may be a useful new avenue of investigation by a surgeon or gastroenterologist. I usually see these undiagnosed patients every 3–6 months, and reinvestigate them during acute exacerbations if it seems indicated. Any laboratory or radiologic abnormality is a signal that the disorder is not merely functional and that further work-up should be performed.

Non-ulcer dyspepsia patients with a completely negative diagnostic evaluation should be reassured that they do not have a serious organic disease, and that they will almost certainly improve with time (1–2 years). They should be reviewed at 3–6-month intervals after that, and examined carefully whenever exacerbations occur. Patients will accept this approach if they have received a careful and thorough initial consultation, appropriate investigations have excluded treatable diseases, and malignancy has been ruled out.

References

1 Marks, G, & Beatty, WK. *The Precious Metals of Medicine (bibliography).* New York: Charles Scribner's Sons, 1975.

2 Ogle, JW. Effervescing bismuth water. *Br. Med. J.* 1864;**1**:249–50.

3 Osler, W. *The Principles and Practice of Medicine.* New York: Appleton, 1920.

4 Robert, AE, & Sauton, B. *Ann. Inst. Pasteur* 1916; **30**:261.

5 Martin, DF, May, SJ, Tweedle, DE, Hollanders, D, Ravenscroft, MM, & Miller, JP. Difference in relapse rates of duodenal ulcer healing with cimetidine or tripotassium dicitrato-bismuthate. *Lancet* 1980;**i**:7–10.

6 Gregory, MA, Moshal, MG, & Spitaels, JM. The effect of tripotassium dicitrato-bismuthate on the duodenal mucosa during ulceration. An ultrastructural study. *S. Afr. Med. J.* 1982;**62**:52–5.

7 Marshall, BJ, Armstrong, JA, Francis, GJ, Nokes, NT, & Wee, SH. The antibacterial action of bismuth in relation to *Campylobacter pyloridis* colonization and gastritis. *Digestion* 1987; **37**(suppl 2):16–30.

8 Goodwin, CS, Armstrong, JA, & Marshall, BJ. *Campylobacter pyloridis,* gastritis, and peptic ulceration. *J. Clin. Pathol.* 1986;**39**:353–65.

9 Borody, TJ, Carrick, J, & Hazell, SL. Symptoms improve after the eradication of gastric *Campylobacter pyloridis* (letter). *Med. J. Aust.* 1987;**146**:450–51.

10 Bayerdorffer, E, & Ottenjann, R. The role of antibiotics in *Campylobacter pylori*-associated peptic ulcer disease. *Scand. J. Gastroenterol.* 1988; **142**(suppl):93–100.

11 Glupczynski, Y, Delmee, M, Bruck, C, Labbe, M, Avesani, V, & Burette, A. Susceptibility of clinical isolates of *Campylobacter pylori* to 24 antimicrobial and anti-ulcer agents. *Eur. J. Epidemiol.* 1988;**4**:154–7.

12 McNulty, CA, & Dent, JC. Susceptibility of clinical isolates of *Campylobacter pylori* to twenty-one antimicrobial agents. *Eur. J. Clin. Microbiol. Infect. Dis.* 1988;**7**:566–9.

13 McNulty, CA, Dent, JC, Ford, GA, & Wilkinson, SP. Inhibitory antimicrobial concentrations against *Campylobacter pylori* in gastric mucosa. *J. Antimicrob. Chemother.* 1988;**22**:729–38.

14 Langenberg, W, Rauws, EA, Widjojokusumo, A, Tytgat, GN, & Zanen, HC. Identification of *Campylobacter pyloridis* isolates by restriction endonuclease DNA analysis. *J. Clin. Microbiol.* 1986;**24**:414–17.

15 Marshall, BJ, Goodwin, CS, Warren, JR, *et al.* A prospective double-blind trial of duodenal ulcer relapse after eradication of *Campylobacter pylori*. *Lancet* 1988;**ii**:1437–42.
16 Rauws, EA, Langenberg, W, Houthoff, HJ, Zanen, HC, & Tytgat, GN. *Campylobacter pyloridis*-associated chronic active antral gastritis. A prospective study of its prevalence and the effects of antibacterial and antiulcer treatment. *Gastroenterology* 1988;**94**:33–40.
17 Marshall, BJ, & Surveyor, I. ^{14}Carbon urea breath test for the diagnosis of *Campylobacter pylori*-associated gastritis. *J. Nucl. Med.* 1988;**29**:11–16.
18 Oderda, G, Vaira, D, Holton, J, Ainley, C, Altare, F, & Ansaldi, N. Amoxycillin plus tinidazole for *Campylobacter pylori* gastritis in children: assessment by serum IgG antibody, pepsinogen I, and gastrin levels. *Lancet* 1989;**i**:690–2.
19 Stiel, D, Murray, DJ, & Peters, TJ. Uptake and subcellular localization of bismuth in the gastrointestinal mucosa of rats after short term administration of colloidal bismuth subcitrate. *Gut* 1985;**26**:364–8.
20 Coghill, SB, Hopwood, D, McPherson, S, & Hislop, S. The ultrastructural localization of DeNol in the upper gastrointestinal tract of man and rodents following oral and instrumental administration. *J. Pathol.* 1983;**139**:105–14.
21 Albert, A, Falk, JE, & Rubbo, SD. Antibacterial action of arsenic. *Nature* 1944;**153**:712.
22 Lehninger, AL, Ammonia excretion. In: Lehninger, AL, *Biochemistry*. New York: Worth, 1978, pp. 428–9.
23 Sarosiek, J, Bilski, J, Murty, VL, Slomiany, A, & Slomiany, BL. Colloidal bismuth subcitrate (DeNol) inhibits degradation of gastric mucus by *Campylobacter pylori* protease. *Am. J. Gastroenterol.* 1989;**84**:506–10.
24 Slomiany, BL, Kasinathan, C, & Slomiany, A. Lipolytic activity of *Campylobacter pylori*: effect of colloidal bismuth subcitrate (DeNol). *Am. J. Gastroenterol.* 1989;**84**:1273–7.
25 Graham, DY, Klein, PD, Opekun, AR, *et al. In vivo* susceptibility of *Campylobacter pylori*. *Am. J. Gastroenterol.* 1989;**84**:233–8.
26 Weil, J, & Bell, GD. Detection of *Campylobacter pylori* with the ^{14}C-breath test. In: Rathbone, BJ, & Heatley, RV, (eds), *Campylobacter pylori and Gastroduodenal Disease*. Oxford: Blackwell Scientific Publications, 1989, pp. 83–93.
27 Lanza, FL, Skoglund, ML, Rack, MF, & Yardley, JH. The effect of bismuth subsalicylate on the histologic gastritis seen with *Campylobacter pylori*: a placebo-controlled, randomized study. *Am. J. Gastroenterol.* 1989;**84**:1060–64.
28 DuPont, HL. Bismuth subsalicylate in the treatment of diarrheal disease. *Drug Intell. Clin. Pharm.* 1987;**21**:687–93.
29 McNulty, CA, Gearty, JC, Crump, B, *et al. Campylobacter pyloridis* and associated gastritis: investigator blind, placebo controlled trial of bismuth salicylate and erythromycin ethylsuccinate. *Br. Med. J. (Clin. Res.)* 1986;**293**:645–9.
30 Marshall, BJ, Valenzuela, JE, McCallum, RW, *et al.* A placebo controlled clinical trial of bismuth subsalicylate for the treatment of *Helicobacter pylori* associated gastritis (abstract). *Gastroenterology* 1990;**98**(2):A83.
31 Lee, FI, Samloff, IM, & Hardman, M. Comparison of tripotassium dicitrato-bismuthate tablets with ranitidine in healing and relapse of duodenal ulcers. *Lancet* 1985;**i**:1299–1302.
32 Coghlan, JG, Gilligan, D, Humphries, H, *et al. Campylobacter pylori* and recurrence of duodenal ulcers — a 12-month follow-up study. *Lancet* 1987;**ii**:1109–11.
33 Rauws, EA, & Tytgat, GN. Cure of duodenal ulcer associated with eradication of *Helicobacter pylori*. *Lancet* 1990;**335**:1233–5.
34 Moshal, MG, Spitaels, JM, & Khan, F. Tripotassium dicitrato-bismuthate chewing tablets and cimetidine tablets in the treatment of duodenal ulcers. A double-blind double-dummy comparative study. *S. Afr. Med. J.* 1981;**60**:420–23.
35 Nwokolo, CU, Gavey, CJ, Smith, JTL, & Pounder, RE. The absorption of bismuth from oral doses of tripotassium dicitrato bismuthate. *Aliment. Pharmacol. Therap.* 1989;**3**:29–39.
36 Lechat, P, & Kisch, R. Bismuth induced encephalopathies: reappraisal of risks. *Gastroenterol. Clin. Biol.* 1986;**10**:562–9.
37 Mendelowitz, PC, Hoffman, RS, & Weber, S. Bismuth absorption and myoclonic encephalopathy during bismuth subsalicylate therapy. *Ann. Intern. Med.* 1990;**112**:140–41.
38 Playford, RJ, Matthews, CH, Campbell, MJ, *et al.* Bismuth induced encephalopathy caused by tripotassium dicitrato-bismuthate in a patient with chronic renal failure. *Gut* 1990;**31**:359–60.
39 Hudson, M, Ashley, N, & Mowat, G. Reversible toxicity in poisoning with colloidal bismuth subcitrate. *Br. Med. J.* 1989;**299**:159.
40 Taylor, EG, & Klenerman, P. Acute renal failure after colloidal bismuth subcitrate overdose (letters to the Editor). *Lancet* 1990;**335**:670–1.
41 Goodwin, CS, Marshall, BJ, Blincow, ED, Wilson, DH, Blackbourn, S, & Phillips, M. Prevention of nitroimidazole resistance in *Campylobacter pylori* by co-administration of colloidal bismuth subcitrate: clinical and *in vitro* studies. *J. Clin. Pathol.* 1988;**41**(2):207–10.
42 Glupczynski, Y, Burette, A, De Koster, E, *et al.* Metronidazole resistance in *Helicobacter pylori* (letter). *Lancet* 1990;**335**:976–7.
43 Marshall, BJ, Dye, KR, Plankey, M, *et al.* Eradication of *Campylobacter pylori* infection with bismuth subsalicylate and antibiotic combinations (abstract). *Am. J. Gastroenterol.* 1988;**83**:1035.

44 Marshall, BJ, Barrett, LJ, McCallum, RW, & Guerrant, RL. *C. pylori* therapy: is *in vitro* disc testing with metronidazole worthwhile? (poster) *Vth International Workshop on Campylobacter Infections, Puerto Vallarta, Mexico,* February 1989.

45 Cooreman, M, Krausgrill, P, Schumacher, B, & Hengels, KJ. Amoxycillin concentrations in antrum, corpus and fundus after single oral application. *Klin. Wochenschr.* 1989;**67**(suppl XVIII): 12–13.

46 Unge, P, Gad, A, Gnarpe, H, & Olsson, J. Does omeprazole improve antimicrobial therapy directed towards gastric *Campylobacter pylori* in patients with antral gastritis? A pilot study. *Scand. J. Gastroenterol.* 1989;**167**(suppl):49–54.

47 Lamouliatte, H, Megraud, F, de Mascarel, A, (abstract) *Klin. Wochenschr.* 1989;**67**(suppl XVIII): 37.

48 Coelho, LGV, Passos, MCF, Queiroz, DMM, *et al.* Five days triple therapy and 15 days double therapy on *C. pylori* eradication (abstract). *Klin. Wochenschr.* 1989;**67**(suppl XVIII):11.

49 Ericsson, CD, Feldman, S, Pickering, LK, & Cleary, TG. Influence of subsalicylate bismuth on absorption of doxycycline. *JAMA* 1982;**247**: 2266–7.

50 Morris, A, & Nicholson, G. Ingestion of *Campylobacter pyloridis* causes gastritis and raised fasting gastric pH. *Am. J. Gastroenterol.* 1987;**82**:192–9.

51 Unge, P, & Gnarpe, H. Pharmacokinetic, bacteriological and clinical aspects of the use of doxycycline in patients with active duodenal ulcer associated with *Campylobacter pylori. Scand. J. Infect. Dis.* 1988;**53**(suppl):70–73.

52 Meshkinpour, H, Thrupp, LD, Shiffler, P, Kitts, D, & Fisher, J. Reflux gastritis syndrome. Role of upper gastrointestinal microflora. *Arch. Surg.* 1981;**116**:1148–52.

53 Kibwage, IO, Verbruggen, A, Hoogmartens, J, & Vanderhaeghe, H. Thin layer chromatographic study of the metabolites of erythromycins in the Wistar rat. *J. Chromatol.* 1988;**434**:177–86.

54 Kucers, A, & Bennett, N.McK. *The Use of Antibiotics*, 4th edn. Philadelphia: J. B. Lippincott Co., 1987, pp. 1249–68.

55 Glupczynski, Y, & Burette, A. Failure of azythromycin to eradicate *Campylobacter pylori* from the stomach because of acquired resistance during treatment (letter). *Am. J. Gastroenterol.* 1990;**85**:98–9.

56 Lamouliatte, H, Megraud, F, DeMascarel, A, *et al.* Étude controlée de la josamycine dans les gastrites associées au *Campylobacter pylori* (abstract). *Gastroenterol. Clin. Biol.* 1988;**12**:A156.

57 Hardy, DJ, Hanson, CW, Hensey, DM, *et al.* Susceptibility of *Campylobacter pylori* to macrolides and fluoroquinolones. *J. Antimicrob. Chemother.* 1988;**22**:631–6.

58 Mandell, GL. The antimicrobial activity of rifampicin: emphasis on the relation to phagocytes. *Rev. Infect. Dis.* 1983;**5**(suppl 3):463.

59 Babiour, BM. Oxygen dependent killing by phagocytes. *N. Engl. J. Med.* 1978;**298**:659–68.

60 Bayerdorffer, E, Kasper, G, Pirlet, T, *et al.* Ofloxacin in the therapy of *Campylobacter pylori* positive duodenal ulcer. A prospective randomised study. *Dtsch. Med. Wochenschr.* 1987;**11**: 1407–11.

61 Zheng, ZT, Wang, ZY, Chu, YX, *et al.* Double-blind short-term trial of furazolidone in peptic ulcer (letter). *Lancet* 1985;**i**:1048–9.

62 Morgan, D, Kraft, W, Bender, M, & Pearson, A. Nitrofurans in the treatment of gastritis associated with *Campylobacter pylori.* The Gastrointestinal Physiology Working Group of Cayetano Heredia and The Johns Hopkins Universities. *Gastroenterology* 1988;**95**:1178–84.

63 Borsch, G, Mai, U, & Muller, KM. Monotherapy or polychemotherapy in the treatment of *Campylobacter pylori*-related gastroduodenal disease. *Scand. J. Gastroenterol.* 1988;**142**(suppl):101–6.

64 Borody, TJ, Cole, P, Noonan, S, *et al.* Recurrence of duodenal ulcer and *Campylobacter pylori* infection after eradication. *Med. J. Aust.* 1989; **151**:431–5.

65 George, LL, Borody, TJ, Andrews, P, *et al.* Cure of duodenal ulcer after eradication of *Helicobacter pylori. Med. J. Aust.* 1990;**153**:145–9.

66 McNulty, CAM, Eyre-Brook, IA, Uff, JS, Dent, JC, & Wilkinson, SP. Triple therapy is not always 95% effective (poster P2–73). *Vth International Workshop on Campylobacter Infections, Puerto Vallarta, Mexico,* February 1989.

67 Graham, DY, Klein, PD, Opekun, AR, *et al. In vivo* susceptibility of *Campylobacter pylori. Am. J. Gastroenterol.* 1989;**84**:233–8.

68 Marshall, BJ, Dye, KR, Plankey, M, *et al.* Eradication of *Campylobacter pylori* infection with bismuth subsalicylate and antibiotic combinations (abstract). *Am. J. Gastroenterol.* 1988;**83**:1035.

69 Langenberg, W, Rauws, EA, Oudbier, JH, & Tytgat, GN. Patient-to-patient transmission of *Campylobacter pylori* infection by fiberoptic gastroduodenoscopy and biopsy. *J. Infect. Dis.* 1990;**161**:507–11.

70 Martin, DF, Montgomery, E, Dobek, AS, Patrissi, GA, & Peura, DA. *Campylobacter pylori*, NSAIDS, and smoking: risk factors for peptic ulcer disease. *Am. J. Gastroenterol.* 1989;**84**: 1268–72.

71 Borkent, MV, & Beker, JA. Treatment of ulcerative reflux esophagitis with colloidal bismuth subcitrate in combination with cimetidine. *Gut* 1988;**29**:385–9.

72 Flook, D, & Stoddard, CJ. Gastro-oesophageal reflux and oesophagitis before and after vagotomy

for duodenal ulcer. *Br. J. Surg.* 1985;**72**:804–7.

73 Earlam, RJ, Amerigo, J, Kakavoulis, T, & Pollock, DJ. Histological appearances of oesophagus, antrum and duodenum and their correlation with symptoms in patients with a duodenal ulcer. *Gut* 1985;**26**:95–100.

74 Dye, KR, Marshall, BJ, Frierson, HF, Barrett, LJ, Guerrant, RL, & McCallum, RW. Is CLOtest alone adequate to diagnose *Campylobacter pylori*? (abstract). *Am. J. Gastroenterol.* 1988;**83**:1032.

75 Marshall, BJ, Caldwell, SH, Yu, ZJ, Darr, F, Chang, T, & McCallum, RW. Prevalence of *C. pylori* and history of upper GI investigation in healthy Virginians (abstract). *Gastroenterology* 1989;**96**(5 suppl 2):A321.

76 Spiro, HM. Moynihan's disease? The diagnosis of duodenal ulcer. *N. Engl. J. Med.* 1974;**291**:567–9.

77 Rokkas, T, Pursey, C, Uzoechina, E, *et al.* Non-ulcer dyspepsia and short term DeNol therapy: a placebo controlled trial with particular reference to the role of *Campylobacter pylori. Gut* 1988; **29**:1386–91.

78 Lambert, JR, Dunn, K, Borromeo, M, Korman, MG, & Hansky, J. *Campylobacter pylori* — a role in non-ulcer dyspepsia. *Scand. J. Gastroenterol.* 1989;**160**(suppl):7–13.

79 Kang, JY, Tay, HH, Wee, A, Guan, R, Math, MV, & Yap, I. Effect of colloidal bismuth subcitrate on symptoms and gastric histology in non-ulcer dyspepsia. A double blind placebo controlled study. *Gut* 1990;**31**:476–80.

80 Loffeld, RJ, Potters, HV, Stobberingh, E, Flendrig, JA, van Spreeuwel, JP, & Arends, JW. *Campylobacter*-associated gastritis in patients with non-ulcer dyspepsia: a double blind placebo controlled trial with colloidal bismuth subcitrate. *Gut* 1989;**30**:1206–12.

81 Marshall, BJ, Valenzuela, JE, McCallum, RW, *et al.* A placebo controlled clinical trial of bismuth subsalicylate for the treatment of *Helicobacter pylori*-associated gastritis (abstract). *Gastroenterology* 1990;**98**(5 part 2):A83.

82 Marshall, BJ, Hoffman, S, Boyd, C, & McCallum, RW. Does eradication of *H. pylori* have a long-term benefit in patients with dyspepsia and gastritis? (abstract). *Am. J. Gastroenterol.* 1990; **85**:89.

83 Talley, NJ, Fung, LH, Gilligan, IJ, McNeil, D, & Piper, DW. Association of anxiety, neuroticism, and depression with dyspepsia of unknown cause. A case control study. *Gastroenterology* 1986; **90**:886–92.

84 Talley, NJ, Ellard, K, Jones, M, Tennant, C, & Piper, DW. Suppression of emotions in essential dyspepsia and chronic duodenal ulcer. A case control study. *Scand. J. Gastroenterol.* 1988;**23**: 337–40.

85 Colin-Jones, DG. Management of dyspepsia: report of a working party. *Lancet* 1988;**i**:576–79.

86 Colin-Jones, DG. *Practical Approaches to the Management of Dyspepsia.* Langhorne, Pennsylvania: The Medicine Group USA, 1989.

87 Colin-Jones, DG. Management of dyspepsia: report of a working party. *Lancet* 1988;**i**:576–9.

14: Nausea, vomiting, and Helicobacter pylori

R.W. McCALLUM, S.H. CALDWELL &
B.J. MARSHALL

Introduction

The many causes of nausea and vomiting are summarized in Fig. 14.1. Although all of these conditions are potential etiologies in the acute setting, a longer history of episodic or cyclical symptoms will usually narrow the differential diagnosis. Usually such patients have received various empiric therapeutic trials and only resistant chronic cases present to the consulting gastroenterologist.

In general, we define "chronic" as persistent symptoms for 3 months or longer. Commonly, patients who fit into this category describe recurring bouts of nausea and vomiting with intermittent periods of normal or near-normal function. Such patients are often diagnostic and therapeutic challenges. Many fall into the realm of non-ulcer dyspepsia, and about half of these are found to harbor chronic bacterial gastritis. Below, we will review the spectrum of chronic nausea and vomiting with attention to the possible role of *Helicobacter pylori* in this setting.

Nausea and vomiting

Nausea is an unpleasant, upper abdominal sensation that usually, but not always, precedes the act of vomiting or forceful expulsion of the gastric contents. Nausea is a component of the involuntary autonomic nervous system and is usually associated with tachy- or bradycardia, tachypnea, hypersalivation, and pupillary dilation. It may be associated with frank abdominal pain. The subsequent act of vomiting is a coordinated interaction of the viscera and central nervous system (CNS), which results in increased pyloroduodenal tone, elevation of the gastric cardia, loss of the normal pressure gradient between the stomach and esophagus, and forceful sustained contraction of the abdominal muscles (Fig. 14.2). Distinguished from vomiting is the act of gastroesophageal reflux, which is seldom associated with nausea, and involves movement of the gastric contents into the esophagus or pharynx as a result of less forceful, sometimes passive, changes in the gastroesophageal pressure gradient.

A related condition is regurgitation and rumination. The latter term describes the effortless regurgitation of food within minutes of its ingestion and without accompanying nausea. Rumination is not forceful, although it may lead to continued "vomiting," even to a dehydration level, but not accompanied by esophagitis. It is to be distinguished from bulimia, which is vomiting induced by the patient, often in a secretive manner.

The nature of the patient's complaints and the medical history usually provide important clues as to the etiology of recurrent nausea and vomiting. A history of prior psychiatric illness is helpful but seldom adequate to draw firm conclusions. Neurosis is common among patients with chronic gastrointestinal symptoms, but it is rarely clear which problem is "cause" and which is "effect," so that psychosomatic disorders are best left as a diagnosis of exclusion.

Obviously, a history of prior ulcer disease or gastric surgery is significant and may have bearing on both diagnostic and therapeutic strategies. The medical history should also emphasize other medical illnesses for which the patient may be on potentially toxic medications, such as theophylline preparations or digoxin. Often, by the time these patients

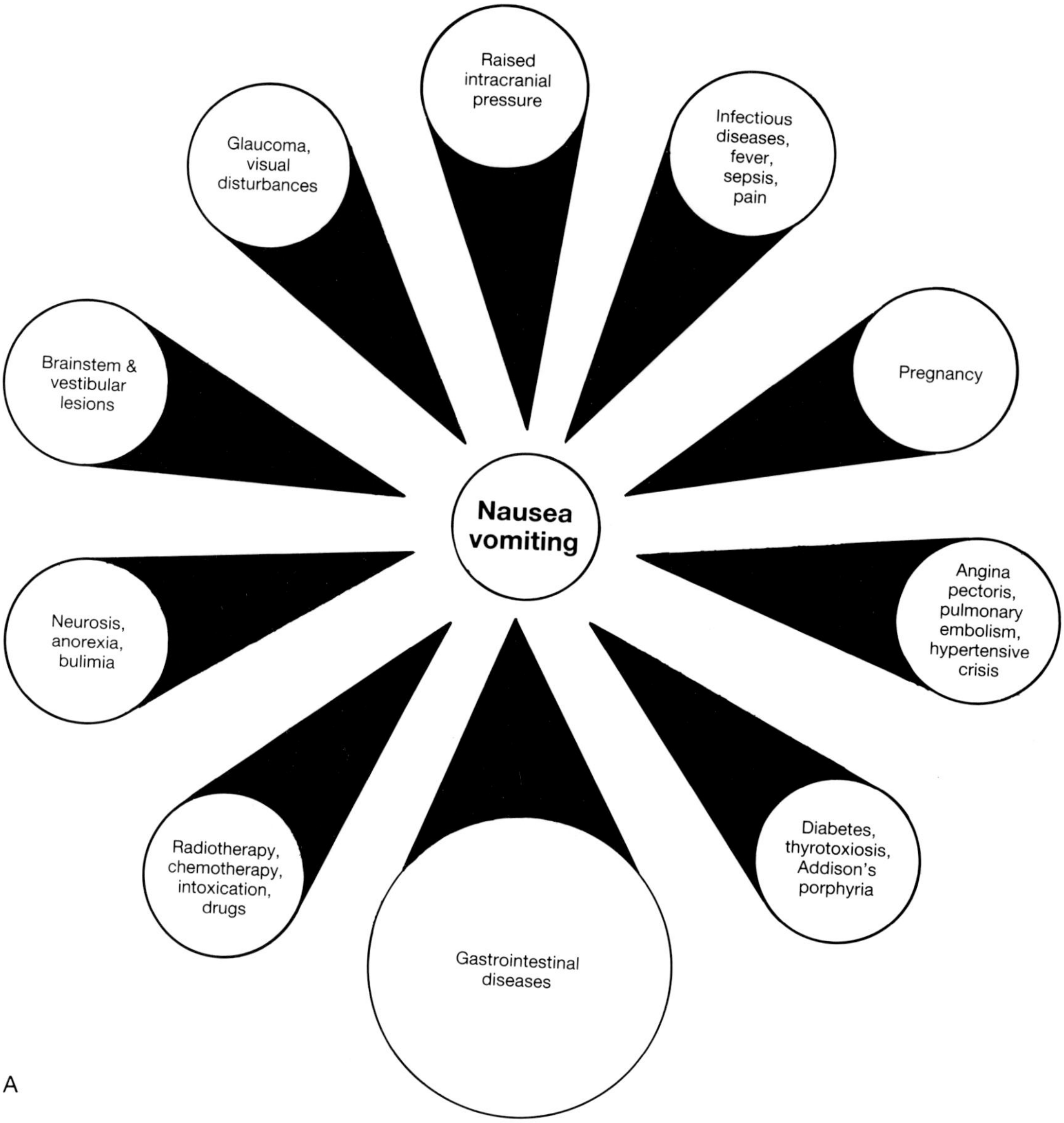

A

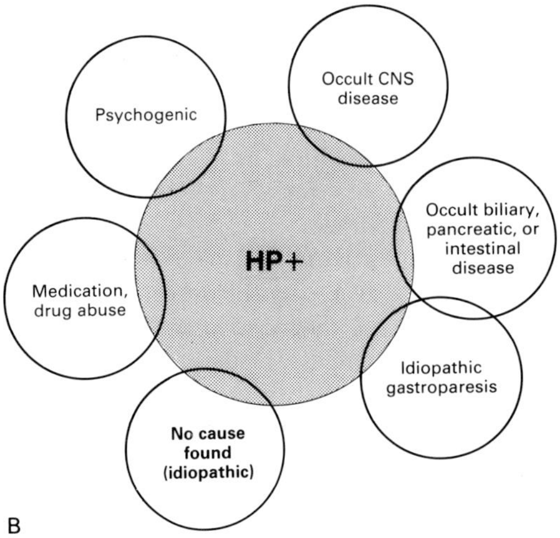

B

Fig. 14.1 Etiology of nausea and vomiting. A, main causes of vomiting. B, likely diagnoses and association with *H. pylori* in patients with chronic symptoms.

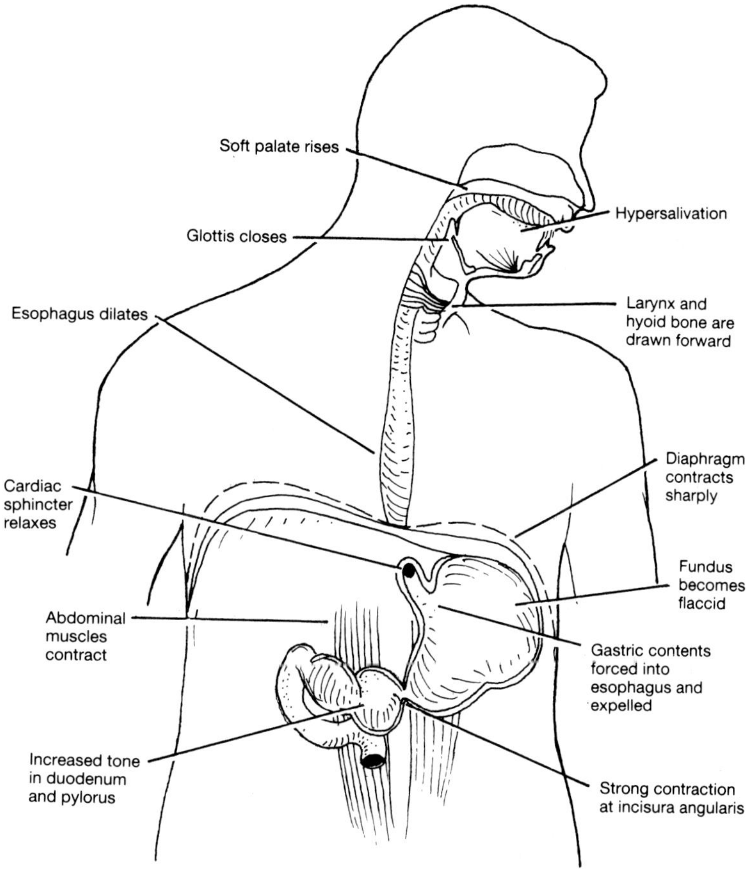

Fig. 14.2 The act of vomiting in man.

reach the gastroenterologist, they are on numerous medications, and a few minutes spent reviewing the side-effects of these drugs can be rewarding.

Once the patient's background has been established, special attention to the details of their symptoms should be given. In particular, the character of the vomitus, associated symptoms, the relation to abdominal pain, and especially the relation to meals, are important variables. Prominent symptoms of headache, vertigo, or visual disturbance indicate a problem outside of the gastrointestinal tract, as do exertional symptoms, association with shortness of breath, or frank chest pain, which suggest a cardiopulmonary disorder.

The appearance of the vomitus is often indicative of the underlying problem. The presence of undigested food is suggestive of a mechanical problem, such as gastric outlet obstruction or stricture. Grossly bloody vomitus may be the result of peptic ulcer or of a Mallory–Weiss tear. Foul-smelling and partially fermented food suggests either a mechanical obstruction or a gastric motility disorder. In rare cases, fistulae between colon and proximal gut can cause this. Pain may be associated with peptic ulcer, biliary tract disease or pancreatitis, particularly when there is a close association between meals, upper abdominal pain, and recurrent nausea and vomiting. Prominent morning symptoms are seen with pregnancy and, perhaps more commonly, with chronic alcoholism, although the latter may also be associated with chronic *H. pylori* infection [1].

The examination and laboratory evaluation of the patient should be directed by the medical history (see also Fig. 14.3). Of particular importance is the need to assess the

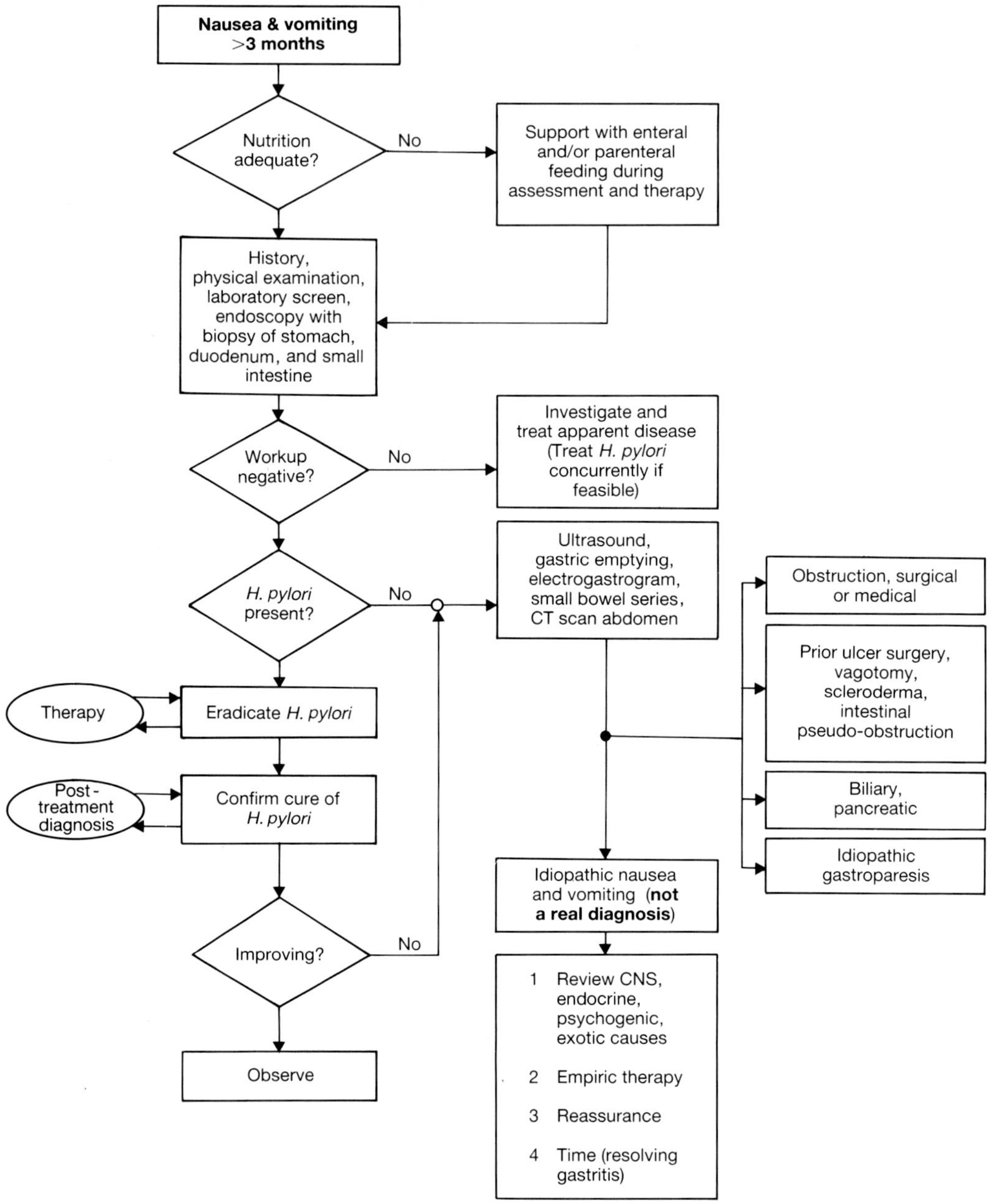

Fig. 14.3 Management of chronic nausea and vomiting.

nutritional status of the patient, as this may be severely compromised and often dictates the need for direct supportive measures prior to, or during, the initial work-up. A brief neurologic examination, with attention to the cranial nerves and optic fundi, may reveal a previously unrecognized CNS lesion. The abdominal examination should determine the presence of distension, a gastric succussion splash, tenderness, or organomegaly, which may require various imaging studies to characterize further. Fecal occult blood may offer a clue to underlying peptic ulcer or malignancy, but is often non-specific and may be unrelated to the presenting symptoms.

In general, we perform screening laboratory tests to assess serum electrolytes (sometimes a clue to the severity of the symptoms or an underlying adrenal disorder), cortisols, blood glucose, liver transaminases, blood counts, sedimentation rate, thyroid function, nutritional indices, and pancreatic enzymes, as well as drug levels if necessary. Sometimes, tests for alcohol or occult drug use are helpful. A chest X-ray, to exclude the possibility of a paraneoplastic syndrome related to small cell carcinoma of the lung, is appropriate where paraneoplastic syndrome is being considered in a middle-aged or older patient. Abdominal flat plate X-rays can identify dilated loops of bowel in pseudo-obstruction settings. Beyond these initial diagnostic measures, further evaluation often includes endoscopic studies, gastric motility tests, and/or abdominal and biliary imaging tests.

Non-ulcer dyspepsia

Many patients with chronic nausea and vomiting fall into the category of non-ulcer dyspepsia (NUD). Among patients with the latter syndrome, approximately 25% have, as prominent symptoms, nausea and vomiting [2] and, at this hospital, about 9% of NUD patients have these symptoms as major complaints. Dyspepsia refers to vague upper abdominal discomfort which is often meal-related. The term "non-ulcer dyspepsia" refers to the presence of these symptoms in the absence of peptic ulcer, and excluding other obvious abnormalities of the pancreas or biliary tree. Aside from anatomic abnormalities, however, many of these patients have *H. pylori* infection, histologic gastroduodenitis and, in some, gastric motility disorders. These three entities, and their possible relationships to each other and to chronic nausea and vomiting, are discussed below.

The spectrum of NUD

Non-ulcer dyspepsia has been conceptually divided into five groups [3, 4]. Among these, the first four are diagnostic categories and the last comprises the 25% or so of individuals who cannot be classified into a distinct category. The first group consists of patients with prominent symptoms of acid reflux, with meal-related or positional epigastric or retrosternal burning, which may be relieved with antacids. The second group has symptoms of classic duodenal ulcer without a demonstrable ulcer crater, i.e. Moynihan's disease. The third group consists of patients with prominent bloating during meals, early satiety, and distension, which are suggestive of a primary dysmotility disorder. The fourth group consists of patients with various mixed upper and lower gastrointestinal symptoms, overlapping with the irritable bowel syndrome and including aerophagia, bloating, distension, abdominal colic, food intolerances, and altered bowel habit.

Although these categories are useful to conceptualize the clinical problem, their relationship to underlying pathophysiologic mechanisms has not yet been fully refined. The NUD syndrome is discussed further in Chapter 13.

H. pylori, motility and non-ulcer dyspepsia

Helicobacter pylori has been implicated in a number of upper gastrointestinal illnesses. Persistent infection after duodenal ulcer healing increases the risk of ulcer relapse [5]. In NUD patients, gastric infection with *H. pylori* occurs in 30–50% [6]. Infection with *H. pylori* is strongly associated with histologic antral gastritis [7]. Eradication of the organism may improve symptoms in a significant number of patients with chronic dyspepsia [8]. Many of these patients complain of chronic nausea, or even intermittent vomiting, associated with their dyspepsia; however, the mechanism by which chronic bacterial gastritis might cause symptoms has not been elucidated. Studies before the discovery of *H. pylori* suggested a relationship between chronic histologic gastritis and gastric hypomotility [9], and recently an association between *H. pylori* infection and delayed orocecal transit time has been reported among patients with NUD [10]. On the other hand, *H. pylori* is not more

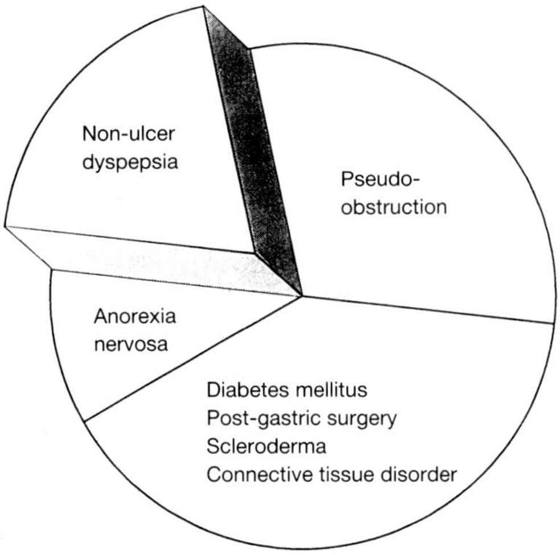

Fig. 14.4 Gastric motor disorders; associated conditions.

Table 14.1 Twenty consecutive patients presenting with known gastroparesis were prospectively evaluated for *H. pylori* infection. The prevalence of *H. pylori* infection in this group was not different to that of 21 age-, sex-, and race-matched patients presenting for routine upper endoscopy for symptoms of dyspepsia

	Gastroparetics	Consecutive endoscopies
n	20	21
Age	43 ± 10	47 ± 13
Range	26–74 years	28–73 years
Females	20	21
HP+	4 (20%)	7 (33%)

common in patients with symptomatic gastroparesis than in dyspeptic controls [11, 12].

Delayed gastric emptying may be a cause of upper abdominal pain [13]. Abnormal gastric motility has been found to be common among patients with dyspepsia [14]. About 20% of patients with delayed gastric emptying have symptoms which allow them to be classified into a category of NUD (Fig. 14.4) and, in our population, about one-third of patients with NUD have delayed gastric motor function. Vomiting is often a prominent symptom among these patients.

Is chronic *H. pylori* infection associated with gastroparesis?

We have recently reported our findings in two groups of patients — one with idiopathic gastroparesis associated with recurrent nausea, vomiting, and abdominal discomfort, and another group of patients with NUD and *H. pylori* infection [15]. The groups were studied for the presence of infection, and underwent gastric emptying studies using a ^{99m}Tc–sulfur–

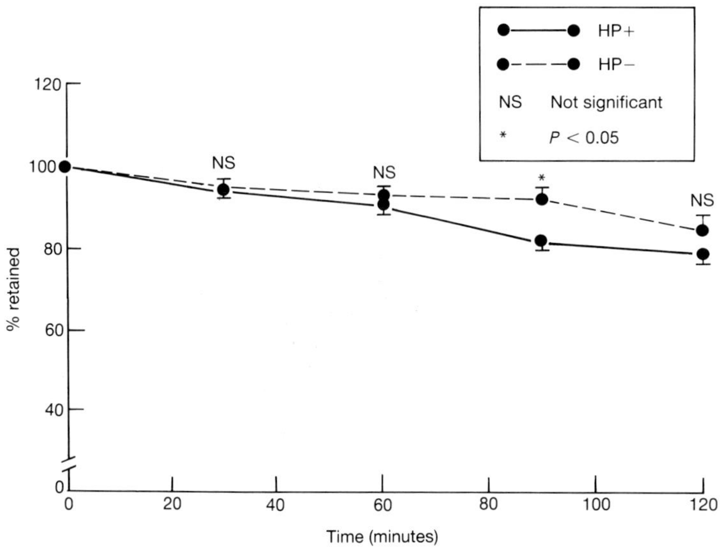

Fig. 14.5 The percentage of retained isotope (^{99m}Tc) among infected ($n = 4$; HP+) versus uninfected ($n = 16$; HP−) consecutive gastroparetic patients. There was no significant difference at 30, 60, and 120 minutes ($P > 0.1$, Student's T-test). At 90 minutes, the infected patients retained significantly less isotope ($P < 0.05$, Student's T-test).

Table 14.2 Nineteen consecutive patients with chronic dyspepsia and *H. pylori* infection underwent ^{99m}Tc-labeled chicken-liver gastric emptying tests. The results of the solid-phase gastric emptying tests were compared to 16 uninfected, asymptomatic volunteers

	HP+ (dyspeptics)	HP− (normals)
n	19	16
Age	38 ± 9	24 ± 4
Range	24–55 years	20–40 years
Females	12	11

colloid-labeled chicken-liver test meal. Among 20 consecutive patients with idiopathic gastroparesis (Table 14.1), four (20%) were infected with *H. pylori*. Solid-phase gastric emptying was delayed in all patients, but less so in the infected group (Fig. 14.5). Symptom scores were similar between infected and uninfected patients, and the prevalence of *H. pylori* in this group was not significantly different from a group of age-matched patients presenting with NUD.

In another group of 19 patients with proven *H. pylori* infection and NUD (Table 14.2), solid-phase gastric emptying was significantly more rapid in infected patients compared to 16 healthy, uninfected controls (Fig. 14.6). This relationship persisted when this group of patients was reanalyzed, using only male patients and controls to exclude possible menstrual cycle effects. Although orocecal transit time may be prolonged in *H. pylori* infection [10], our data and those of others [11, 12, 15] do not suggest an association between *H. pylori* and delayed gastric emptying. On the contrary, our results suggest increased emptying of solids among infected, symptomatic patients. These findings have yet to be correlated to the extent of underlying histologic disease, and they have not been reconciled with the apparent frequent presence of recurrent vomiting among symptomatic patients, as discussed further below. However, decreased gastric compliance related to chronic gastritis accompanying the *H. pylori* infection could be a contributing factor.

Evidence for a relationship between *H. pylori* and vomiting

The usual division between NUD and peptic ulcer disease may be invalid in patients with *H. pylori*, because many such NUD patients give a history of prior ulcer disease, and some go on to develop peptic ulcer disease [16]. In addition, ulcer patients sometimes have milder but persistent dyspeptic symptoms, even nausea and vomiting, in between actual clinical ulcer episodes [17, 18]. These authors believe that gastritis in NUD is the more benign end of the *H. pylori* clinical spectrum, which starts asymptomatic gastritis, includes NUD syn-

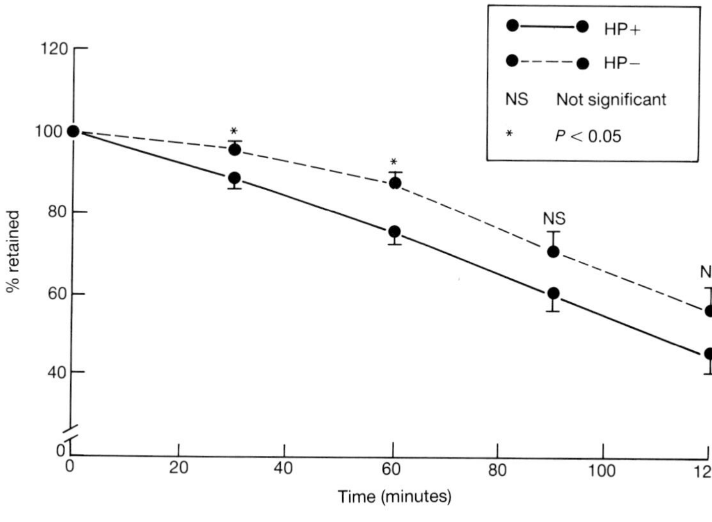

Fig. 14.6 The percentage of retained isotope (^{99m}Tc) in 19 dyspeptic patients with *H. pylori* infection (HP+) versus 16 uninfected, asymptomatic volunteers (HP−). Gastric emptying in the infected group was significantly faster in the early post-prandial period ($P < 0.05$, Wilcoxon Rank Sum).

drome, and ends with severe mucosal ulceration of the duodenum and/or stomach.

At the turn of the century, when acute *H. pylori* infections may have been common in children, Osler described acute gastritis with hypochlorhydria as a short-lived vomiting illness, which at times progressed to chronic dyspepsia [19]. Subsequent reports of acute gastritis with hypochlorhydria [20], now known to be due to *H. pylori*, usually describe a transient illness consisting of epigastric pain, nausea, and vomiting. In the epidemic of *H. pylori* reported by Ramsey *et al.* [21], the onset of hypochlorhydria was accompanied by an upper gastrointestinal illness lasting a week or so. In the self-administration experiment reported by Marshall *et al.* [22], early morning nausea and concurrent gnawing hunger pains were felt. These symptoms are very similar to those reported by patients with duodenal ulcer, who often have nausea and epigastric gnawing relieved by eating small snacks. In the self-administration experiment reported by Morris & Nicholson [23], nausea and vomiting occurred from day 4 until around day 7 after ingestion of the bacterium. Similarly, nausea and vomiting were prominent in apparent acute *H. pylori* episodes reported by several other authors [24, 25, 26].

Children with *H. pylori* often present with unexplained vomiting [27]. Pediatric *H. pylori* may also cause radiologic enlargement of the gastric folds [28] and a Menetrier-like protein-losing enteropathy [29], which responds well to eradication of the bacterium.

Recent reports suggest that *H. pylori* is a common cause of chronic nausea and vomiting. Mohiuddin *et al.* [30] studied 10 consecutive patients with unexplained intractable symptoms. The mean duration of the syndrome was 12 months (range 5–60) and no cause had been found after exhaustive work-up. Many of the patients carried a psychiatric diagnosis, reflecting an absence of discernible organic disease. Endoscopy was normal in the 10, but nine were found to have active gastritis and *H. pylori* on biopsy. Suppressive therapy with bismuth subsalicylate resulted in complete remission in six patients and substantial improvement in the other three. Those patients who had lost weight immediately regained it once the vomiting had ceased.

In a double-blind study of *H. pylori* treatment in duodenal ulcer disease, Marshall *et al.* [31] reported that three patients continued to have nausea and vomiting after healing of their ulcer. All three had received H2 receptor antagonists and *H. pylori* had not been eradicated. They immediately responded to antibacterial therapy with colloidal bismuth subcitrate, and achieved permanent remission after eradication of the bacterium. Although this was a small subset of patients, and not statistically significant, it did suggest that in patients with duodenal ulcer disease, vomiting may be related to *H. pylori* and gastritis and not always to the ulcer crater.

At the University of Virginia, we have seen six patients with intractable vomiting in whom *H. pylori* was the only abnormality detected after extensive work-up. In these patients, therapy for *H. pylori* resulted in symptomatic cure, except for one patient subsequently found to have small intestinal Crohn's disease.

Pathogenic effects of *H. pylori*

The pathogenic aspects of the *H. pylori* organism have been reviewed elsewhere [32]. *H. pylori* organisms colonize the gastric epithelium in vast numbers and the majority of isolates are toxigenic [33]. *In vitro*, 30–60% of isolates from NUD patients will cause vacuolation of cultured epithelial cells [34]. Vacuolation also occurs when such cells are incubated with high concentrations of ammonia, or *H. pylori* (urease) and urea [35]. Ammonia collects in the gastric juice of patients with *H. pylori* and can reach concentrations of 50 mM, about 1000 times higher than that of the blood [36].

Other enzymes produced by *H. pylori* may also damage the gastric mucosa. Proteases digest the gastric mucus layer [37], phospholipases compromise the integrity of the mucus layer and may damage epithelial cell membranes [38], and a toxin inhibits acid production by parietal cells [39]. This "hypochlorhydric" toxin may be relevant to gastric emptying delays, because slower emptying is known to occur in hypochlorhydric states, such as drug-induced hypochlorhydria or pernicious anemia [40].

Finally, the presence of bacterial proteins incites an immune response, giving rise to activated complement, inflammatory mediators, and superoxide radicals generated from phagocytic cells [41]. It is possible that the nausea and vomiting present in patients with *H. pylori*-associated disease are the normal response to stimulation of local chemoreceptors designed to trigger the expulsion of noxious gastric contents.

Management of nausea and vomiting

Chronic nausea and vomiting are a therapeutic challenge, since many patients cannot take the oral medication prescribed and in severe cases even the investigation of the problem is difficult. The flow chart in Fig. 14.3 suggests a management plan.

Initially, obvious known causes should be ruled out and *H. pylori* should be excluded. If no mucosal abnormality is found, further investigation may reveal a gastric motility disorder. In general, chronic nausea and vomiting associated with an identifiable motility disorder are more difficult to treat, and may never resolve. In some cases, underlying diseases such as diabetes, scleroderma, previous gastric surgery, or intestinal myoneuropathy will be irreversible causes. Therapy for these is a stepwise increase in measures starting with:

1 Low-residue soft or liquid diet, frequent small oral feeds, erect posture to assist gastric drainage.

2 Oral or parenteral antiemetic medications, known and experimental prokinetic agents (see Table 14.3).

3 Frequent small feeds, soft naso–gastric–jejunal feeding tube.

4 Percutaneous gastrostomy feeding tube, either into the stomach or via gastrostomy into the jejunum (depends on the amount of nausea

Table 14.3 Drugs used for the treatment of nausea and vomiting

Drug name	Mode of action	Dosage and administration	Side-effects
Metoclopramide, "Reglan", "Octamide"	Dopamine antagonist and anticholinergic with peripheral and central action. Speeds gastric emptying, increases LES tone, antinauseant	Oral, 10 mg t.i.d. 30–60 minute ac; SC or IV = 5–10 mg t.i.d.; for chemotherapy, infuse 2 mg kg^{-1} IV 2 hourly for 5 doses in 24 hours (2–3 hourly); halve dose in renal failure	Sedation, extrapyramidal reactions (give 50 mg diphenhydramine, "Benadryl," IM), amenorrhea, lactation
Chlorpromazine, "Thorazine"	The prototype phenothiazine, anticholinergic, dopamine antagonist, weak serotonin antagonist, central antiemetic, peripheral alpha blocker, psychotropic	Oral, 10–25 mg 4–6 hourly (may increase if no side-effects); suppositories, 100 mg 6–8 hourly; IM, 25–50 mg 4–6 hourly (deep IM); IV, 25–50 mg, dilute to 1 mg ml^{-1} as 1 mg $minute^{-1}$	Anticholinergic, alpha blocking, sedation, dopamine antagonist, galactorrhea, gynecomastia, cholestatic jaundice, extrapyramidal effects
Prochlorperazine, "Compazine"	A phenothiazine, some anticholinergic action, dopamine antagonist, central antiemetic, peripheral alpha blocker	Oral, IM, IV, 5–10 mg t.i.d., maximum dose around 40 mg day^{-1}; also available as suppositories, 25 mg b.i.d.	Sedation, extrapyramidal reactions, tardive dyskinesia (long-term use), amenorrhea, lactation, orthostatic hypotension, cholestatic jaundice
Thiethylperazine, "Torecan"	Related to phenothiazine, a centrally acting antiemetic	Oral, 10 mg t.i.d.; suppositories, 10 mg t.i.d.; IM, 10 mg t.i.d.	As for phenothiazines; anticholinergic, alpha blocking, dopamine antagonist, sedation, extrapyramidal effects

Table 14.3 (*continued*)

Drug name	Mode of action	Dosage and administration	Side-effects
Scopolamine, "Transderm Scop"	Centrally acting antiemetic via anticholinergic effect on vomiting center. Peripheral (GI) actions also present. 75% reduction in motion sickness. About 40-minute delay before effect is evident	Cutaneous patch attaches behind ear. One patch releases 0.5 mg scopolamine over 73 hours	Anticholinergic. Dry mouth, sedation (20%), blurred vision, glaucoma. Temporary exacerbation of symptoms after withdrawal
Diphenhydramine, "Benadryl," and diphenhydrinate, "Dramamine"	Antihistamine, anticholinergic, central antiemetic action	Oral, IM, and IV dose is 50 mg 3–6 hourly, maximum dose 400 mg day^{-1}	Anticholinergic, sedative, photosensitivity, GI side-effects, glaucoma
Promethazine, "Phenergan"	Phenothiazine derivative, an antihistamine, very weak dopaminergic action. Central antiemetic, sedative, weakly anticholinergic	Oral, 12.5–50 mg 4–6 hourly; suppository, same dose; IM, 25–50 mg 4–6 hourly (can cause gangrene if intraarterial, or necrosis if given SC); IV, 25–50 mg as 25 mg ml^{-1} or less, best if IV solution running, repeat 4–6 hourly	Sedation, dry mouth, blurred vision, glaucoma, hyper or hypotension, allergic reaction, photosensitivity, GI upset
Meclizine, "Antivert," "Bonine"	Antihistamine with weak anticholinergic action. Central antiemetic	Oral, 25–100 mg daily, as b.i.d. dose	Sedative, anticholinergic, glaucoma
Cyclizine, "Marezine"	Antihistamine, anticholinergic, central antiemetic	Oral, IM, or IV 50 mg 4–6 hourly	Sedative, anticholinergic, glaucoma
Hydroxyzine, "Vistaril"	Antihistamine, unrelated chemically to the phenothiazines, sedative, anticholinergic, central antiemetic action	Oral, 25–100 mg q.i.d. Well absorbed, onset of action 15–30 minutes	Anticholinergic, sedative
Benzquinamide, "Emete-con"	A benzoquinolizine chemically unrelated to phenothiazines. Central antiemetic. Antihistamine, weak anticholinergic, sedative. Half-life 40 minutes, used to prevent post-operative nausea and vomiting in anesthesiology. Has caused hypertension when given IV	IM, 50 mg repeated 3–4 hourly. Not usually used for a prolonged period. Halve dose in the elderly. IV, give 25 mg initially, then use IM (do not give IV to patients with cardiovascular disease)	Hypertension, hypotension, anticholinergic effects, arrhythmias, drowsiness, GI upset, fatigue, chills, fever

Table 14.3 (*continued*)

Drug name	Mode of action	Dosage and administration	Side-effects
Trimethobenzamide, "Tigan"	Central antiemetic with anticholinergic, dopamine antagonist and sedative effects	Oral, 250 mg 3–4 times daily; suppositories, 200 mg 3–4 times daily; IM, 200 mg 3–4 times daily (not recommended for intravenous use)	Extrapyramidal reactions, drowsiness, allergic reactions, convulsions, masking of other CNS signs. Injection is painful
Domperidone, "Motilium"	Peripherally acting dopamine antagonist. Prokinetic action (similar to metoclopramide) but less central effects	Oral, 20 mg ac and at bedtime	Some central action allows dopamine antagonism with consequent gynecomastia, and galactorrhea. Can be used (with caution) in Parkinson's disease
Cisapride	Facilitates acetylcholine release from gut myenteric plexus, also serotonin antagonism, very little central action, no dopamine antagonism and minimal anticholinergic action. Not primarily an antiemetic. Increases GI motility from stomach to colon. Half-life 7–10 hours	Oral 10–20 mg 6 hourly; IM, 4–8 mg (not yet available in the United States, consult *Physicians Desk Reference* (PDR))	Abdominal cramps, GI discomfort, diarrhea
δ-9-THC, "Marinol"	The active agent in cannabis. Central action. Psychotropic and antiemetic	Oral, 5–10 mg repeated at 2–4 hour intervals for 4–6 doses per day; mainly used in chemotherapy	About twice the side-effects of prochlorperazine in comparative studies. Drowsiness, dizziness, euphoria, dry mouth, ataxia, visual, hypotension. Psychological dependence
Nabilone, "Cesamet"	"	Oral, 1–2 mg b.i.d.	"
Erythromycin "Eryc," "Erythromycin base filmtabs"	Erythromycin base is a motilin receptor agonist. It enhances gastric motor activity *in vitro* and *in vivo*. Use as a prokinetic agent is being investigated	Oral, 250 mg q.i.d.; IV, 150–300 mg t.i.d. Experimental in this prokinetic role, clinical efficacy not proven. Not an antinauseant	Abdominal cramps, allergies, nausea. Omeprazole ramitidine may decrease side-effects

ac, *ante cebum*; GI, gastrointestinal; IM, intramuscular; IV, intravenous; LES, lower esophageal sphincter; SC, subcutaneous.

present, and necessary only in persons who cannot maintain adequate oral intake).

5 Surgical feeding jejunostomy, necessary when gastric emptying is very poor and enteric feeds are vomited.

Table 14.3 lists the drugs and doses used for the treatment of nausea and vomiting. The table includes some new "prokinetic" agents (i.e. they increase gastric motility), which are experimental and not yet fully evaluated in the United States. An interesting new agent is erythromycin, which stimulates motilin receptors in the upper gastrointestinal tract and increases gut peristalsis [42]. The clinical relevance of this effect is presently under investigation. Prokinetic drugs are not necessarily antiemetic, so their use is best restricted to those patients with documented gastroparesis.

Unlike *H. pylori*-negative (HP−) nausea and vomiting, *H. pylori*-positive (HP+) cases often respond well, albeit slowly, to antibacterial therapy. These patients may give a history of vomiting several times per week for months or even years, sometimes starting in childhood. Usually a psychiatric diagnosis has been entertained by previous physicians.

Since 20% of patients with known gastroparetic syndromes will have *H. pylori* (i.e. the usual population prevalence after age 30), one must keep in mind that eradicating *H. pylori* in this setting will not necessarily change the underlying gastric motor disturbance, and that symptoms of gastroparesis will continue.

Nevertheless, we have seen three patients with *H. pylori*-associated gastroparesis and vomiting who responded symptomatically to antibiotic therapy. In two of these, gastric emptying returned to normal; in a third it remained slightly delayed after 1 year.

Figure 14.7 shows the response to therapy in NUD patients at this hospital who had nausea and/or vomiting as a major symptom. Of 26 patients with nausea at least once per week, one worsened, seven were unchanged, and 18 (70%) improved. Of these 18, 11 had symptoms less than once per month at follow-up 15 months later.

For reasons unknown, most patients with nausea and vomiting are women. They are very well motivated and will attempt to complete even the most difficult antibiotic therapy.

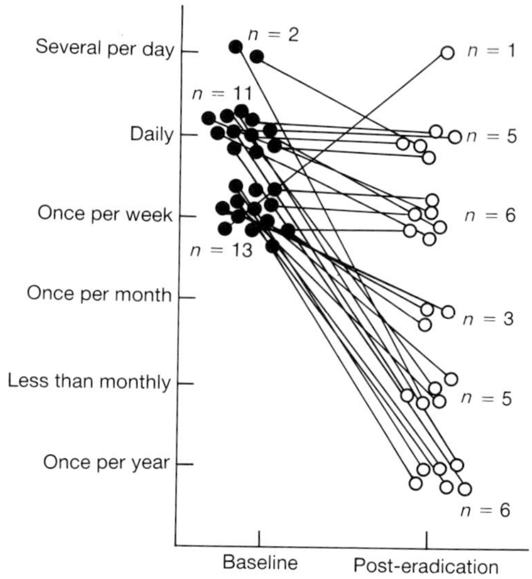

Fig. 14.7 Nausea and vomiting: symptom response in 26 patients after eradication of *H. pylori*.

As with all antibacterial therapy, the aim is to eradicate the underlying organism which, in the case of *H. pylori*, may involve more than one cycle of treatment. Nauseated patients may refuse a second course of antibiotic therapy if the first fails to eradicate *H. pylori*. Therefore, to ensure maximum success of the initial antibiotic course, we attempt to obtain culture and sensitivity of the organism prior to therapy, and may even ask the patient to return for endoscopic biopsy to achieve this purpose.

If the organism is sensitive to metronidazole, simple dual therapy usually eradicates *H. pylori* with minimum discomfort to the patient. If the organism is resistant to metronidazole (30% of cases), then alternative antibiotics are used in the first instance.

When medication is likely to be vomited back up, we recommend starting with liquid BSS in frequent small doses, and maintaining this until a partial clinical response is observed, when other agents can be added one by one. Metronidazole should be added last, since it is ineffective unless bacterial suppression is achieved with the initial therapeutic agents.

After treatment of *H. pylori* for 10–14 days (see Chapter 13), the patient and the physician must resist the temptation to give extra antibiotic therapy if a clinical response has not occurred, because further antibiotic therapy will produce false-negative diagnostic tests for *H. pylori*. Negative endoscopic biopsy or breath test 1 month later is strong evidence for bacteriologic cure, but testing earlier than this is unreliable. The exception is the very unwell patient, in whom endoscopy and multiple biopsies for histology and culture at an earlier time may be worthwhile, since absence of *H. pylori* and healing of gastritis will prevent further unnecessary antibiotic treatment.

In our clinic, patients remain on their usual antiemetic therapy during antibacterial treatment, and may continue this after completing therapy for *H. pylori*. One month later a breath test is performed. If this is negative, we repeat it 3 months later to confirm long-term eradication of *H. pylori*.

After eradication of *H. pylori*, symptoms improve in many patients, although exacerbations and remissions often cause further concern. If a non-invasive *H. pylori* test is available, a negative result is reassuring and no extra intervention is necessary. If a breath test is unavailable, then endoscopy and biopsy should be repeated. Half of the patients successfully treated will improve immediately, while the others respond gradually over 3–12 months. Eventually, clinical relapses become uncommon and 75% cease their antiemetic medication. Older women, who may have had symptoms all their lives, seem to be the slowest to respond.

In patients with severe *H. pylori*-associated syndromes we routinely screen the spouse for the infection, and advise antibacterial therapy if infection is present. Because of the relapsing and remitting nature of the symptoms, fewer investigations will be performed during clinical relapses if we know the spouse is free of *H. pylori*.

References

1 Laine, L, Marin Sorensen, M, & Weinstein, WM. *Campylobacter pylori* in alcoholic hemorrhagic "gastritis". *Dig. Dis. Sci.* 1989;**34**:677–80.

2 McCallum, RW. Motor function of the stomach in health and disease. In: Sleisenger, MH, & Fordtran, JS (eds), *Gastrointestinal Disease: Pathophysiology, Diagnosis, Management, Vol.1*, 4th edn. Philadelphia: W.B. Saunders, 1989, pp. 675–713.

3 Colin-Jones, DG. Management of dyspepsia: report of a working party. *Lancet* 1988;**i**:576–9.

4 Colin-Jones, DG. *Practical Approaches to the Management of Dyspepsia*. Langhorne, Pennsylvania: The Medicine Group USA, 1989.

5 Marshall, BJ, Goodwin, CS, Warren, JR, *et al.* Prospective double-blind trial of duodenal ulcer relapse after eradication of *Campylobacter pylori*. *Lancet* 1988;**ii**:1439–42.

6 Marshall, BJ, McGechie, DB, Rogers, PA, & Glancy, RJ. Pyloric *Campylobacter* infection and gastroduodenal disease. *Med. J. Aust.* 1985;**142**: 439–44.

7 Dooley, CP, & Cohen, H. The clinical significance of *Campylobacter pylori*. *Ann. Intern. Med.* 1988; **108**:70–79.

8 Borody, TJ, Carrick, J, & Hazell, SL. Symptoms improve after the eradication of gastric *Campylobacter pyloridis* (letter). *Med. J. Aust.* 1987;**146**:450–1.

9 Fink, SM, Barwick, KW, DeLuca, V, Sanders, FJ, Kandathil, M, & McCallum, RW. The association of histologic gastritis with gastroesophageal reflux and disorders of gastric emptying. *J. Clin. Gastroenterol.* 1984;**6**:301–9.

10 Wilberg, S, Pieramico, O, & Malfertheiner, P. Role of antral inflammation on orocecal transit time in patients with non-ulcer dyspepsia. *Klin. Wochenschr.* 1989;**67**(suppl XVIII):72.

11 Wegener, M, Borsch, G, Schaffstein, J, *et al.* Are dyspeptic symptoms in patients with *Campylobacter pylori*-associated type B gastritis linked to delayed gastric emptying. *Am. J. Gastroenterol.* 1988;**83**:737–40.

12 Barnett, JL, Behler, EM, Appelman, HD, & Elta, GH. *Campylobacter pylori* is not associated with gastroparesis. *Dig. Dis. Sci.* 1989;**34**:1677–80.

13 Rees, WD, Miller, LJ, & Malagelada, JR. Dyspepsia, antral motor dysfunction and gastric stasis of solids. *Gastroenterology* 1980;**78**:360–65.

14 Malagelada, JR, & Stranghellini, V. Manometric evaluation of functional upper gut symptoms. *Gastroenterology* 1988;**88**:1223–31.

15 Caldwell, SH, Valenzuela, G, Marshall, BJ, Hoffman, SR, Plankey, MW, & McCallum, RW. *Campylobacter pylori* (CP) gastritis does not slow solid-phase ^{99}Tc gastric emptying. *Am. J. Gastroenterol.* 1989;**84**:1155.

16 Thompson, WO, Robertson, AG, Imrie, CW, Joffe, SN, Lee, FD, & Blumgart, LH. Is duodenitis a dyspeptic myth? *Lancet* 1977;**i**:1197.

17 Spiro, HM. Moynihan's disease? The diagnosis of duodenal ulcer. *N. Engl. J. Med.* 1974;**291**:567.

18 Sol, AH, & Isenberg, JI. Duodenal ulcer disease. In: Sleisenger MH, & Fordtran JS (eds), *Gastrointestinal Disease*. Philadelphia: WB Saunders, 1983, p. 647.

19 Osler, W. *The Principles and Practice of Medicine*.

New York: Appleton, 1920.
20 Graham, DY, Alpert, LC, Smith, JL, & Yoshimura, HH. Iatrogenic *Campylobacter pylori* infection is a cause of epidemic achlorhydria. *Am. J. Gastroenterol.* 1988;**83**:974–80.
21 Ramsey, EJ, Carey, KV, Peterson, WL, *et al.* Epidemic gastritis with achlorhydria. *Gastroenterology* 1979;**76**:1449–57.
22 Marshall, BJ, Armstrong, JA, McGechie, DB, & Glancy, RJ, Attempt to fulfil Koch's postulates for pyloric *Campylobacter. Med. J. Aust.* 1985;**142**: 436–9.
23 Morris, A, & Nicholson, G. Ingestion of *Campylobacter pyloridis* causes gastritis and raised fasting gastric pH. *Am. J. Gastroenterol.* 1987;**82**:192–9.
24 Salmeron, M, Desplaces, N, Lavergne, A, & Houdart, R. *Campylobacter*-like organisms and acute purulent gastritis (letter). *Lancet* 1986;**ii**: 975–6.
25 Weirsinga, WM, & Tytgat, GN. Clinical recovery owing to parietal cell failure in a patient with Zollinger–Ellison syndrome. *Gastroenterology* 1977;**73**:1413–17.
26 Frommer, DJ, Carrick, J, Lee, A, & Hazell, SL. Acute presentation of *Campylobacter pylori* gastritis. *Am. J. Gastroenterol.* 1988;**83**:1168–71.
27 Cadranel, S, Glupczinsky, Y, Labbe, M, & De-Prez, C. *Campylobacter pylori* in children. In: Menge, H, Gregor, M, Tytgat, GNJ, & Marshall, BJ (eds), *Campylobacter pylori*. Berlin: Springer-Verlag, 1988, p. 110.
28 Morrison, S, Dahms, BB, Hoffenberg, E, & Czinn, SJ. Enlarged gastric folds in association with *Campylobacter pylori* gastritis. *Radiology* 1989; **171**:819–21.
29 Hill, ID, Sinclair Smith, C, Lastovica, AJ, Bowie, MD, & Emms, M. Transient protein-losing enteropathy associated with acute gastritis and *Campylobacter pylori. Arch. Dis. Child.* 1987; **62**:1215–19.
30 Mohiuddin, J, Sloane, BE, Langdale Brown, B, & Rhodes, JM. *Campylobacter* gastritis and vomiting (letter). *Lancet* 1988;**ii**:1502.
31 Marshall, BJ, Goodwin, CS, Warren, JR, *et al.* Prospective double-blind trial of duodenal ulcer relapse after eradication of *Campylobacter pylori. Lancet* 1988;**ii**:1439–42.
32 Marshall, BJ. Virulence and pathogenicity of *Helicobacter pylori. J. Gastroenterol. Hepatol.* 1991;**6**:121–4.
33 Cover, TL, Dooley, CP, & Blaser, MJ. Characterization of and human serologic response to proteins in *Helicobacter pylori* broth culture supernatants with vacuolizing cytotoxin activity. *Infect. Immun.* 1990;**58**:603–10.
34 Leunk, RD, Johnson, PT, David, BC, Kraft, WG, & Morgan, DR. Cytotoxic activity in broth-culture filtrates of *Campylobacter pylori. J. Med. Microbiol.* 1988;**26**:93–9.
35 Xu, Jia-k, Goodwin, CS, Cooper, M, & Robinson, J. Intracellular vacuolization caused by the urease of *Helicobacter pylori. J. Infect. Dis.* 1990;**161**: 1302–4.
36 Marshall, BJ, & Langton, SR. Urea hydrolysis in patients with *Campylobacter pyloridis* infection. *Lancet* 1986;**i**:965–6.
37 Slomiany, BL, Bilski, J, Sarosiek, J, *et al. Campylobacter pyloridis* degrades mucin and undermines gastric mucosal integrity. *Biochem. Biophys. Res. Commun.* 1987;**144**:307–14.
38 Slomiany, BL, Nishikawa, H, Piotrowski, J, Okazaki, K, & Slomiany, A. Lipolytic activity of *Campylobacter pylori*: effect of sofalcone. *Digestion* 1989;**43**:33–40.
39 Cave, DR, & Vargas, M. Effect of a *Campylobacter pylori* protein on acid secretion by parietal cells. *Lancet* 1989;**ii**:187–9.
40 Minami, H, & McCallum, RW. The physiology and pathophysiology of gastric emptying in humans. *Gastroenterology* 1984;**86**:1592–610.
41 Barbour, BM. Oxygen dependent microbial killing by phagocytes. *N. Engl. J. Med.* 1978;**298**:659–68.
42 Janssens, J, Vantrappen, G, Urbain, JL, *et al.* The motilin agonist erythromycin normalizes impaired gastric emptying in diabetic gastroparesis. *Gastroenterology* 1989;**96**:A237.

15: Pharmacology of colloidal bismuth subcitrate ("DeNol") and use in non-ulcer dyspepsia

J.R. LAMBERT & A. McLEAN

Introduction

Bismuth salts have been used as medicinal agents for nearly 200 years, mainly for the treatment of gastrointestinal disorders (Table 15.1). Their use gradually declined with the advent of the newer generation potent antacids. Renewed interest in bismuth salts arose as the recognition of the unique properties of colloidal bismuth subcitrate (CBS, "DeNol") became apparent.

Colloidal bismuth subcitrate is an effective agent in healing both gastric [1–3] and duodenal [4–7] ulcer disease when compared to placebo. Prolonged remission from duodenal ulcer disease occurs after initial healing with CBS, which is associated with its ability to eradicate *Helicobacter pylori* [8–10] and improve the gastroduodenitis [10–13] (Fig. 15.1).

As well as an effect on *H. pylori*-associated gastroduodenitis, CBS has many other actions on the gastroduodenal mucosa (Table 15.2). In an acid environment, CBS precipitates from the solution phase, yielding fine crystals of bismuth citrate and bismuth oxychloride. These small particles have been found coating the ulcer crater in experimental models [16]. CBS also complexes with mucus, thus decreasing the barrier function of mucus to H^+ back-diffusion [18]. Furthermore, CBS stimulates endogenous gastric prostaglandin synthesis [25] as well as markedly reducing pepsin output and activity [21, 22].

Finally, CBS may bind epidermal growth factor and hence provide higher concentrations in the ulcer base [26]. The role of local versus systemic (absorbed) bismuth from CBS in achieving these actions is unclear.

Colloidal bismuth subcitrate is now available for prescription in countries all over the world. The safety record of these products over a long period of time is exceptionally favorable. Confusion still prevails regarding the safety of CBS, as a lingering aftermath of the historical misuse of many of the other salts of bismuth [27–31]. In this chapter the local and systemic pharmacokinetics of CBS are discussed, followed by a review of its use in non-ulcer dyspepsia.

Pharmacokinetics

CBS acts locally on the upper gastroduodenal mucosa, as well as potentially exerting systemic effects as a result of gastrointestinal absorption (less than 2% of the ingested dose). Different formulations/preparations of CBS have been used clinically and include liquid as well as chew and swallow tablets. Minor differences in first dose pharmacokinetics are noted between the chew and swallow tablets; however, this is not evident with chronic dosing [32, 33].

Topical gastroduodenal pharmacokinetics

Bismuth concentrations measured in human gastric and duodenal mucosa at different times after single doses of CBS tablets reveal a rapid increase in mucosal levels, reaching a peak at 30–60 minutes [19]. Levels fall rapidly in the first 4 hours after ingestion (Fig. 15.2). In antral mucus the *in vitro* minimum inhibitory concentration (MIC) of CBS against *H. pylori* (range 2–16 $\mu g\,ml^{-1}$) [34] was exceeded in the first 2 hours, but not after 4 hours following the CBS dose (Fig. 15.2). The apparent initial half-lives of bismuth were 0.54, 0.69, 0.88, and 0.90 hours for gastric juice, gastric mucus, duodenal mucosa, and antral mucosa respectively.

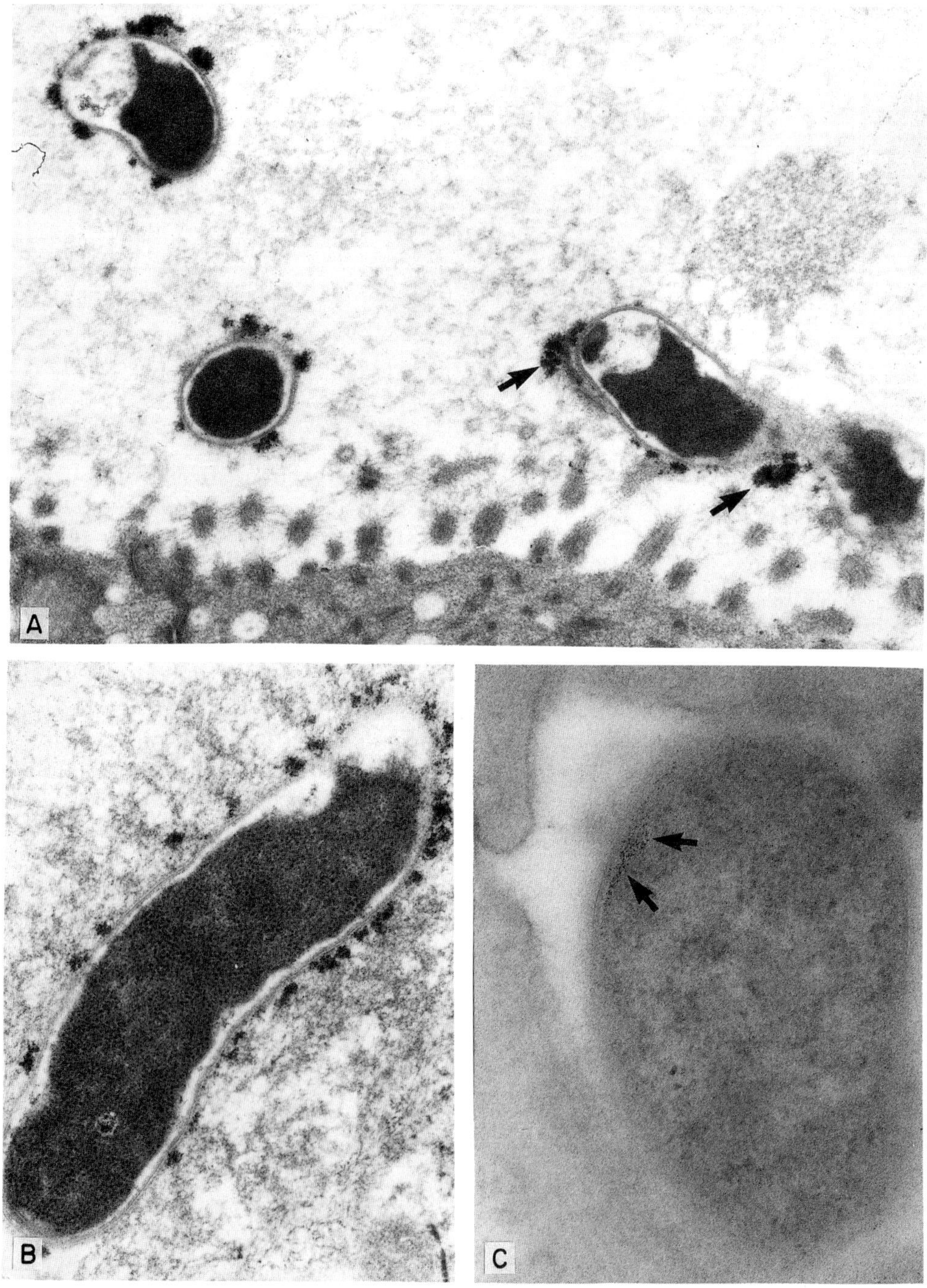

Fig. 15.1 Appearance of *H. pylori* bacteria as found in biopsy specimens between 30 and 150 minutes after oral "DeNol". A, Deformed and vacuolated *H. pylori* with opaque aggregates of bismuth complex deposited on the cell walls (←): biopsy 70 minutes after a single dose of liquid "DeNol". ×24 000. B, Typical longitudinal profile of structurally degraded organism, free in the gastric mucus 95 minutes after commencing "DeNol" treatment. Note irregular retraction of bacterial contents, surrounding cavitation, and external bismuth deposits. ×40 000. C, Focal penetration of particulate bismuth complex (←) under the cell wall of a residual (still intact) organism 60 minutes after "DeNol" liquid ingestion. Section is unstained. ×75 000.

Table 15.1 Historical uses of bismuth salts — past and present

Bismuth compound	Indication
Bismuth subnitrate	Irritable colon, gastric disorders, constipation
Bismuth subgallate	Improving stool consistency and odor in colostomy and ileostomy patients
Bismuth phosphate, aluminate and subcarbonate	Various gastrointestinal disorders
Bismuth subsalicylate	Traveler's diarrhea (prevention), dyspepsia
Colloidal bismuth subcitrate	Gastric and duodenal ulcers, ?non-ulcer dyspepsia

Further pharmacokinetic studies of bismuth in the mucosa after chronic dosing are needed to optimize local delivery of CBS.

Systemic absorption

Following oral intake of CBS, a significant increase in blood concentration of bismuth occurs with estimates of bioavailability ranging from 0.16 to 1.5% of the ingested dose [32]. Table 15.3 summarizes plasma concentrations during ingestion of CBS after 4 or more weeks of therapy [32, 33, 35–38].

A rapidly occurring peak in blood bismuth concentration is noted 15–60 minutes after a single oral dose of CBS. Peak values differ between different formulations. With chew "DeNol" tablets, values are less than $58\,\mu g\,l^{-1}$ [38], whereas with the "DeNol" swallow tablets the peak plasma concentrations range from 3 to $530\,\mu g\,l^{-1}$ [33]. These first dose differences between preparations are not evident with chronic dosing [32]. Figure 15.3 shows the first dose and 8-week dose pharmacokinetics after therapy with CBS swallow tablets in a single patient. Bismuth absorption with the swallow tablets is subject to high intra- and inter-individual variation. Considerable care should be taken in relating the chronic toxicity described for other bismuth compounds with the peak concentrations in blood and plasma shortly after ingestion of CBS.

Table 15.2 Postulated mechanisms of action of colloidal bismuth subcitrate

Action	Reference
Protect gastric mucosa	[14, 15]
Eradication of *H. pylori*	[8–13]
Binding ulcer base and mucus	[16–19]
Binds bile acids	[20]
Reduces pepsin output and activity	[21, 22]
Improves mucosal ultrastructure	[23, 24]
Increases endogenous prostaglandin and alkali secretion	[25]
Binding epidermal growth factor	[26]

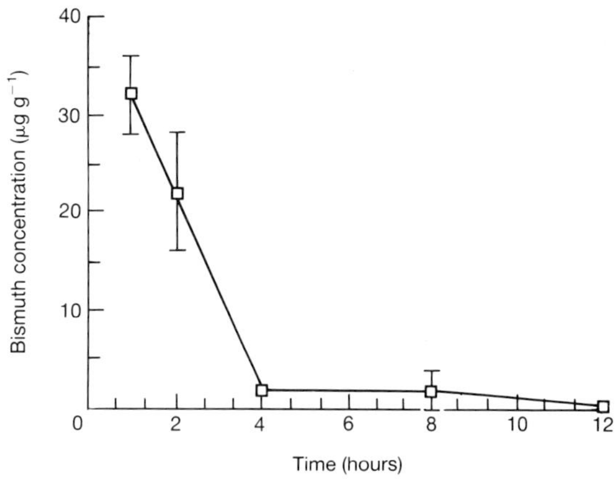

Fig. 15.2 Bismuth concentration in human antral gastric mucus after ingestion of "DeNol" at time 0 hours.

The large interindividual variation in bismuth absorption may be due to many factors, including differences in dissolution of tablets, gastric pH, gastrointestinal motility, and chemical form of bismuth [35, 39, 40].

Steady-state concentrations and bismuth clearance

Multiple-dosing studies with both CBS tablet preparations show an apparent steady state reached by 3–4 weeks [32, 35, 38]. Mean bismuth steady-state concentrations ranged from 3 to $58\,\mu g\,l^{-1}$ as shown in Table 15.3, following standard doses of CBS over 4–18 weeks.

Accumulation in plasma depends on the clearance of bismuth. The elimination half-life

Table 15.3 Plasma concentration after 4 or more weeks' therapy with colloidal bismuth subcitrate

Reference	No. of subjects	Therapy duration (weeks)	Formulation	Range peak plasma/blood* concentration ($\mu g\ l^{-1}$)	Range steady-state concentration ($\mu g\ l^{-1}$)
Lee [35]	24	4–6	Liquid	2–35	3–35
Hamilton *et al.* [36]	20	6	Chew tablet 4×1	Not reported	5–51
Dekker *et al.* [37]	76	4	Chew tablet 4×1	3–34*	Not reported
	67	4	Swallow (coated) 4×1	2–21*	Not reported
Froomes *et al.* [38]	12	6–8	Chew tablet 4×1	8–58	8–58
Gavey *et al.* [32]	9	6	Swallow (coated) 2×2	Not reported	4–38
Nwokolo *et al.* [33]	6	4–18	Swallow (coated) 2×2	3–530 (1st dose)	2–12

after steady state was reached was between 20 and 30 days for urine and plasma, for all CBS preparations studied [32, 38].

Elimination of bismuth from the body is via both the urine and fecal route, with the proportional contribution of each route yet to be determined in man. Bismuth present in feces after cessation of oral therapy is excreted partly via the bile and partly via intestinal secretion. Preliminary evidence has suggested an enterohepatic circulation of the bismuth pool [35, 41].

Studies have suggested a two- or three-compartment model to describe the elimination kinetics of bismuth from the blood in humans [42] and animal models [21, 43]. In a three-compartment model, as proposed by Hespe (personal communication), the first half-life ($t_{\frac{1}{2}}$ = 4 hours) accounts for 4.8% of the area under the curve (AUC); the second half-life ($t_{\frac{1}{2}}$ = 11 days) 67.9% of AUC; and the 72-day half-life 27.3%. The AUC is a measure of CBS bioavailability.

Distribution

In humans and animals receiving bismuth compounds, the highest concentration per gram net weight was always found in the kidney [44–47]. After 14 months of CBS administered to rats, the concentrations of bismuth in the organs,

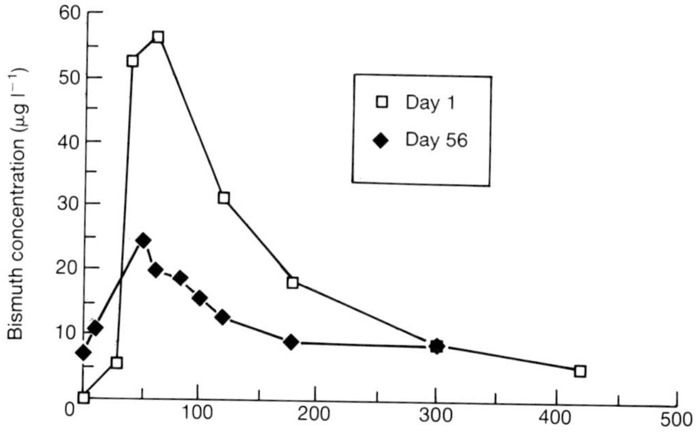

Fig. 15.3 Plasma bismuth concentrations vs time after initial (day 1) and final (day 56) stages of treatment with swallow "DeNol" tablets (2×420 mg day^{-1}). AUC (area under curve): day 1, 8033.2 µl minute^{-1}; day 56, 4033 µl minute^{-1}.

ranging from high to low, were: kidney, lung, spleen, brain (very low), and muscle (very low) [48]. Values ranged between 13.9 $\mu g\, g^{-1}$ net wt in kidney and 0.13 $\mu g\, g^{-1}$ in muscle.

The volume of distribution of bismuth from CBS in the body is unknown. Assuming clearance in the range of 50–85 ml $minute^{-1}$ and the predominant plasma half-life of 10 days, the volume of distribution can be estimated to range between 900 and 1250 l.

Toxicity in humans

Bismuth toxicity involving brain, kidneys, liver, and bones has been reported with most bismuth salts except for CBS and bismuth subsalicylate [27–31]. In subjects with encephalopathy, blood bismuth levels are usually more than 100 $\mu g\, l^{-1}$ with most having levels greater than 500 $\mu g\, l^{-1}$ at time of presentation [27, 49].

The Hillemand [50] safety levels of 50–100 $\mu g\, l^{-1}$, often quoted as warning levels of toxicity, are not justified on current knowledge. This range was based on earlier French studies, where the accuracy of analytical methods was uncertain and the sampling times of toxic subjects not specified.

As anticipated from the pharmacokinetics of CBS, there have been no reports of toxic effects in normal subjects taking therapeutic doses for recommended periods. The range of steady-state plasma bismuth concentrations are 1.5–5% of the concentrations reported from subjects with encephalopathy (see Table 15.3).

There is no basis for relating transient plasma peaks to clinical toxicity in general and neurologic toxicity in particular. Concern related to first-dose peaks [33] is not supported by any objective database. Calculations, using the Hespe model which assumes a constant occurrence of the peak, indicate that significant accumulation will not occur upon multiple dosing of the drug, as only some 5% of body load is involved in the peaking process.

Clinical use of CBS

In controlled clinical studies, CBS in liquid, tablet, and swallow (coated) preparations is effective in healing duodenal [1, 4–7] and gastric [1–3] ulcer disease, after 4 and 8 weeks of therapy when compared to placebo. In duodenal ulcer disease, comparison with cimetidine [51–53], ranitidine [54], and sucralfate [55] shows equal or improved healing rates with CBS after 8 weeks of therapy.

Non-ulcer dyspepsia

Non-ulcer dyspepsia (NUD) is defined as chronic (>4 weeks) upper abdominal or retrosternal pain, discomfort, heartburn, nausea, vomiting, or other symptoms referrable to the proximal alimentary tract, unrelated to exercise, for which no focal lesion or systemic disease can be identified [56]. Several recent reviews have highlighted problems with definition and etiology [57, 58]. The term "essential dyspepsia" has been suggested [57] to cover the group in whom all diseases, including irritable bowel syndrome, gastroesophageal reflux, aerophagy, and gallstones, have been excluded.

The prevalence of dyspepsia is between 20 and 30% [59], with NUD at least three times as common as peptic ulcer disease. Despite being a common disease, the precise etiology is unclear with many factors previously assessed, including heredity, environmental influences, hormonal changes, abnormal gastric acid secretion, psychological factors, and abnormal motility. No consistent abnormalities have been identified in this disorder. Moreover, no therapy has been universally effective. These have included antacids, H2 receptor antagonists, anticholinergics, and agents improving gastric motility [60–63].

The discovery of *H. pylori* has led to a re-emergence of interest in the pathogenesis and treatment of NUD. Between 50 and 70% of patients with NUD have *H. pylori*-associated gastritis [64–67]. Unfortunately, in most studies no significant differences in symptoms between *H. pylori*-positive (HP+) and -negative (HP−) subjects could be detected [67–69]. The symptoms were more severe in HP+ subjects in a study of 83 subjects with NUD [66].

Does *H. pylori* clearance or eradication result in symptomatic improvement? The results of studies currently available are summarized in Table 15.4, which suggests that symptomatic improvement occurs with eradication of *H. pylori* and resolution of the gastritis. Differ-

Table 15.4 Effect of *H. pylori* eradication on histologic gastritis and symptoms in non-ulcer dyspepsia

Therapy (dose, mg)	Duration (weeks)	No. of subjects	*H. pylori* clearance (%)	Histologic gastritis	Symptoms	Reference
Amoxicillin (120 q.i.d.)	4	22	68	Improved	Improved	[70]
Amoxicillin (1000 b.i.d.)	1	22	91	Improved	No change	[71]
Erythromycin (500 q.i.d.)	2	15	7	No change	No difference	[72]
Bismuth subsalicylate + metronidazole	3	10	—	—	No difference	[73]
CBS (120 q.i.d.) + amoxicillin (375 t.i.d.)	4	20	90	Improved	Improved	[70]
CBS (120 q.i.d.)	4	67	45	Improved	Improved	[70]
CBS (120 q.i.d.)	4	83	73	Improved	Improved	[69]
CBS (120 q.i.d.)	4	43	74	Improved	Improved	[74]
CBS (120 q.i.d.)	8	66	83	Improved	Improved	[75]
CBS (120 q.i.d.)	8	51	88	Improved	Improved	[76]

ences in methodology, duration and type of therapy, bacterial detection methods, and symptom assessment make interpretation of the findings of many studies difficult. Moreover, long-term bacterial eradication and symptoms were not assessed in most studies.

In the placebo-controlled trials, in which CBS was used for either 4 or 8 weeks treatment, histological assessment showed consistent improvement in gastritis, associated with eradication of *H. pylori* [12, 74–76]. Symptoms of abdominal pain were also significantly improved in these patients in all three studies, and in one study, post-prandial abdominal distension and nausea were also improved [74].

Despite the obvious limitations of most studies in evaluating the efficacy of CBS in the treatment of NUD, the therapy has been beneficial in the majority. Long-term follow-up of symptoms, antral histology, and *H. pylori* in subjects with essential NUD, following effective and specific therapy directed against *H. pylori*, will be necessary to confirm the role of this organism.

Conclusions

Colloidal bismuth subcitrate is an effective agent in healing gastric and duodenal ulcer disease. The low relapse of duodenal ulcer closely correlates with its ability to eradicate *H. pylori* and to improve the associated histologic gastroduodenitis. Despite limitations in definition, and problems in conducting controlled clinical trials in NUD subjects, the published data support the clinical efficacy of CBS in HP+ subjects with moderate to severe symptoms.

All currently available preparations of CBS are safe when used according to therapeutic guidelines. Based on the use of sensitive bismuth assays, the bioavailability of bismuth following oral intake of CBS ranges from 0.16 to 1.5% of the ingested dose. Clearance of bismuth is via the kidney and biliary systems, with a probable enterohepatic circulation. The apparent steady state is reached by 3–4 weeks, with mean bismuth steady-state concentrations in blood/plasma ranging from 2 to 58 $\mu g\,l^{-1}$.

Toxicity in humans with CBS has not been reported. This is not unexpected from what is known of the steady-state concentrations and current understanding of the pharmacokinetics. Previous concern over potential plasma peaks, following initial dosing with the swallow (coated) tablet, appears unwarranted when the relationship between initial peaks and steady-state dosing levels is considered (Table 15.3).

Further understanding of the local pharmacokinetics and modes of action of CBS in both ulcer healing and *H. pylori* eradication is necessary to optimize delivery of CBS into the gastroduodenal mucosa.

References

1 Lee, SP, & Nicholson, GI. Increased healing of gastric and duodenal ulcers in a controlled trial using tripotassium dicitrato-bismuthate. *Med. J. Aust.* 1977;**1**:808–12.

2 Glover, SC, Cantlay, JS, Weir, J, & Mowat, NAG. Oral tripotassium dicitrato-bismuthate in gastric and duodenal ulceration: a double-blind controlled trial. *Dig. Dis. Sci.* 1983;**28**:13–7.

3 Morales, A, Antezana, C, Roman, I, & Hurtado, C. Effecto de un derivado del bismuto (DeNol) en la cicatrizacion de ulceras gastricas y duodenales. *Revista Medica de Chile* 1982;**110**:959–63.

4 Coughlin, GP, Kupa, A, & Alp, MH. The effect of tripotassium dicitrato-bismuthate (DeNol) on the healing of chronic duodenal ulcers. *Med J Aust.* 1977;**1**:294–8.

5 Vissoulis, C, Vissoulis, G, Golfis, G, & Psimenos, G. Endoscopic evaluation of TDB in the treatment of duodenal ulcer. *Iatrica Chronica* 1977;**17**: 157–64.

6 Shreeve, DR. A double-blind study of tripotassium dicitrato-bismuthate in duodenal ulcer. *Postgrad. Med. J.* 1975;**51**(suppl 5):33–6.

7 Wilson, P, & Alp, MH. Colloidal bismuth subcitrate tablets and placebo in chronic duodenal ulceration: a double-blind, randomised trial. *Med. J. Aust.* 1982;**1**:222–3.

8 Marshall, BJ, Goodwin, CS, Warren, JR, Murray, R, Blincow, ED, Blackbourn, SJ, Phillips, M, Waters, TE, & Sanderson, CR. Prospective double-blind trial of duodenal ulcer relapse after eradication of *Campylobacter pylori. Lancet* 1988;**ii**:1437–42.

9 Coghlan, JG, Gilligan, D, & Humphries, H. *Campylobacter pylori* and recurrence of duodenal ulcers — a 12-month follow-up study. *Lancet* 1987;**ii**:1109–11.

10 Lambert, JR, Borromeo, M, Korman, MG, Hansky, J, & Eaves, ER. Effect of colloidal bismuth (DeNol) on healing and relapse of duodenal ulcers — role of *Campylobacter pyloridis. Gastroenterology* 1987; **2**:1489.

11 Borody, TJ, Cole, P, Noonans, S, *et al.* Recurrence of duodenal ulcer and *Campylobacter pylori* after eradication. *Med. J. Aust.* 1989;**151**:431–4.

12 Rauws, EAJ, Langenberg, W, Houthoff, HJ, Zanen, HC, & Tytgat, GNJ. *Campylobacter pyloridis*-associated chronic active antral gastritis: a prospective study of its prevalence and the effects of antibacterial and antiulcer treatment. *Gastroenterology* 1988;**94**:229–38.

13 Lambert, JR, Dunn, KL, Turner, H, & Korman, MG. Effect on histological gastritis following eradication of *Campylobacter pyloridis. Gastroenterology* 1986;**90**:1509.

14 Hall, DWR, & van den Hoven, WE. Gastric mucosa protective effects of colloidal bismuth subcitrate (DeNol). *Int. J. Tissue Reactions* 1987; **9**:427–32.

15 Konturek, SJ, Radecki, T, Piastucki, I, & Drozdowicz, D. Advances in the understanding of the mechanism of cytoprotective action by colloidal bismuth subcitrate. *Scand. J. Gastroenterol.* 1986;**21**(suppl 122):6–10.

16 Koo, J, Ho, J, Lam, SK, Wong, J, & Ong, GB. Selective coating of gastric ulcer by tripotassium dicitrato-bismuthate in the rat. *Gastroenterology* 1982;**82**:864–70.

17 Lee, SP. A potential mechanism of action of colloidal bismuth subcitrate; diffusion barrier to hydrochloric acid. *Scand. J. Gastroenterol.* 1982; **17**(suppl 80):17–21.

18 Tasman-Jones, C, Maher, C, Thomsen, L, Lee, SP, & Vanderwee, M. Mucosal defences and gastroduodenal disease. *Digestion* 1987;**37**(suppl 2):1–7.

19 Lambert, JR, Way, DJ, King, RG, Eaves, ER, Liancas, K, & Wan, A. DeNol vs Pepto-Bismol bismuth pharmacokinetics in human gastric mucosa. *Gastroenterology* 1989;**96**:A284.

20 Stiel, D, & Peters, TJ. Tripotassium dicitrato-bismuthate (DeNol) binds conjugated bile acids *in vitro* — a possible mechanism in gastric ulcer healing. *Proc. Aust. Soc. Med. Res.* 1983;**16**:18.

21 Roberts, NB, & Taylor, WH. The effect of tripotassium dicitrato-bismuthate (DeNol) upon the individual human pepsins. *Scand. J. Gastroenterol.* 1982;**17**(suppl 78):114.

22 Baron, JH, Barr, J, Batten, J, Sidebotham, R, & Spencer, J. Acid, pepsin, and mucus secretion in patients with gastric and duodenal ulcer before and after colloidal bismuth subcitrate (DeNol). *Gut* 1986;**27**:486–90.

23 Moshal, MG, Gregory, MA, Pillay, C, & Spitaels, JM. Does the duodenal cell ever return to normal? A comparison between treatment with cimetidine and DeNol. *Scand. J. Gastroenterol.* 1979;**14**(suppl 54):48–51.

24 Gregory, MA, Moshal, MG, & Spitaels, JM. The effect of tripotassium dicitrato-bismuthate on the duodenal mucosa during ulceration; an ultrastructural study. *S. Afr. Med. J.* 1982;**62**:52–5.

25 Konturek, SJ, Bilski, J, Kwiecien, N, *et al.* DeNol stimulates gastric and duodenal alkaline secretion through prostaglandin dependent mechanism. *Gut* 1987;**28**:1557–63.

26 Slomiany, BL, Bilski, J, Sarosiek, J, Liau, YH, &

Slomianyu, A. Colloidal bismuth subcitrate inhibits peptic degradation of epidermal growth factor. *Gastroenterology* 1988;**94**:A431.
27 Buge, A, Supino-Viterbo, V, Rancurel, G, H *et al.* Correlations evolutives: cliniques electroencephalographiques, tomodensitometriques et toxicologiques, dans cinq cas d'encephalopathies bismuthiques. *Sem. Hop. Paris* 1979;**55**:1466–72.
28 Burns, RJ, Thomas, DW, & Barron, VJ. Reversible encephalopathy possibly associated with bismuth subgallate ingestion. *Br. Med. J.* 1974;**1**:220–3.
29 Guard, O, Soichot, P, Dumas, R, Besancenot, J-B, & Gaudet, M. Reflexions à propos de dix observations d'encephalopathie bismuthique. *J. Med. Lyon* 1977;**58**:403–16.
30 Randall, RE, Osherhoff, RJ, Bakerman, S, & Setter, JG. Bismuth nephrotoxicity. *Ann. Int. Med.* 1972; 77:481–2.
31 Slikkerveet, A, & de Wolff, FA. Pharmacokinetics and toxicity of bismuth compounds. *Med. Toxicol. Adv. Drug Exp.* 1989;**4**:303–23.
32 Gavey, CJ, Szeto, M-L, Nwokolo, CU, Sercombe, J, & Pounder, RE. Bismuth accumulates in the body during treatment with tripotassium dicitratobismuthate. *Aliment. Pharm. Therap.* 1989; **3**: 21–8.
33 Nwokolo, CU, Gavey, CJ, Smith, JTL, & Pounder, RE. The absorption of bismuth from oral doses of tripotassium dicitrato-bismuthate. *Aliment. Pharm. Therap.* 1989;**3**:29–39.
34 Goodwin, CS, Blake, PK, & Blincow, ED. The minimum and bactericidal concentrations of antibiotics and antiulcer agents against *Campylobacter pyloridis. Chemotherapy* 1989; **17**:309–14.
35 Lee, SP. Studies on the absorption and excretion of tripotassium dicitrato-bismuthate in man. *Res. Commun. Chem. Path. Pharm.* 1981;**34**:359–64.
36 Hamilton, I, Worsley, BW, O'Connor, HJ, & Axon, ATR. Effects of tripotassium dicitrato-bismuthate (TDB) tablets or cimetidine in the treatment of duodenal ulcer. *Gut* 1983;**24**:1148–51.
37 Dekker, W, Dal Monte, PR, Bianchi Porro, G, *et al.* An international multi-clinic study comparing the therapeutic efficacy of colloidal bismuth subcitrate coated tablets with chewing tablets in the treatment of duodenal ulceration. *Scand. J. Gastroenterol.* 1986;**21**(suppl 122):46–50.
38 Froomes, PRA, Wan, AT, Keech, AC, McNeil, JJ, & McLean, AJ. Absorption and elimination of bismuth from oral doses of tripotassium dicitratobismuthate. *Eur. J. Clin. Pharm.* 1989; **37**:533–6.
39 Conso, F, Bourdon, R, & Gaultier, M. Bismuth sanguin et urinaire après traitement bref par differents sels "insolubles" de bismuth. *Eur. J. Toxicol.* 1975;**8**:137–41.
40 Hespe, W, Staal, HJM, & Hall, DWR. Bismuth absorption from the colloidal subcitrate. *Lancet* 1988;**ii**:1258.
41 McLean, AJ, Islam, S, & Lambert, JR. Anomalous short plasma elimination half life in a patient intoxicated with bismuth citrate. *Gut* 1990;**31**: 1086.
42 De Bray, J-M, Emile, J, Moreau, R, *et al.* Pathogenie des encephalopathies bismuthiques: étude preliminaire a l'aide du ^{206}bismuth chez l'homme. *Nouv. Press. Med.* 1977;**6**:1394.
43 Vienet, R, Bouvet, P, & Istin, M. Cinetique et distribution du ^{206}Bi chez le rat et le lapin: un modele. *Int. J. Appl. Rad. Isot.* 1983;**34**:747–53.
44 Russ, GA, Bigler, RE, Tilbury, RS, Woodard, HQ, & Laughlin, JS. Metabolic studies with radiobismuth. I:Retention and distribution of ^{206}Bi in the normal rat. *Rad. Res.* 1975;**63**:443–54.
45 Hall, RJ, & Farber, T. Drug residues in animal tissues: determination of bismuth in body tissues and fluids after administration of controlled doses. *J. Assoc. Anal. Chem.* 1972;**55**:639–42.
46 Hursh, JB, & Brown, C. Tissue distribution of ^{212}Bi in rats. *Proc. Soc. Exp. Biol. Med.* 1969;**131**: 116–20.
47 Sollman, T, Cole, HN, & Henderson, K. Clinical excretion of bismuth. VII: The autopsy distribution of bismuth in patients after clinical bismuth treatment. *Am. J. Syphilis Gonor. Vener. Dis.* 1938;**22**:555–83.
48 Lee, SP, Lim, TH, Pybus, J, & Clarke, AC. Tissue distribution of orally administered bismuth in the rat. *Clin. Exp. Pharm. Physiol.* 1980;**7**: 319–24.
49 Bes, A, Caussanel, JP, Geraud, G, Jauzac, PH, & Geraud, J. Encephalopathie toxique par les sels de bismuth. *Rev. Med. Toulouse* 1976;**12**:801–13.
50 Hillemand, P, Palliere, M, Laquais, B, & Bouvet, P. Traitement bismuthique et bismuthemie. *Sem. Hop. Paris.* 1977;**53**:1663–9.
51 Martin, DF, Hollanders, D, May, SJ, *et al.* Difference in relapse rates of duodenal ulcer after healing with cimetidine or tripotassium dicitratobismuthate. *Lancet* 1981;**i**:7–10.
52 Moshal, MG, Spitaels, JM, & Khan, F. Tripotassium dicitrato-bismuthate chewing tablets and cimetidine tablets in the treatment of duodenal ulcers: a double-blind double-dummy comparative study. *S. Afr. Med. J.* 1981;**60**:420–3.
53 Kang, JY, & Piper, DW. Cimetidine and colloidal bismuth in treatment of chronic duodenal ulcer: comparison of initial healing and recurrence after healing. *Digestion* 1982;**23**:73–9.
54 Parente, F, Lazzaroni, M, Petrillo, M, & Bianchi Porro, G. Colloidal bismuth subcitrate and ranitidine in the short-term treatment of benign gastric ulcer: an endoscopically controlled trial. *Scand. J. Gastroenterol.* 1986;**21**(suppl 122): 42–5.
55 Dang, ZD, Wang, KT, Tao, JY, Zhu, LF, & Hu, XE. A clinical trial comparing colloidal bismuth subcitrate (DeNol liquid) with sucralfate in the treatment of peptic ulceration. *Clin. Trials J.*

1986;**23**:235–41.
56 Colin Jones, DG. Management of dyspepsia: report of a working party. *Lancet* 1988;**i**:576–9.
57 Talley, NJ, & Phillips, SF. Non-ulcer dyspepsia: potential causes and pathophysiology. *Ann. Int. Med.* 1988;**108**:865–79.
58 Heatley, RV, & Rathbone, BJ. Dyspepsia: a dilemma for doctors. *Lancet* 1987;**ii**:779–81.
59 Tibblin, G. Introduction to the epidemiology of dyspepsia. *Scand. J. Gastroenterol.* 1985;**109**: 29–33.
60 Nyren, O, Adami, HO, Bates, S, *et al.* Absence of therapeutic benefit from antacids or cimetidine in non-ulcer dyspepsia. *N. Engl. J. Med.* 1986; **314**:339–43.
61 Johnson, AG. Controlled trial of metoclopramide in the treatment of flatulent dyspepsia. *Br. Med. J.* 1971;**2**:25–6.
62 Nagler, J, & Miskovitz, P. Clinical evaluation of domperidone in the treatment of chronic postprandial idiopathic upper gastrointestinal distress. *Am. J. Gastroenterol.* 1981;**76**:495–9.
63 Rosch, W. Cisapride in non-ulcer dyspepsia. Results of a placebo-controlled trial. *Scand. J. Gastroenterol* 1987;**22**:161–4.
64 Wyatt, JI, Rathbone, BJ, Heatley, RV, & Losowsky, MS. *Campylobacter pylori* and the History of dyspepsia in healthy blood donors. *Gut* 1988;**29**: A706–7.
65 Marshall, BJ. Nervous dyspepsia (letter). *Med. J. Aust.* 1985;**142**:704.
66 Lambert, JR, Dunn, K, Borromeo, M, Korman, MG, & Hansky, J. *Campylobacter pylori* — a role in non-ulcer dyspepsia? *Scand. J. Gastroenterol.* 1989;**24**:7–13.
67 Anderson, LP, Elsborg, L, & Justesen, T. *Campylobacter pylori* in peptic ulcer disease. III: Symptoms and paraclinical and epidemiological findings. *Scand. J. Gastroenterol.* 1988;**23**: 347–50.
68 Jeena, CP, Simjee, KE, Pettengell, JM, *et al.* Comparison of symptoms in *Campylobacter pylori*-positive and -negative patients presenting with dyspepsia for upper gastrointestinal endoscopy. *Afr. Med. J.* 1988;**73**:659.
69 Borsch, G, Wegener, M, & Reitemeyer, E. Clinical and histologic factors associated with *Campylobacter pylori* colonisation. *Proc. Eur. Assoc. Gastroenterol. Endosc.* **1988**;A23.
70 Rauws, EAJ, Langenberg, W, Houthoff, HJ, Zanen, HC, & Tytgat, GNJ. *Campylobacter pyloridis*-associated chronic active antral gastritis. A prospective study of its prevalence and the effects of antibacterial and antiulcer treatment. *Gastroenterology* 1988;**94**:33–40.
71 Glupczynski, Y, Burette, A, Labbe, M, Deprez, C, De Reuck, M, & Deltenre, M. *Campylobacter pylori*-associated gastritis: a double-blind placebo-controlled trial with amoxycillin. *Am. J. Gastroenterol.* 1988;**84**(4):365–73.
72 McNulty, CAM, Gearty, JC, Crump, B, *et al.* *Campylobacter pyloridis* and associated gastritis: investigator-blind, placebo-controlled trial of bismuth salicylate and erythromycin ethylsuccinate. *Br. Med. J.* 1986;**293**:645–9.
73 Murphy, R, Behler, EM, Appleman, HD, Barnett, JL, & Elta, GH. Four-year follow-up of gastroduodenitis and its association with *Campylobacter pylori. Gastroenterology* 1988;**94**(2):A317.
74 Borody, T, Hennessy, W, Daskolopoulos, G, *et al.* Double-blind trial of DeNol in non-ulcer dyspepsia associated with *Campylobacter pyloridis* gastritis. *Gastroenterology* 1987;**92**: 1324.
75 Rokkas, T, Pursey, C, Uzoechina, E, *et al.* Non-ulcer dyspepsia and short term DeNol therapy: a placebo-controlled trial with particular reference to the role of *Campylobacter pylori. Gut* 1988;**29**: 1386–91.
76 Kang, JY, Tay, HH, Wee, A, Guan, R, Math, MV, & Yap, I. The effect of colloidal bismuth subcitrate on symptoms and gastric histology in non-ulcer dyspepsia — a double blind placebo-controlled study (abstract). *Gut* 1988;**29**:1440.

16: Pediatric Helicobacter pylori infection

S. CADRANEL

Introduction

Since the original report [1] in 1983 of the presence of curved S-shaped Gram-negative microorganisms in the antral mucosa of adults, the association of *Helicobacter pylori* with peptic ulcers is well documented. Its association with histologic evidence of gastritis has been widely reported in adults and, subsequently, a great interest has arisen in the study of *H. pylori* (its detection, characteristics, treatments aimed at its eradication, epidemiology, etc.) among gastroenterologists, microbiologists, pathologists, immunologists, and epidemiologists.

More recently, in 1986, the first cases of *H. pylori* infection in children were published [2, 3] and were followed by other reports from several authors [4–6], stressing the similitude of findings in pediatric and adult patients. Secondary ulcers are not uncommon in children, whereas primary ulcers are infrequent [7]; on the other hand, in this age group, secondary gastritis, due to a known precipitating cause, is often clinically diagnosed but rarely fully documented, whereas primary gastritis is most often underdiagnosed.

The availability of adapted miniaturized endoscopes has led pediatric gastroenterologists to give more attention to the possibility of gastric lesions in children complaining of chronic abdominal pain, a very common complaint in childhood [8]. More and more pediatricians are becoming aware of the possible role of chronic gastritis as a cause of recurrent abdominal pain and, in consequence, of the possible role of *H. pylori* in childhood. Information is now gathering about the incidence of *H. pylori* in the pediatric population in various parts of the world.

Since children are seldom exposed to the harmful effects of alcohol, tobacco, or other aggressive factors commonly encountered in adult life, the occurrence of *H. pylori* infection in childhood might help to understand better the role of this microorganism as a pathogen in the gastric mucosa. Although many questions remain unsolved concerning the sources and routes of contamination, the study of *H. pylori* infection in children gives an opportunity to understand better the natural history of this infection, and its role in the development and persistence of gastric lesions and disease in the child himself, but also in his family and environment, in relation with such important factors as social and ethnic backgrounds, and general hygiene.

Clinical features

Symptoms

As with adults, a strong correlation between primary ulcer or gastritis and the presence of *H. pylori* in (or on) the antral mucosa has also been found in the first reports of *H. pylori* infection in children [2–5]. *H. pylori* seems to be associated with mucosal lesions in the child in the same fashion that it is in the adult. However, indications for endoscopy are not as frequent in children as in adults.

As chronic recurrent abdominal pain is a very frequent complaint among children, the cause is thought, in the overwhelming majority of cases, to be "functional," and further endoscopic investigation is either not considered or replaced by the more usual barium meal. For this reason, it might be difficult to evaluate the true incidence of symptoms related to *H. pylori* infection in childhood. However, when these symptoms are spectacular (such as hematemesis or melena), or when their characteristics point clearly towards the epigastric region, or when they are somehow related to meals, indication for an endoscopy is becoming popular among pediatricians, and therefore more and more cases of *H. pylori*-associated gastritis and ulcers are being reported in small series from various centers in Italy [9], Poland [10], United Kingdom [11], and Spain [12].

In a recent workshop on *H. pylori* infections in children, held in Budapest by the European Society for Paediatric Gastroenterology and Nutrition, pediatric cases have been reported to us from centers in Belgium, France, Spain, Italy, Greece, Yugoslavia, Israel, and Japan [13]. Four larger series have been reported in the literature, from Canada [14], Belgium [15], England [16], and Italy [17], in which the authors have conducted prospective systematic detections of *H. pylori* in all children undergoing upper gastrointestinal endoscopy or analyzed the data retrospectively. The clinical features of these four series are summarized in Table 16.1. It is difficult to make a comparison between them because the indications may vary according to local medical attitudes. On the other hand, the authors usually give far more detail on the clinical presentation of children positive for *H. pylori* (HP+) compared to the *H. pylori*-negative (HP−) ones included in their endoscopic series; there is not a clear-cut separation between indications for endoscopy, symptoms, and findings. However, epigastric pain seems to be one of the most frequent clinical symptoms found in 38–78% of the HP+ patients according to the series.

Many questions remain unsolved:

1 How often is epigastric pain present in HP− children?

An interesting clue is given by Mahony *et al.* [16] who carried out a retrospective study of the biopsy material of 38 out of 111 children undergoing upper gastrointestinal endoscopy, and showed that seven out of 10 children com-

Table 16.1 Symptoms in children with *H. pylori* infection

	Drumm *et al.* [5]	Cadranel *et al.* [15]	Mahony *et al.* [16]	Oderda *et al.* [17]
No. of patients	71	114	111	42
Data available	67	114	38	42
Type of study	Prospective, unselected		Retrospective, unselected	Prospective, selected
Indications for endoscopy				
Recurrent abdominal pain	39	26	19	15
Vomiting and gastroesophageal reflux	23	27	16	—
Hematemesis, anemia, or occult blood	18	—	2	—
History of peptic disease	—	11	—	18
History of esophagitis	—	9	—	9
Dysphagia	—	7	1	—
Crohn's disease	7	3	—	—
Varia	—	31	—	—
Symptoms in HP+				
No. of patients	12	43	9	42
Epigastric pain	7	19	7	16
Vomiting	—	7	1	7
Nausea or dysphagia	—	5	—	2
Anorexia	—	—	—	1
Hematemesis (or anemia)	—	2	1	1
Peptic disease (or follow up)	5	3	—	—
Asymptomatic	?	7	?	?

plaining of epigastric pain harbored *H. pylori* in the antrum; on the contrary, not one of the 13 complaining of periumbilical pain was infected with *H. pylori*.

2 Is the pain typical?

In our experience the symptoms do not differ very much from those reported in adults, except that pain is perhaps less severe and more vague. However, epigastric pain is the most common feature, usually immediately after the meal and sometimes severe enough to reduce the food intake. Nocturnal pain is found in seven out of 10 patients in the Drumm *et al.* series [18], and tends to be more severe in those with ulcers than in those with gastritis: six out of the 10 patients with duodenal ulcers in the same series had a symptom score of 4, whereas none with gastritis alone reached that score. However, one must be aware that pain is an essentially subjective symptom, especially in children and adolescents.

In our experience, belching is not often present, while abdominal distension is a very frequent symptom, sometimes lasting until the next meal. Tenderness of the epigastric region is present in more than 80% of our 103 patients with antral *H. pylori* infection. Nausea and heartburn have been reported by all the authors previously mentioned, but are difficult to evaluate; they do not seem to be frequent in our series, while bad breath is very common. More than half of our patients with gastritis did not eat breakfast, and experienced pain and abdominal distension only with their first meal later in the course of the day. Post-prandial symptoms are the first to be alleviated, about 7 days after initiation of treatment. As many of our patients are Muslims, it is interesting to discover that symptoms are not aggravated during the month of their ritual day-fasting (Ramadan).

3 How many HP+ children are still asymptomatic?

The prevalence of *H. pylori* in healthy individuals is uncertain because most investigators have evaluated tissue obtained from symptomatic patients. In the three series reporting *H. pylori* infection in healthy volunteers, the Amsterdam group [19] found *H. pylori* infection in six out of 25 (24%) young medical students with a mean age of 27 years; Barthel *et al.* [20] in four out of 20 (25%) members of a medical staff with a mean age of 30 years; and Peterson *et al.* [21] in nine out of 23 (39%) volunteers at Dallas Veterans Administration Medical Center. What happens in children? Little is known about the possibility of asymptomatic infection in children. Some information has been given by epidemiologic studies, but usually this emerges from serologic mass screening, and clinical features are seldom reported.

Some interesting information can be drawn from children undergoing frequent endoscopic follow-up investigations. In our unit, nine children have been endoscoped repeatedly for monitoring of sequelae of caustic ingestion at the ages of 2–4 years, and data are available over a period of 3–12 years: seven are HP+ and two HP−. None of the seven HP+ children has severe complaints, although three of them have occasional dysphagia and sensation of abdominal distension, unrelated to the esophageal dysmotility. When did these children acquire their *H. pylori* infection? And how? Is the frequent contact with contaminated instruments — probably not the endoscopes — responsible for it? On the other hand most of these children have HP+ parents (see section on Epidemiology, below), who may be the source of contamination.

The further observation of the modification of the gastric mucosa in these patients might be interesting in order to understand the natural evolution of this infection in children. Indeed, asymptomatic or pauci-symptomatic children are rarely investigated endoscopically, except for very young infants with gastroesophageal reflux, who are very seldom HP+ (see section on Age, below), and do not require repeated long-term follow-up. Another interesting group is formed by nine children with celiac disease: only three of them are HP+, this finding being probably more related to ethnic origin than to the underlying disease.

4 Are there other clinical features associated with *H. pylori* infection in children?

Hill *et al.* [22] reported three children from South Africa aged respectively 2, 3, and 4 years, with a history of acute-onset protein-losing enteropathy due to gastritis. In these three cases, *H. pylori* was identified in the gastric mucosa and cultured in two of them; healing of the protein-losing enteropathy, which occurred rapidly in the two cases treated with erythromycin, and within 2 months in the third case not treated with antibiotics, coincided with the disappearance of *H. pylori* from the stomach. To our knowledge, these are the first cases of protein-losing enteropathy in children in which *H. pylori* is also present. However, a direct responsibility of *H. pylori* in the pathogenesis of protein-losing enteropathy in these children is not proved, since the incidence of *H. pylori* infection in this age group might be very high in developing countries, as reported from other parts of Africa and South America (see section on Epidemiology, below): they might have had a previous *H. pylori* infection and developed protein-losing enteropathy following another aggressive agent, or as a consequence of malnutrition. On the other hand, if erythromycin is not effective *in vivo*, then *H. pylori* was cleared spontaneously and these patients have had acute gastritis related to *H. pylori*.

In a similar case of protein-losing enteropathy due to acute gastritis, observed in our department in a 9-month-old caucasian girl, *H. pylori* was not identified; both gastritis and protein-losing enteropathy cured spontaneously in 4 weeks. Further reports of acute *H. pylori* infections in young infants from developing countries could be particularly helpful in understanding the pathogenicity of *H. pylori*.

Age

The various larger prospective series generally include children ranging in age from less than 1 year to adolescence. These limits may vary largely from one country to the other, since some pediatric centers accept only infants and schoolchildren, whereas others also include adolescents and, in some cases, young adults with chronic diseases followed up since their childhood, for such diseases as cystic fibrosis, diabetes, or thalassemia.

In our series, the HP+ patients range from 2 to 16 years, with nine extra older patients included because they were still followed up for chronic diseases initiated in infancy (Table 16.2). The most numerous are to be found in the 9–16 years age group, although as many as 14 children under the age of 5 years were HP+. The youngest child in our series is a Moroccan infant aged 4 months with a severe esophagitis with hiatal hernia, in whom a Nissen fundoplication was performed. We do not know yet if he is still HP+. Another very young Belgian child was 2 years and 3 months old when *H. pylori* gastritis was diagnosed; however, this child already had the same symptoms of colicky pain and poor appetite since age 8 months, which was attributed to cow's milk allergy. A family history of peptic ulcers was present in both children.

Table 16.2 Age of *H. pylori*-positive (HP+) children

Age (years)	0–5*	6–10	10–16	>16
No. of patients	14*	27	52	9

* <1 year, $n = 1$; <2 years, $n = 2$; <3 years, $n = 3$; <4 years, $n = 7$; <5 years, $n = 2$.

The ages of children investigated endoscopically, and a comparison of HP+ children with HP− ones, were published previously [15], and are given in Fig. 16.1.

Ethnic origins

The large Turin series [17] is composed of Italians, probably from South Italy and Sicily because of the large immigration from these regions to this industrial city. No information is given about ethnic origin in the Toronto series [5]. We know that most children included in the northern England series [16] are from British origin, although some of them are from Indian and Caribbean immigrant parents. It is noteworthy to point out that *H. pylori* infection is rare in children from southern England and London, where numerous Indians and Pakistanis are settled (J.A. Walker-Smith, personal communication).

The ethnic origin of the patients in our own series [15] is given in Table 16.3. More than half of our HP+ children are of Moroccan origin, and the incidence of *H. pylori* infection was as high as 57% in Moroccan children investigated. The same proportion is found in children from Turkish and Yugoslavian origins. These are children from low social class background and their parents are first-generation immigrants. The Bantu children, on the contrary, come from

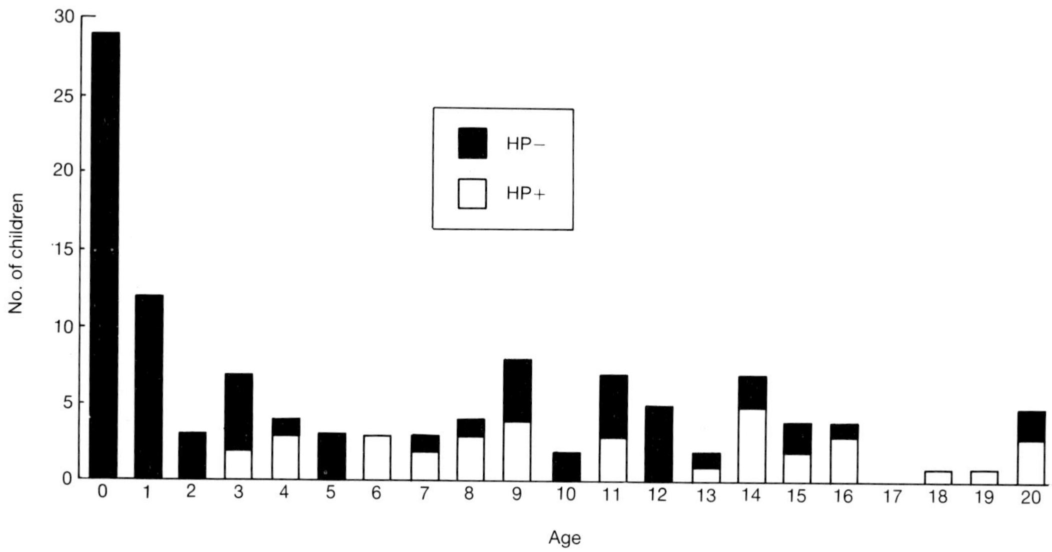

Fig. 16.1 Distribution of the patients according to the age. $n = 114$; HP+, 36; HP−, 78.

a different social environment, their parents being usually Zairese students, fellows of different Belgian universities. However, the incidence of *H. pylori* infection also seems to be very high in this population. Therefore, there is a high incidence of 58% of *H. pylori* infection in symptomatic children living in Belgium, and whose parents come from three different regions of the world, contrasting with an incidence of only 24% in symptomatic children of western European parents.

Endoscopic findings

Ulcers

Primary ulcers are far less frequent in childhood than in adulthood; however, the long-term prognosis for patients with peptic ulcers beginning in their teens is not favorable, and progression towards chronic relapsing peptic disease in adulthood is noted in a large proportion of them [23]. The same association between primary ulcers and *H. pylori* occurs in children as in adults, as reported by Drumm *et al.* [18] in 10 out of 10 cases, by Mahony *et al.* [16] in two out of two cases, by Socha *et al.* [10] in six out of eight children, and by Oderda *et al.* [17] in 18 out of 18 cases. Little is said about the clinical presentation of these patients.

In our own series, during the last 4 years, seven teenagers (six boys and one girl) aged 11–19 years, were diagnosed with a duodenal ulcer (in five cases with gastric ulcerations as well), and all of them had HP+ culture of antral, fundic, and in five cases duodenal, biopsies. Furthermore, eight further children (four boys and four girls), aged 4–18 years, investigated previously for *H. pylori*-associated gastritis, developed small shallow ulcerations in the antrum or the duodenal bulb: in all cases *H. pylori* was cultured from antral biopsies. The clinical symptoms in children with peptic ulcer do not differ from their presentation in the adult. Three main symptoms are prominent: bleeding, vomiting and, most frequently, epigastric pain. In their 1986 series, Czinn *et al.* [4] report five children with HP+ cultures: three of them presented with pain while the two others had hematemesis as chief symptom; four of them had a gastric or duodenal ulcer and all of them had gastritis.

Thus, it seems that, although relatively rare in childhood, primary ulcers are also associated with the presence of *H. pylori*. Does the microorganism colonize the gastric mucosa because of the ulceration or is it, at least partly, responsible for the lesion? Authors of pediatric series have not speculated on this question; however, the finding of small ulcerations in eight of our children who were known to already have an *H.*

Table 16.3 Ethnic origins of *H. pylori*-positive (HP+) children

Origin	No. HP+	No. receiving endoscopy	HP+ (%)
Moroccan	57	100	57
Belgian	23		
Italian	2	191	14
Portuguese	2		
Turkish	8	17	58
Yugoslavian	2		
Latin American	1	1	/
Bantu	7	12	58
Total	102	321	

pylori-associated gastritis is of interest, and supports the second hypothesis.

Micronodular gastritis

In all the pediatric series already mentioned, ulcers are less frequent than gastritis, which is documented by histologic studies. Is there a particular endoscopic pattern predictive of *H. pylori* infection? While Hill *et al.* [2] report mainly ulcerations in their six HP+ children, our first report in 1986 [3] insisted on a micronodular aspect of the antrum in six HP+ patients and three HP− ones. This endoscopic aspect is referred to as "lymphoid nodular hyperplasia" in three out of six childen with active gastritis from northern England [24]; or as "nodular antral gastritis" or "antral nodularity" in four out of five children from Cleveland [4]; or as "nodular antritis" in 23 out of 42 patients from Turin [17]; or as "antral micronodular pattern" in 19 out of 36 children from Brussels [15]. It is noteworthy that only two children of the latter series presenting with this particular pattern had an HP− culture of the biopsy of the antral mucosa.

All these reports strongly support the observation that this endoscopic finding is very frequently, if not always, associated with the presence of *H. pylori* in the antrum, as suggested by Oderda *et al.* [25]. In an abstract submitted (but not accepted) to the 1979 meeting of the European Society for Paediatric Gastroenterology and Nutritian (ESPGAN) in London, we had identified such an endoscopic lesion, described as "pseudopolypoid antral gastritis" in 20 children aged 6–15 years; surprisingly, there were 15 girls and five boys; elevated values of fasting gastrinemia were found in two cases, and low values of maximal acid output following pentagastrin stimulation occurred in three out of 11 [26].

A similar description of "granular antral aspect" has been given in the Spanish literature in 1978 by Beltran *et al.* [27], who also found decreased maximal acid output in some cases. In their series as well as in ours, this endoscopic feature was often associated with abdominal or, more specifically, epigastric pain.

In describing this endoscopic finding, one should avoid reference to histologic features such as "lymphoid hyperplasia" or to pathologic lesions such as the redundant "pseudopolypoid" or "polypoid."

How "micro" is the nodularity of the antrum in these cases? In double-contrast barium X-ray studies (Fig. 16.2), the nodularity is clearly shown and corresponds to elevations of the mucosa in the antral region. Endoscopically they appear, even when the antrum is fully insufflated, as clearly distinguishable irregularities of the mucosal surface ranging from 0.5 to 2 mm wide (Fig. 16.3), sometimes without any other sign of inflammation, but more often associated with erythema or, in some cases, with small erosions (Fig. 16.4).

The lesions are usually found in the antrum, and are better seen with a reduced intensity of the endoscope light and a tangent incidence of the beam. Occasionally, these lesions may also involve the body of the stomach; in our experience, this fundic involvement is rare and usually the lesions are restricted to the antrum, even in cases with severe inflammation. How-

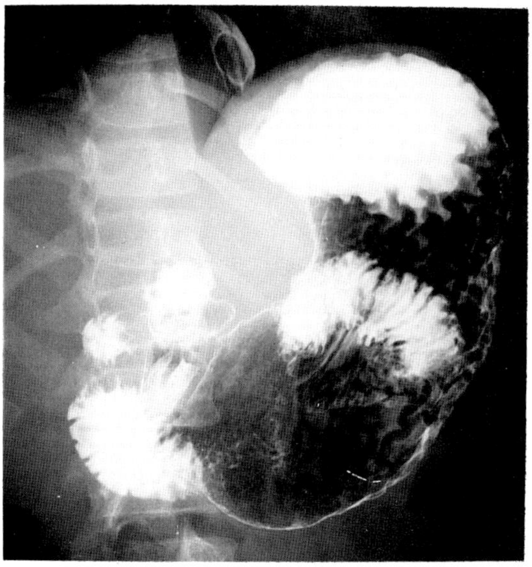

Fig. 16.2 A double-contrast barium meal, given in 1977, showing the granular aspect of the antral region of a 10-year-old boy.

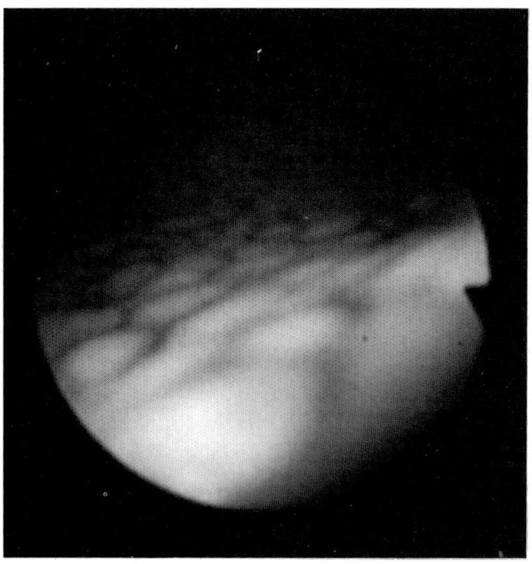

Fig. 16.3 Endoscopic aspect of the antrum in a 14-year-old boy with a relapsing duodenal ulcer and an *H. pylori*-associated chronic gastritis: the relief is finely micronodular.

ever, Hill *et al.* [22] report a severe acute gastritis predominantly affecting the body of the stomach in the three children in his study with protein-losing enteropathy. De Giacomo *et al.*

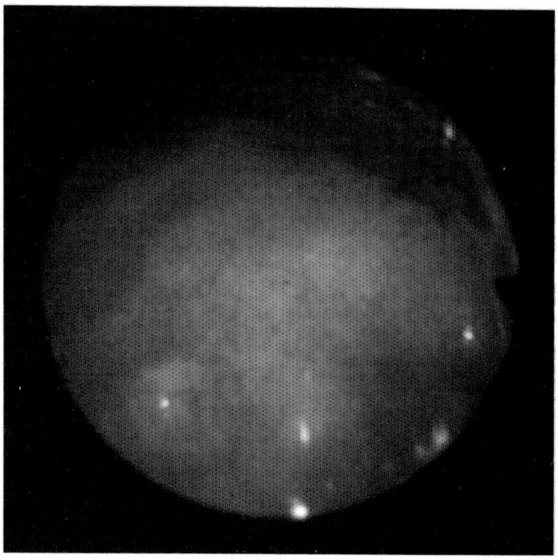

Fig. 16.4 Antral nodularity in a 13-year-old girl with *H. pylori*-associated chronic gastritis: note that the nodules are larger than in Fig. 16.3 and there are small shallow erosions.

[28] reported the presence of *Campylobacter*-like organisms in a Barrett's ulcer in an 8-year-old boy. Usually this micronodular aspect is improved following treatment, especially when associated with inflammation, but the irregularities do not disappear; how they progress without treatment in the adult is insufficiently known.

Erythema

This finding is reported by all authors in all the previously quoted series. However, it is difficult, in many cases, to give much credit to color-limited changes, since they are rather subjective and unspecific.

Endoscopically normal mucosa

In our previous series [15], a normal aspect of the antrum was found in only five HP+ children, although only one of these mucosae was histologically normal. The same coincidence of normal endoscopy with abnormal pathology has been widely reported in both adults and children [5, 24, 29] and stresses the need for systematic biopsies [16].

Histology

There are no particular differences between histologic features of *H. pylori* infection in children and adults, so much so that most authors describe the lesions as "abnormalities typical of gastritis" [14]. The following comprehensive description was given by Czinn *et al.* [4], regarding the five patients in their study:

> "The lamina propria was uniformly crowded with a mixture of lymphocytes, plasma cells and histiocytes. Acute inflammation was lacking, although occasional polymorphonuclear leukocytes were present in two patients, and rare eosinophils in one. Gastric glands were intact, although at times widely separated by the surrounding inflammatory infiltrate. Occasional glands contained intraepithelial lymphocytes, but there was no active glandular destruction or glandular abcess formation. Two patients had a well-formed lymphoid follicle in the mucosa. The surface epithelium was intact and well differentiated in all patients."

Our findings do not differ from this picture except that signs of acute inflammation, although less frequent than signs of chronic inflammation, are not so rare in our patients. The finding of lymphoid follicles in the gastric antral mucosa may be relevant to the micronodular endoscopic aspect. Transmission electron microscopy studies have not shown any specific lesion in children compared to adults.

Epidemiology

Little is known about the source and spread of *H. pylori*. Most authors reporting pediatric cases of *H. pylori* infection, whether associated with primary ulcers or primary gastritis, usually report the high incidence of a family history of peptic diseases [15, 17].

How often do we find an *H. pylori* infection in the family contacts of these children? How often are they symptomatic? What is the incidence of *H. pylori* infection in the pediatric age group? As systematic endoscopy is not an acceptable method for epidemiologic studies, data rely mostly on serologic studies or on breath tests using either ^{14}C- [30] or ^{13}C-labeled urea [31].

The most popular technique is the assay of anti-*H. pylori* IgG and IgM antibodies using the enzyme-linked immunosorbent assay (ELISA) technique. Mahony & Littlewood [32] showed, in an endoscopically validated study, that there was a good correlation between IgG antibodies to *H. pylori* and endoscopic findings. Similar results were obtained by Thomas *et al.* [33]. From the latter group, using a serologic method in 361 Gambian children, the prevalence rate of *H. pylori* infection was estimated to be 14% of children under the age of 20 months, rising to 46% in those up to 60 months of age. The prevalence rate of *H. pylori* infection was 53% in 77 children under 3 years of age with chronic diarrhea and malnutrition, significantly more frequent than in age-matched healthy controls (26%) or in children with marasmus without diarrhea (24%); the authors speculate on the possible role of *H. pylori* as an indirect agent, precipitating the diarrhea through its achlorhydric effect on the stomach in these malnourished Gambian children. Also, elevated titers of IgG to *H. pylori* were found in nine of 14 family contacts of four children in Australia [34].

In a mass screening of 1000 sera from France, Algeria, Ivory Coast, and Vietnam, Megraud *et al.* [35] showed evidence for a worldwide distribution of *H. pylori* infection and a high prevalence in developing countries, where 50% of the population was HP+ by the age of 10 years, rising to 75% from the third decade on.

The same high prevalence was found in Peruvian children by Klein *et al.* [36] using a ^{13}C-urea breath test: 54% of children aged 1–10 years and 90% of parents from low income families were HP+, contrasting with "only" 30% of children and 78% of parents from high income families.

For epidemiologic purposes we have been using a modified technique of the ^{14}C-urea breath test, using 1 μCi (37 kBq) [37, 38] in the families of our HP+ gastritis children. The

Table 16.4 ^{14}C-urea breath test in 42 families of *H. pylori*-positive (HP+) gastritis children

	Fathers		Mothers		Siblings	
Total no.	35		38		102	
Symptomatic	19		15		19	
Asymptomatic		16		23		83
^{14}C-urea positive	19	14	13	14	16	15*
Breath test negative	0	2	0	6	0	5
Not done	—	—	2	3	3	63**

* 10 > 15 years.
** 32 > 15 years.
Reference: [37].

results are given in Table 16.4. 90% of the fathers and 80% of the mothers, whether symptomatic or not, had a positive ^{14}C-urea breath test, meaning that the incidence of *H. pylori* infection was, indeed, very high in this population. The same was true for young adult siblings in which the test was performed. In about half of the parents, an endoscopic or X-ray study had been performed elsewhere: peptic ulcers were very frequent in the fathers; gastritis was more frequent in the mothers; in investigated siblings, primary peptic ulcers were almost as frequent as chronic gastritis (Table 16.5).

^{14}C- labeled isotopes are used with some reluctance in children because of the theoretical radiation hazards. Although our modified technique delivers a very low radiation dose, it is not a suitable technique for routine epidemiologic investigation in asymptomatic children. However, it can be used as an alternative, in order to avoid too frequent endoscopies, in the follow-up and treatment evaluation of most cases of adolescents and young adults. We are now planning to investigate the prevalence rate of *H. pylori* infection in "healthy" schoolchildren using a ^{13}C-urea breath test, more suitable for asymptomatic children and for mass screening: the only disadvantage is the high cost of this technique.

Treatment

Attempts to eradicate *H. pylori* in adults have often been hampered by a high rate of recolonization. In a very well designed study from Amsterdam, Rauws *et al.* [38] showed that *H. pylori* did not disappear spontaneously from the gastric mucosa. Treatment with amoxicillin, colloidal bismuth subcitrate (CBS, "DeNol"), or a combination of both drugs, was effective in eradicating *H. pylori* from 68%, 45%, and 90% respectively of patients with non-ulcer dyspepsia. Recolonization with the same bacterial subtype was frequent during the first month after the discontinuation of the therapy.

Almost every pediatric research group has been trying to eradicate *H. pylori*, either with amoxicillin alone [17, 39, 40], or with CBS alone [18], or a combination of both [18, 39], or a combination of amoxicillin with tinidazole [40], or, as in our own series, with metronidazole.

A triple therapy for children has not yet been reported. As a matter of fact, it is very difficult, at the present moment, to compare all these studies, since the drugs used, their combination, the doses given, and the regimens adopted, vary greatly. In addition, long-term follow-up is currently not available in these pediatric series.

We have been treating a series of 22 children with amoxicillin for 1 week and CBS for 1 month. Disappearance of *H. pylori* occurred in only half of the cases, but compliance was very poor. We are currently treating with a combination of amoxicillin ($50\,mg\,kg^{-1}\,day^{-1}$) and metronidazole ($20\,mg\,kg^{-1}\,day^{-1}$), and the

Table 16.5 Endoscopic findings in symptomatic family members of children with *H. pylori*-positive (HP+) gastritis

	Fathers	Mothers	Siblings
Symptomatic	19	16	19
Investigated	16	10	16
Findings			
Peptic ulcer	10	0	3
Acute gastritis	1	4	3
Chronic gastritis	5	6	4
Normal	0	0	6

preliminary results in 20 children show a very high eradication rate after 1 month (95%). The recolonization rate is not yet known but could be reduced by repeating short periods (1 week) of treatment every 2 or 3 months.

Low socioeconomic background and rapid relief of painful symptoms, together with a reluctance to undergo frequent endoscopic reevaluations are, to our opinion, the main reasons for the non-compliance encountered with the series. Practical details, such as palatability, side-effects, and number of doses also play a role: for instance, many children complained about the bad taste of the CBS solution, or about the difficulty of taking their antibiotic medication as a fluid solution while attending school, or about nausea following ingestion of metronidazole.

In order to avoid constant recontamination from family contacts, an attempt aimed at eradication of *H. pylori* in children, designed as a simultaneous treatment of all the members of the family, is currently under study in our unit.

Conclusions

There is now proof that *H. pylori* is associated with gastric antral lesions in the child. The possibility of lesions appearing in an acute-onset pattern, as in cases with protein-losing enteropathy gastritis, has currently been reported by only one group. A chronic-type onset and lesions are more commonly documented. However, as recurrent abdominal pain is very common in infancy and childhood, it is likely that this type of acute-onset disease could be easily missed or misdiagnosed.

The epidemiology of *H. pylori* infection in the pediatric population might possibly be a rewarding area of study for the understanding of the role of this common microorganism, which probably lives in the stomach of more than half of the world's population over the age of ten.

What is the most appropriate therapy in symptomatic children? Collaborative multicenter therapeutic trials are now planned in different centers throughout Europe, Asia, and Africa, in order to test an important series of pediatric cases over a short period with different drugs and combinations of drugs. In any case, attempts aimed at eradication of *H. pylori* should always be augmented by a full investigation of the *H. pylori* infection status of other members of the family, in order to evaluate the possibility of continuous reinfection.

Is eradication of the infection in asymptomatic children a necessity? In other words should we try so hard to eradicate *H. pylori* from these patients or does a symbiotic adaptation occur when infection is acquired early in life?

Answering these questions is a stimulating challenge for epidemiologists and pediatric gastroenterologists.

References

1 Warren, JR, & Marshall, BJ. Unidentified curved bacilli on gastric epithelium in active chronic gastritis. *Lancet* 1983;**i**:1273–5.

2 Hill, R, Pearman, J, Worthy, P, Caruso, V, Goodwin, S, & Blincow, E. *Campylobacter pyloridis* and gastritis in children. *Lancet* 1986; **i**:387.

3 Cadranel, S, Goossens, H, De Boeck, M, Malengreau, P, Rodesch, P, & Butzler, JP. *Campylobacter pyloridis* in children. *Lancet* 1986;**i**:735.

4 Czinn, S, Dahms, BB, Jacobs, GH, Kaplan, B, & Rothstein, FC. *Campylobacter*-like organisms in association with symptomatic gastritis in children. *J. Pediatr.* 1986;**109**:80–3.

5 Drumm, B, Sherman, P, Cutz, E, & Kharmali, M. Association of *Campylobacter pylori* on the gastric mucosa with antral gastritis in children. *N. Engl. J. Med.* 1987;**316**:1557–61.

6 Mahony, MJ, Wyatt, J, & Littlewood, JM. *Campylobacter*-associated gastritis in children. *Gut* 1987;**28**:A1357.

7 Hermier, M, Descos, B, & Foasso, MF. Les ulceres gastro-duodenaux primaires de l'enfant. Etude multicentrique de 58 cas de diagnostic endoscopique ou chirurgical. *Arch. Fr. Pediatr.* 1983;**40**:681–7.

8 Apley, J. *The Children with Abdominal Pains.* Oxford: Blackwell Scientific Publications, 1975.

9 Bonamico, M, Chiesa, C, Carpino, F, *et al.* *Campylobacter pylori* in children. A preliminary study. *Pediatr. Res.* 1988;**24**:A416.

10 Socha, J, Celinska-Cedro, D, Teisseyre, M, & Rasinski, A. *Campylobacter pyloridis* in children. *Pediatr. Res.* 1988;**24**:A416.

11 Mahony, MJ, Littlewood, MJ, Rathbone, BJ, & Wyatt, J. *Campylobacter pylori*-associated gastritis in children. In: Megraud, F, & Lamouliatte, H. (eds) *Proceedings of the Workshop on Gastroduodenal Pathology and Campylobacter pylori*, Bordeaux, October 1988, p. 142.

12 de Rafael, L, Vascones, F, Camarero, C, Perdomo, M, Suarez, L, & Escobar, H. *Campylobacter pylori* and recurrent abdominal pain in children. In: *Proceedings of the Workshop on Gastroduodenal Pathology and Campylobacter pylori*, Bordeaux, October 1988, p. 143.
13 Cadranel, S, De Giacomo, C, Droy, M, Oderda, G, & Thomas, JE. *Workshop on Campylobacter Pylori Infection in Paediatrics. XXII Annual Meeting, Eur. Soc. Paediatr. Gastroenterol. Nutr., Budapest*, 1989.
14 Drumm, B, O'Brien, A, Cutz, E, & Sherman, P. *Campylobacter pyloridis*-associated primary gastritis in children. *Pediatrics* 1987;**80**:192–5.
15 Cadranel, S, Glupczinski, Y, Labbe, M, & De Prez, C. *Campylobacter pylori* in children. In: Menge, H, Gregor, M, Tytgat, GNJ, & Marshall, BJ (eds), *Campylobacter pylori*. Berlin: Springer-Verlag, 1988, pp. 110–7.
16 Mahony, MJ, Wyatt, JI, & Littlewood, MJ. *Campylobacter pylori* gastritis. *Arch. Dis. Child.* 1988;**63**:654–5.
17 Oderda, G, Dell'Olio, D, Morra, I, & Ansaldi, N. *Campylobacter pylori* gastritis: long-term results of treatment with amoxycillin. *Arch. Dis. Child.* 1989;**64**:326–9.
18 Drumm, B, Sherman, P, Chiasson, D, Karmali, M, & Cutz, E. Treatment of *Campylobacter pylori*-associated antral gastritis in children with bismuth subsalicylate and ampicillin. *J. Pediatr.* 1988;**113**:908–12.
19 Langenberg, ML, Tytgat, GNJ, Schipper, MEJ, Rietra, PJGM, & Zanen, HC. *Campylobacter*-like organisms in the stomach of patients and healthy individuals. *Lancet* 1984;**i**:1348.
20 Barthel, JS, Westbloom, U, Havey, AD, Gonzalez, F, & Everett, ED. Gastritis and *Campylobacter pylori* in healthy, asymptomatic volunteers. *Arch. Intern. Med.* 1988;**148**:1149–51.
21 Peterson, WL, Lee, E, & Feldman, M. Relationship between *Campylobacter pylori* and gastritis in healthy humans after administration of placebo or indomethacin. *Gastroenterology* 1988;**95**:1185–9.
22 Hill, JD, Sinclair-Smith, C, Lastovica, AJ, Bowie, MD, & Emms, M. Transient protein-losing enteropathy associated with acute gastritis and *Campylobacter pylori. Arch. Dis. Child.* 1987;**62**:1215–9.
23 Murphy, MS, & Eastham, EJ. Peptic ulcer disease in childhood: long-term prognosis. *J. Pediatr. Gastroenterol. Nutr.* 1987;**6**:721–4.
24 Eastham, EJ, & Elliott, TSM. *Campylobacter pyloridis* in children. *Arch. Dis. Child.* 1987;**62**:652.
25 Oderda, G, Lerro, P, Poli, E, & Tavassoli, K. Childhood nodular antritis and *Campylobacter pylori. Endoscopy* 1988;**20**:86.
26 Unpublished personal data.
27 Beltran, S, Varea, V, Vilar, P, Cusi, V, Vila, J, & Farre, C. Gastritis cronica infantil. *An. Esp. Pediatr.* 1978;**11**:383.
28 De Giacomo, C, Fiocca, R, Villani, L, Bertolotti, L, & Maggiore, M. Barrett's ulcer and *Campylobacter*-like organisms infection in a child. *J. Pediatr. Gastroenterol. Nutr.* 1988;**7**:766–8.
29 Oderda, G, Vaira, D, Holton, J, Dowsett, JF, & Ansaldi, N. Serum pepsinogen I and IgG antibody to *Campylobacter pylori* in non-specific abdominal pain in childhood. *Gut* 1989;**30**:912–16.
30 Marshall, BJ, & Surveyor, I. ^{14}Carbon-urea breath test for the diagnosis of *Campylobacter pylori*-associated gastritis. *J. Nucl. Med.* 1988;**29**:11–16.
31 Graham, DY, Evans, DJ, Alpert, LC, Klein, PD, Evans, DG, Opekun, AR, & Boutton, TW. *Campylobacter pylori* detected by the ^{13}C-urea breath test. *Lancet* 1987;**i**:1174–7.
32 Mahony, MJ, & Littlewood, JM. Diagnosis of *Campylobacter pylori* gastritis by IgG ELISA. *Pediatr. Res.* 1988;**24**:416.
33 Thomas, JE, Eastham, EJ, Elliott, TSJ, Berkely, D, & Jones, D. *Campylobacter pylori* gastritis can be diagnosed serologically. *Arch. Dis. Child.* 1988;**63**:696.
34 Mitchell, HM, Bohane, TD, Berkowicz, J, Hazell, SI, & Lee, A. Antibody to *Campylobacter pylori* in families of index children with gastrointestinal illness due to *C. pylori. Lancet* 1987;**ii**:681–2.
35 Megraud, F, Brassens Rabbe, MP, Denis, F, Belbouri, A, & Hoa, DQ. Seroepidemiology of *Campylobacter pylori* infection in various populations. *J. Clin. Microbiol.* 1989;**27**:1870–3.
36 Klein, PD, Graham, DY, Opekun, AR, Sekeley, S, Evans, DG, & Evans, DJ. High prevalence of *Campylobacter pylori* infection in poor and rich Peruvian children determined by ^{13}C-urea breath test. *Gastroenterology* 1989;**96**:A260.
37 Verhas, M, Cadranel, S, Conti, S, *et al.* Accuracy of ^{14}C-urea breath test in detection of *Campylobacter pylori*. In: Schattauer, P, (ed), *Trends and Possibilities in Nuclear Medicine. Eur. Nucl. Med. Congress, Milan*, 1988, pp. 376–9.
38 Rauws, EAJ, Langenberg, W, Houthoff, J, Zanen, HC, & Tytgat, GNJ. *Campylobacter pyloridis*-associated chronic active gastritis. *Gastroenterology* 1988;**94**:33–40.
39 De Giacomo, C, Maggiore, G, Licardi, G, Scotta, MS, & Fiocca, R. Effects of antibacterial treatment of *Campylobacter pylori*-associated gastritis in children. *Gastroenterology* 1988;**95**:1699.
40 Oderda, G, Vaira, D, Holton, J, Ainley, C, Altare, F, & Ansaldi, N. Amoxycillin plus tinidazole for *Campylobacter pylori* gastritis in children: assessment by serum IgG antibody, pepsinogen I, and gastrin levels. *Lancet* 1989;**i**:690–92.

Index

Page numbers in *italic* refer to figures or plates; those in **bold** refer to tables.